User's Guide to the Book

Introductory pages:
- The introductory pages provide all relevant anatomical informations concerning the subject of the chapter. Important details and connections are explained easily to understand.
- The Dissection Link for each chapter comprises brief and concise tips essential for the dissection of the respective body region.
- Exam Check Lists provide all keywords for possible exam questions.

Atlas pages:
- The menu bar on top indicates the topics of each chapter, the bold print shows the subject of the respective pages.
- Important anatomical structures in the figures are highlighted in bold print.
- Small supplement sketches located next to complex views show visual angles and intersecting planes and, thus, facilitate orientation.
- Detailed figure captions explain the relationships of anatomical structures.

- Bulleted lists in figure captions as well as in tables help structuring complex facts and provide a better overview.
- Figures, tables, and text boxes are interconnected by cross-references.
- Cross-references link the figures to the separate Table Booklet with tables of muscles, joints, and nerves, thus providing a sufficient anatomical knowledge for the exam.
- Clinical Remarks boxes provide clinical background knowledge concerning the anatomical structures illustrated on the page.
- The dissection link on the page indicates if a tip for dissecting the illustrated anatomical region is available on www.e-sobotta.com.

Appendix:
- List of abbreviations, general terms of direction and position can be found at the end of the book.

Perfect Orientation – the New Navigation System

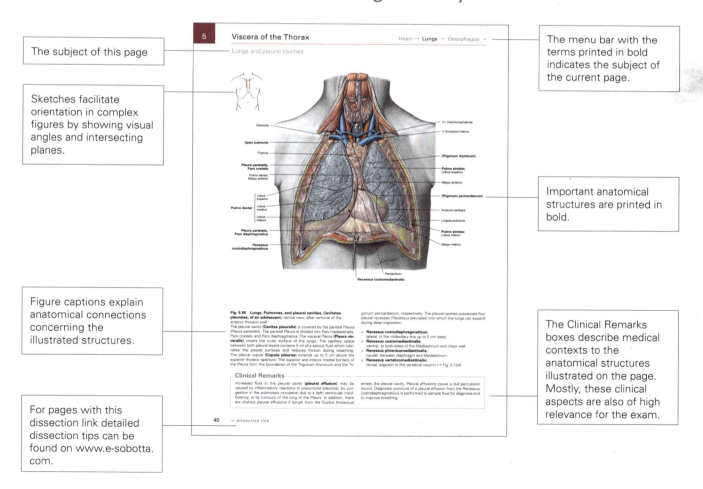

- The subject of this page
- Sketches facilitate orientation in complex figures by showing visual angles and intersecting planes.
- Figure captions explain anatomical connections concerning the illustrated structures.
- For pages with this dissection link detailed dissection tips can be found on www.e-sobotta.com.
- The menu bar with the terms printed in bold indicates the subject of the current page.
- Important anatomical structures are printed in bold.
- The Clinical Remarks boxes describe medical contexts to the anatomical structures illustrated on the page. Mostly, these clinical aspects are also of high relevance for the exam.

The following contents can be found in the other two volumes:

Vol. 1 — General Anatomy and Musculoskeletal System

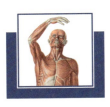

1 General Anatomy
Orientation on the Body → Surface Anatomy → Development → Muskuloskeletal System → Vessels and Nerves → Imaging Techniques → Integumentary System

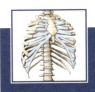

2 Trunk
Surface Anatomy → Development → Skeleton → Imaging → Muscles → Vessels and Nerves → Topography, Back → Female Breast → Topography, Abdomen and Abdominal Wall

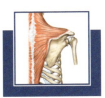

3 Upper Extremity
Surface Anatomy → Development → Skeleton → Imaging → Muscles → Topography → Sections

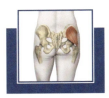

4 Lower Extremity
Surface Anatomy → Skeleton → Imaging → Muscles → Topography → Sections

Vol. 3 — Head, Neck, and Neuroanatomy

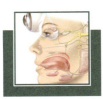

8 Head
Overview → Skeleton and Joints → Muscles → Topography → Vessels and Nerves → Nose → Mouth and Oral Cavity → Salivary Glands

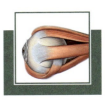

9 Eye
Development → Skeleton → Eyelids → Lacrimal Apparatus → Muscles of the Eye → Topography → Eyeball → Visual Pathway

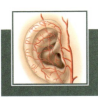

10 Ear
Overview → Outer Ear → Middle Ear → Auditory Tube → Inner Ear → Hearing and Equilibrium

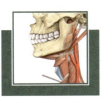

11 Neck
Muscles → Pharynx → Larynx → Thyroid Gland → Topography

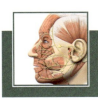

12 Brain and Spinal Cord
General → Meninges and Blood Supply → Brain → Sections → Cranial Nerves → Spinal Cord

Paulsen, Waschke

Sobotta

Atlas of Human Anatomy
Latin Nomenclature

Internal Organs

Translated by
T. Klonisch and S. Hombach-Klonisch

Editors

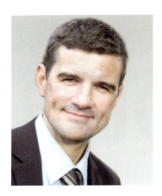

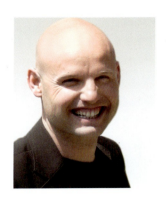

Prof. Dr. Friedrich Paulsen
Dissecting Courses for Students

In his teaching, Friedrich Paulsen puts great emphasis on the fact that students can actually dissect on cadavers of body donors. "The hands-on experience in dissection is extremely important not only for the three-dimensional understanding of anatomy and as the basis for virtually every medical profession, but for many students also clearly addresses the issue of death and dying for the first time. The members of the dissection team not only study anatomy but also learn to deal with this special issue. At no other time medical students will have such a close contact to their classmates and teachers again."
"The dissection links in the atlas lead to online images that are relevant for the dissection. You can print them and take them along. The offered dissection tips are not instructions, but make sure that you are oriented exceptionally well and not 'cutting in the dark'."

Professor Friedrich Paulsen (born 1965 in Kiel) passed the 'Abitur' in Brunswick and trained successfully as a nurse. After studying human medicine in Kiel, he became scientific associate at the Institute of Anatomy, Department of Oral and Maxillofacial Surgery and the Department of Otolaryngology, Head and Neck Surgery of the Christian-Albrechts-Universität Kiel. In 2002, together with his colleagues, he was awarded the Teaching Award for outstanding teaching in the field of anatomy at the Medical Faculty of the University of Kiel. On several occasions he gained work experience abroad in the academic section of the Department of Ophthalmology, University of Bristol, UK, where he did research for several months.

From 2004 to 2010 as a University Professor, he was head of the Macroscopic Anatomy and Prosector Section at the Department of Anatomy and Cell Biology of the Martin-Luther-Universität Halle-Wittenberg. Starting in April 2010, Professor Paulsen became the Chairman at the Institute of Anatomy II of the Friedrich-Alexander-Universität Erlangen. Since 2006, Professor Paulsen is a board member of the Anatomical Society and 2009 he was elected the general secretary of the International Federation of Associations of Anatomy (IFAA).

His main research area concerns the innate immune system. Topics of special interest are antimicrobial peptides, trefoil factor peptides, surfactant proteins, mucins, corneal wound healing, as well as stem cells of the lacrimal gland and diseases such as eye infections, dry eye, or osteoarthritis.

Prof. Dr. Jens Waschke
More Clinical Relevance in Teaching

From March 2011 on, Professor Jens Waschke is Chairman of Department I at the Institute of Anatomy and Cell Biology at the Ludwig-Maximilians-Universität (LMU) Munich. "For me, teaching at the department of vegetative anatomy, which is responsible for the dissection courses of both Munich's large universities LMU and TU, emphasizes the importance of teaching anatomy with clear clinical relevance", says Jens Waschke.
"The clinical aspects in the Atlas introduce students to anatomy in the first semesters. At the same time, it indicates the importance of this subject for future clinical practice, as understanding human anatomy means more than just memorization of structures."

Professor Jens Waschke (born in 1974) habilitated in 2007 after graduation from Medical School and completing a doctoral thesis at the University of Wuerzburg. From 2003 to 2004 he joined Professor Fitz-Roy Curry at the University of California in Davis for a nine months research visit. Starting in June 2008, he became the Chairman at the Institute of Anatomy and Cell Biology III at the University of Wuerzburg. In 2005, together with his colleagues, Professor Waschke was awarded the Albert Koelliker Teaching Award of the Faculty of Medicine in Wuerzburg. In 2006, he was awarded the Wolfgang Bargmann Prize of the Anatomical Society.

His main research area concerns cellular mechanisms that control the adhesion between cells and the cellular junctions establishing the outer and inner barriers of the human body. The attention is focused on the regulations of the endothelial barrier in inflammation and the mechanisms, which lead to the formation of fatal dermal blisters in pemphigus, an autoimmune disease. The goal is to gain a better understanding of cell adhesion as a basis for the development of new therapeutic strategies.

Sobotta

Atlas of Human Anatomy

Internal Organs

15th edition
Edited by F. Paulsen and J. Waschke

Translated by T. Klonisch and
S. Hombach-Klonisch, Winnipeg, Canada

363 Coloured Plates with 441 Figures

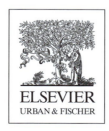

URBAN & FISCHER
München

All business correspondence should be made with:
Elsevier GmbH, Urban & Fischer Verlag, Hackerbrücke 6, 80335 Munich, Germany, mail to: medizinstudium@elsevier.de

Addresses of the editors:
Professor Dr. med. Friedrich Paulsen
Institut für Anatomie II (Vorstand)
Universität Erlangen-Nürnberg
Universitätsstraße 19
91054 Erlangen
Germany

Professor Dr. med. Jens Waschke
Institut für Anatomie
Ludwig-Maximilians-Universität
Pettenkoferstraße 11
80333 München
Germany

Addresses of the translators:
Professor Dr. med. Sabine Hombach-Klonisch
Professor Dr. med. Thomas Klonisch
Faculty of Medicine
Department of Human Anatomy and Cell Science
University of Manitoba
745 Bannatyne Avenue
Winnipeg Manitoba R3E 0J9
Canada

Bibliographic information published by the Deutsche Nationalbibliothek
The Deutsche Nationalbibliothek lists this publication in the Deutsche Nationalbibliografie; detailed bibliographic data are available in the Internet at http://www.d-nb.de.

All rights reserved
15th Edition 2011
© Elsevier GmbH, Munich
Urban & Fischer Verlag is an imprint of Elsevier GmbH.

13 14 15   5 4 3

For copyright concerning the pictorial material see picture credits.

All rights, including translation, are reserved. No part of this publication may be reproduced, stored in a retrieval system, or transmitted in any other form or by any means, electronic, mechanical, photocopying, recording, or otherwise without the prior written permission of the publisher.

Acquisition editor: Alexandra Frntic, Munich
Development editor: Dr. Andrea Beilmann, Munich
Editing: Ulrike Kriegel, buchundmehr, Munich
Production manager: Sibylle Hartl, Munich; Renate Hausdorf, buchundmehr, Gräfelfing
Composed by: Mitterweger & Partner, Plankstadt
Printed and bound by: Firmengruppe appl, Wemding
Illustrators: Dr. Katja Dalkowski, Buckenhof; Sonja Klebe, Aying-Großhelfendorf; Jörg Mair, Munich; Stephan Winkler, Munich
Cover illustration: Nicola Neubauer, Puchheim
Cover design: SpieszDesign, Neu-Ulm
Printed on 115 g Quatro Silk

ISBN 978-0-7234-3732-1

This atlas was founded by Johannes Sobotta †, former Professor of Anatomy and Director of the Anatomical Institute of the University in Bonn, Germany.

German editions:
1st edition: 1904–1907 J. F. Lehmanns Verlag, Munich
2nd–11th edition: 1913–1944 J. F. Lehmanns Verlag, Munich
12th edition: 1948 and following editions
          Urban & Schwarzenberg, Munich
13th edition: 1953, editor H. Becher
14th edition: 1956, editor H. Becher
15th edition: 1957, editor H. Becher
16th edition: 1967, editor H. Becher
17th edition: 1972, editors H. Ferner and J. Staubesand
18th edition: 1982, editors H. Ferner and J. Staubesand
19th edition: 1988, editor J. Staubesand
20th edition: 1993, editors R. Putz and R. Pabst
          Urban & Schwarzenberg, Munich
21st edition: 2000, editors R. Putz and R. Pabst
          Urban & Fischer, Munich
22nd edition: 2006, editors R. Putz and R. Pabst
          Urban & Fischer, Munich
23rd edition: 2010, editors F. Paulsen and J. Waschke
          Elsevier, Munich

Foreign editions:
Arabic edition
Modern Technical Center, Damaskus
Chinese edition (complex characters)
Ho-Chi Book Publishing Co, Taiwan
Chinese edition (simplified Chinese edition)
Elsevier, Health Sciences Asia, Singapore
Croatian edition
Naklada Slap, Jastrebarsko
Czech edition
Grada Publishing, Prague
Dutch edition
Springer Media, Houten
English edition (with nomenclature in English)
Elsevier Inc., Philadelphia
English edition (with nomenclature in Latin)
Elsevier GmbH, Urban & Fischer
French edition
Tec & Doc Lavoisier, Paris
Greek edition (with nomenclature in Greek)
Parisianou, S.A., Athen
Greek edition (with nomenclature in Latin)
Parisianou, S.A., Athen
Hungarian edition
Medicina Publishing, Budapest
Indonesian edition
Penerbit Buku Kedokteran EGC, Jakarta
Italian edition
Elsevier Masson STL, Milan
Japanese edition
Igaku Shoin Ltd., Tokyo
Korean edition
Elsevier Korea LLC
Polish edition
Elsevier Urban & Partner, Wroclaw
Portuguese edition (with nomenclature in English)
Editora Guanabara Koogan, Rio de Janeiro
Portuguese edition (with nomenclature in Latin)
Editora Guanabara Koogan, Rio de Janeiro
Russian edition
Reed Elsevier LLC, Moscow
Spanish edition
Elsevier España S.L.
Turkish edition
Beta Basim Yayim Dagitim, Istanbul
Ukrainian edition
Elsevier Urban & Partner, Wroclaw

Current information by www.elsevier.de and www.elsevier.com

Table of contents

Viscera of the Thorax
Heart 4
Lungs 28
Oesophagus 42
Thymus 50
Topography 52
Sections 62

Viscera of the Abdomen
Development 72
Stomach 74
Intestines 86
Liver and Gallbladder 102
Pancreas 120
Spleen 128
Topography 130
Sections 148

Pelvis and Retroperitoneal Space
Kidney and Adrenal Gland 160
Efferent Urinary System 174
Genitalia 182
Rectum and Anal Canal 220
Topography 228
Sections 236

Translators

Prof. Dr. Thomas Klonisch

Professor Thomas Klonisch (born 1960) studied human medicine at the Ruhr-Universität Bochum and the Justus-Liebig-Universität (JLU) Giessen. He successfully completed his doctoral thesis at the Institute of Biochemistry at the Faculty of Medicine of the JLU Giessen and became a scientific associate at the Institute of Medical Microbiology, University of Mainz (1989–1991). As an Alexander von Humboldt Fellow he joined the University of Guelph, Ontario, Canada, from 1991–1992 and, in 1993–1994, continued his research at the Ontario Veterinary College, Guelph, Ontario. From 1994–1996, he joined the immunoprotein engineering group at the Department of Immunology, University College London, UK, as a senior research fellow. From 1996–2004 he was a scientific associate at the Department of Anatomy and Cell Biology, Martin-Luther-Universität Halle-Wittenberg, where he received his accreditation as anatomist (1999), completed his habilitation (2000), and held continuous national research funding by the German Research Council (DFG) and German Cancer Research Foundation (Deutsche Krebshilfe). In 2004, he was appointed Full Professor and Head at the Department of Human Anatomy and Cell Science at the Faculty of Medicine, University of Manitoba, Winnipeg, Canada, where he is currently serving his second term as department chairman.

His research areas concern the mechanisms employed by cancer cells and their cancer stem/progenitor cells to enhance tissue invasiveness and survival strategies in response to anticancer treatments. One particular focus is on the role of endocrine factors, such as the relaxin-like ligand-receptor system, in promoting carcinogenesis.

Prof. Dr. Sabine Hombach-Klonisch

Teaching clinically relevant anatomy and clinical case-based anatomy learning are the main teaching focus of Sabine Hombach-Klonisch at the Medical Faculty of the University of Manitoba. Since her appointment in 2004, Professor Hombach has been nominated annually for teaching awards by the Manitoba Medical Student Association.

Sabine Hombach (born 1963) graduated from Medical School at the Justus-Liebig-Universität Giessen in 1991 and successfully completed her doctoral thesis in 1994. Following a career break to attend to her two children she re-engaged as a sessional lecturer at the Department of Anatomy and Cell Biology of the Martin-Luther-Universität Halle-Wittenberg in 1997 and received a post-doctoral fellowship by the province of Saxony-Anhalt from 1998–2000. Thereafter, she joined the Department of Anatomy and Cell Biology as a scientific associate. Professor Hombach received her accreditation as anatomist in 2003 by the German Society of Anatomists and by the Medical Association of Saxony-Anhalt and completed her habilitation at the Medical Faculty of the Martin-Luther-Universität Halle-Wittenberg in 2004. In 2004, Professor Hombach was appointed Assistant Professor at the Department of Human Anatomy and Cell Science, Faculty of Medicine of the University of Manitoba. She has been the recipient of the Merck European Thyroid von Basedow Research Prize by the German Endocrine Society in 2002 and received the Murray L. Barr Young Investigator Award by the Canadian Association for Anatomy, Neurobiology and Cell Biology in 2009.

Her main research interests are in the field of cancer research and environmental toxicants. Her focus in cancer research is to identify the molecular mechanisms that regulate cancer cell migration and metastasis. She employs unique cell and animal models and human primary cells to study epigenetic and transgenerational effects facilitated by environmental chemicals.

Preface

In the preface to the first edition of his Atlas, Johannes Sobotta wrote in May 1904: "Many years of experience in anatomical dissection led the author to proceed with the presentation of the peripheral nervous system and the blood vessels such that the illustrations of the book are presented to the student exactly in the same manner as body parts are presented to them in the dissection laboratories, i.e. simultaneous presentation of blood vessels and nerves of the same region. Alternating descriptive and image materials are distinctive features of this atlas. The images are the core piece of the atlas. Apart from table legends, auxiliary and schematic drawings, the descriptive material includes short and concise text parts suitable for use of this book in the gross anatomy laboratory."

As with fashions, reading and study habits of students change periodically. The multimedia presence and availability of information as well as stimuli are certainly the main reasons of ever changing study habits. These developments and changing demands of students to textbooks and atlases, which they utilise, as well as the availability of digital media of textbook contents, is accounted for by editors and publishers. Apart from interviews and systematic surveys of students, the textbook sector is occasionally an indicator enabling the evaluation of expectations of students. Detailed textbooks with the absolute claim of completeness are exchanged in favour of educational books that are tailored to the didactic needs of students and the contents of the study of human medicine, dentistry, and biomedical sciences, as well as the corresponding examinations. Similarly, illustrations in atlases such as the Sobotta, which contain exact naturalistic depiction of real anatomical specimens, fascinate doctors and associated medical professions for many generations throughout the world. However, students sometimes perceive them as too complicated and detailed. This awareness requires the consideration of how the strength of the atlas, which is known for its standards of accuracy and quality during its centennial existence featuring 22 editions, can be adapted to modern educational concepts without compromising the oeuvre's unique characteristics and authenticity. After careful consideration, Elsevier and the editors Professor Reinhard Putz and Professor Reinhard Pabst, who were in charge of the atlas up to its 22nd edition, came to the conclusion that a new editorial team with the same great enthusiasm for anatomy and teaching would meet the new requirements best. Together with the Elsevier publishing house, we are extremely pleased to be charged with the new composition of the 23rd edition of Sobotta. In redesigning, a very clear outline of contents and a didactic introduction to the pictures was taken into account. Not every fashion is accompanied with something entirely new. Under didactical aspects we have revisited the old concept of a three-volume atlas, as used in Sobotta's first edition, with: General Anatomy and Musculoskeletal System (vol. 1), Internal Organs (vol. 2), and Head, Neck, and Neuroanatomy (vol. 3). We have also adopted, although slightly modified, the approach mentioned already in the preface of the first edition, i.e. combining the figures in the atlas with explanatory text which is an old trend being currently back into fashion once more. Each image is accompanied by a short explanatory text, which serves to introduce students to the image, explaining why the particular preparation and presentation of a region was selected. The individual chapters were systematically organised in terms of current subject matter and prevailing study habits; omitted and incomplete illustrations – particularly the systematics of the neurovascular pathways – were supplemented or replaced. The majority of these new figures are conceptualised to facilitate studying the relevant pathways of blood supply and innervation by didactical aspects. We have also reviewed many existing figures, reduced figure legends, and highlighted keywords by bold print to simplify access to the anatomical contents. Numerous clinical examples are used to enhance the "lifeless anatomy", present the relevance of anatomy for the future career to the student, and provide a taste of what's to come. Introductions to the individual chapters received a new conceptual design, covering in brief a summary of the content, the associated clinical aspects, and relevant dissection steps for the covered topic. It serves as a checklist for the requirements of the Institute of Medical and Pharmaceutical Examination Questions (IMPP) and is based on the German oral part of the preclinical medical examination (Physikum). Also new are brief introductions to each topic in embryology and the online connections of the atlas with the ability to download all images for reports, lectures, and presentations.

We want to emphasise two points:
1. The "new" Sobotta in the 23rd edition is not a study atlas, claiming completeness of a comprehensive knowledge and, thus, does not try to convey the intention to replace an accompanying textbook.
2. No matter how good the didactic approach, it cannot relieve the students of studying, but aid in visualisation. Anatomy is not difficult to study, but very time-consuming. Sacrificing this time is worthwhile, since physicians and patients will benefit from it.

The goal of the 23rd edition of Sobotta is not only to facilitate learning, but also to make learning exciting and attracting, so that the atlas is consulted during the study period as well as in the course of professional practice.

Erlangen and Wuerzburg, summer 2010, exactly 106 years after the first edition.

Friedrich Paulsen and Jens Waschke

Acknowledgements

First, we would like to express that the work on the Sobotta was exciting and challenging. During stages, at which one could see the progress of development of individual chapters and newly developed pictures with a slight detachment, one obtained satisfaction, was elated with pride and identified oneself evermore with the Sobotta.

The redesign of Sobotta is obviously not the sole work of two inexperienced editors, but rather requires more than ever a well-attuned team under the coordination of the publisher. Without the long experience of Dr. Andrea Beilmann, who supervised several editions of the Sobotta and exerted the calming influence of the Sobotta team, many things would have been impossible. We thank her for all the help and support. Ms. Alexandra Frntic, who is also part of the four-member Sobotta team, pursued the first major project of her career and tackled it with passion and enthusiasm. Her liveliness and management by motivation have enlivened and cheered the editors. We express our gratitude to Ms. Frntic. We like to reflect back on the Sobotta initialisation week in Parsberg and weekly conference calls, in which Dr. Beilmann and Ms. Frntic supported us in the composition of the Sobotta and presented an admirable way to merge the variety of two personalities to achieve a single layout. Without the assertiveness, the calls for perseverance and the protective hand of Dr. Dorothea Hennessen, who directed the project of the "23rd edition of Sobotta" and always believed in her Sobotta team and the tight schedule, this edition would have not been published. Like a number of previous productions, the routinier Renate Hausdorf led the successful reproduction of the atlas. Other people involved in the editing process and the success of the 23rd edition of the Sobotta and whom we sincerely thank are Ms. Susanne Szczepanek (manuscript editing), Ms. Julia Baier, Mr. Martin Kortenhaus and Ms. Ulrike Kriegel (editing), Ms. Amelie Gutsmiedl (formal text editing), Ms. Sibylle Hartl (internal production), Ms. Claudia Adam and Mr. Michael Wiedorn (formal figure editing and typesetting), Ms. Nicola Neubauer (layout development and refining the typesetting data) and the students Doris Bindl, Derkje Hockertz, Lisa Link, Sophia Poppe, Cornelia Rippl and Katherina and Florian Stumpfe. For the compilation of the index, we express our gratitude to Dr. Ursula Osterkamp-Baust. Special thanks are expressed to the illustrators Dr. Katja Dalkowski, Ms. Sonja Klebe, Mr. Jörg Mair and Mr. Stephan Winkler, who in addition to revising existing illustrations have developed a variety of excellent figures. Priv.-Doz. Dr. rer. nat. Helmut Wicht, Senkenberg Anatomy, Goethe-Universität Frankfurt/Main, has revived the lifelessness of the introductions to the chapters indited by the two editors through his unique style of writing. We express our gratitude to Priv.-Doz. Dr. rer. nat. Wicht.

A big help to us was the advisory council, which in addition to the former editors Prof. Dr. med. Dr. h. c. Reinhard Putz, Ludwig-Maximilians-Universität Munich, and Prof. Dr. med. Reinhard Pabst, Hannover Medical School, and colleagues Prof. Dr. med. Peter Kugler, Julius-Maximilians-Universität Wuerzburg, and Prof. Dr. rer. nat. Gottfried Bogusch, Charité Berlin, supported us strongly with advice and critical comments. We would like to specifically emphasise the effort of Ms. Renate Putz, who corrected the manuscript very carefully; her comments were of crucial importance for the consistency of the work in itself and with the earlier editions.

For support with corrections and revisions, we express our sincere thanks to Ms. Stephanie Beilicke, Dr. rer. nat. Lars Bräuer, Ms. Anett Diker, Mr. Fabian Garreis, Ms. Elisabeth George, Ms. Patricia Maake, Ms. Susann Möschter, Mr. Jörg Pekarsky and Mr. Martin Schicht.

For assistance in creating clinical figures, we express our gratitude to Priv.-Doz. Dr. med. Hannes Kutta, Clinic and Polyclinic for Oto-Rhino-Laryngology at the University Hospital Hamburg-Eppendorf, Prof. Dr. med. Norbert Kleinsasser, University Clinic for Oto-Rhino-Laryngo-Pathology, Julius-Maximilians-Universität Wuerzburg, Prof. Dr. med. Andreas Dietz, Head of Clinic and Polyclinic for Oto-Rhino-Laryngology at the University Leipzig, Dr. med. Dietrich Stoevesandt, Clinic for Diagnostic Radiology at the Martin-Luther-Universität Halle-Wittenberg, Prof. Dr. med. Stephan Zierz, Director of the University Hospital and Polyclinic for Neurology at the Martin-Luther-Universität Halle-Wittenberg, Dr. med. Berit Jordan, Hospital and Polyclinic for Neurology at the Martin-Luther-Universität Halle-Wittenberg, Dr. med. Saadettin Sel, University Hospital for Ophthalmology at the Martin-Luther-Universität Halle-Wittenberg, Mr. cand. med. Christian Schroeder, Eckernförde, and Mr. Denis Hiller, Bad Lauchstädt.

We also would like to express our thanks to our anatomical mentors Prof. Dr. med. Bernhard Tillmann, Christian-Albrechts-Universität Kiel, and Prof. Dr. med. Detlev Drenckhahn, Julius-Maximilians-Universität Wuerzburg, whom we not only owe our anatomical training, the motivation for subject matter, and the sense of mission, but also have been great role models in their design of textbooks and atlases, as well as in their teaching excellence.

Our deepest gratitude to our parents, Dr. med. Ursula Paulsen and Prof. Dr. med. Karsten Paulsen, and also Annelies Waschke and Dr. med. Dieter Waschke, who intensely supported and sustained the Sobotta project. Karsten Paulsen, who passed away in May 2010, studied anatomy as a medical student from the 4th edition of Sobotta. Dieter Waschke used the 16th edition of Sobotta and continues to attain knowledge with medical literature even during retirement. The 23rd edition is dedicated to our fathers.

Last but not least, we thank our wives Dr. med. Dana Paulsen and Susanne Waschke, who not only had to share us with the Sobotta in the last year, but also were on hand with help and advice on many issues and have been strongly supportive.

Viscera of the Thorax

Heart 4

Lungs 28

Oesophagus 42

Thymus 50

Topography 52

Sections 62

The Thorax –
Partly Intricate Organs

The thoracic cage (Cavea thoracis) contains the heart (Cor) and the lungs (Pulmones). In ancient times, it was believed that life spirits along with the inhaled air reached the lungs, mixed with blood in the heart, which was at that time thought to be the seat of the soul, and distributed throughout the whole body by the blood vessels. Even today, the heart is still considered to be the engine of life and in colloquial terms it is also referred to as the centre of emotions. Scientifically, the heart is defined as a hollow muscle which pumps blood through the lesser circulation of the lungs (pulmonary circulation) and the greater circulation of the body (systemic circulation): The **left side of the heart** pumps oxygenated blood into the **systemic circulation** which transports the blood to the organs via arteries (leaving the heart). Blood vessels of the microcirculation branch out to allow the nutrient and gas exchange at the capillary level. The veins return deoxygenated blood to the **right side of the heart** from where the blood is forwarded to the **pulmonary circulation.** Pulmonary arteries transport deoxygenated blood to the lungs. In a network of pulmonary capillaries the deoxygenated blood finally reaches the alveoli, is enriched with oxygen and transferred via pulmonary veins to the left atrium. This completes the blood circulation.

The function of the heart as a pump is especially fascinating: On average the heart rate is 70 beats per minute and with every systolic contraction the heart forces 70 ml of blood into the circulation. Even without further stimulation of the heart in "excitement", it beats more than 100,000 times per day and 36 million times per year. The volume of blood (206,000 m^3), which is pumped by the heart in the course of 80 years, would be sufficient to fill 80 Olympic swimming pools. Conversely, no function of the body would be possible without the heart: in most cases cardiac arrest is an immediate cause of death.

In the dissection course, the opening of the thoracic cavity is perceived with mixed feelings of awe, excitement and interest by teaching professionals and students. The exposure of heart and lungs as well as the entitlement to touch and observe these vital organs is perceived as a great privilege during these training sessions.

The Mediastinum

A sagittal massive separation crosses the Thorax from the rear aspect of the Sternum to the ventral aspect of the thoracic vertebrae. It is called the Mediastinum (from Latin "in medio stans" = "standing in the middle"). Cranially the Mediastinum is continuous without sharp boundaries with the viscera of the neck through the superior thoracic aperture. Caudally it rests on the diaphragm and is sharply defined. The lungs are located within individual pleural cavities (Cavitates pleurales) to both sides of the Mediastinum.

In the Mediastinum, several organs are intertwined. The **Thymus** is located in the **Mediastinum superius** just behind the Sternum. It is an organ of the immune system but soon after puberty regresses to become an adipose body. The V. cava superior is displaced to the right from the median plane. Its tributaries – both Vv. brachiocephalicae – cover the large arterial trunks to the neck and the arms that emerge from the **aortic arch.** The cane-like curved main artery (Aorta) dominates on the left side of the Mediastinum. Hidden beneath the veins and the arch of the Aorta, the **Trachea** descends in the Mediastinum superius and branches into right and left main bronchi, Bronchi principales. The **Oesophagus** descends dorsal of the Trachea and in front of the vertebrae. Between the Oesophagus and the vertebrae there is the delicate **thoracic duct,** the Ductus thoracicus, which carries milky lymph (containing absorbed fats from meals) from the lower body.

The **heart** dominates in the **Mediastinum inferius** which is directed towards the diaphragm. It is located in a separate, thin-walled serous cavity, the Cavitas pericardiaca, and extends the Mediastinum towards the left side. The heart is only exposed after incision or removal of the cavity wall, the pericardium. A large area of the heart rests on the diaphragm with its apex (Apex cordis) pointing to the lower left side towards the left fifth intercostal space. Holding the heart by the apex, it can be freely moved in the cavity. Its only attachments are the large vessels that emerge at the upper pole (Aorta, A. pulmonalis) and enter at the its rear surface (Vv. pulmonales, Vv. cavae superior et inferior). The base of the heart (Basis cordis) with the origin of the blood vessels is opposite to the apex.

Immediately behind the Pericardium – more exactly: behind the left atrium of the heart – the **Oesophagus** descends to the oesophageal hiatus (Hiatus oesophageus) in the diaphragm. Slightly left side to the Oesophagus, also behind the Pericardium, the **Aorta** and the **Ductus thoracicus** descend and pass through the Hiatus aorticus in the diaphragm. The **V. cava inferior** traverses the diaphragm through a separate orifice (Foramen venae cavae), located slightly to the right and dorsal side of the centre of the diaphragm, and enters the pericardium and the Basis cordis from inferior. Additionally, numerous other structures, such as the Aa. thoracicae internae, Nn. phrenici, Nn. vagi, Vv. azygotes, and ganglia and nerves of the sympathetic trunk (part of the autonomic nervous system) descend in the mediastinum.

The Lungs and their Cavities

The larger trilobular right lung and the smaller bilobular left **lung** are located in separate serous cavities (Cavitates pleurales, pleural cavities) to the right and left side of the Mediastinum, respectively. Both lungs are covered by a thin, transparent, serous membrane (Pleura visceralis), through which a black, net-like pigment pattern is visible. This anthracotic pigment consists mainly of soot, the carbon which emanates from exhaust fumes and cigarette smoke. Numerous lymph nodes near the hilum of the lungs (see below) show an abundance of this pigment.

The lungs are supposed to move freely in their pleural cavities. They are attached only at the hilum where the bronchi, the Aa. pulmonales, and the Vv. pulmonales enter the lungs from the Mediastinum. Often, as a result of inflammation, the pleura covering the lungs (Pleura visceralis) adheres to the serous pleura of the ribs (Pleura costalis), the Mediastinum (Pleura mediastinalis), or the diaphragm (Pleura diaphragmatica), all of which comprise the **Pleura parietalis.** In exhaled condition, the parietal pleura is more substantial than the visceral pleura and reaches beyond the margins of the lungs. The virtual spaces in which the lungs may expand during deep inspiration are called the pleural recesses of the Pleura. During respiration, the lungs adapt to the shape of the thoracic wall and diaphragm. The lungs expand and retract as they slide in and out of the recesses. Therefore, adhesions of the Pleura parietalis to the Pleura visceralis restrain lung function.

Clinical Remarks

The **electrocardiogram** (ECG) is a standard diagnostic tool and provides information on the muscular function of the heart and on its size and position. The ECG may be indicative of a stenosis of certain coronary arteries. **Conventional radiography, computed tomography** (CT) and **magnetic resonance tomographic imaging** (MRI) of the Thorax are essential diagnostic tools to identify diseases of the lung and the Mediastinum and provide information on the size and function of the heart. Specific diagnostic procedures, such as **cardiac catheterisation,** require detailed anatomical knowledge. The cardiac catheter is used to inject a contrast agent into the coronary arteries (coronary angiogram) to visualise and potentially dilate stenoses. The **echocardiography** enables visualisation of the cardiac valves and their function. These diagnostic methods are carried out by specialists in internal medicine or radiologists. Cardiothoracic surgery is performed for lung resection (or parts of the lung), treatment of defects of the great vessels, transplantation of the heart or lungs, or other indications.

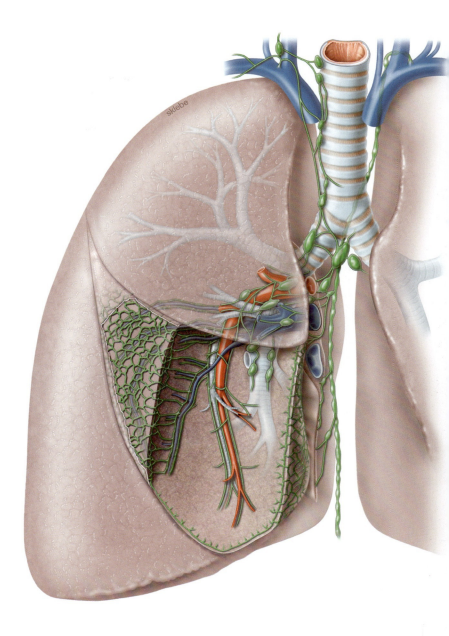

→ *Dissection Link*

The Vasa thoracica interna, which are descending parallel to the Sternum, are presented by fenestration of the intercostal spaces to avoid damage during opening of the thoracic cavity. After removal of the Sternum with the anterior portions of the ribs, the lungs are separated at the hilum and removed. Now, the mediastinum is dissected: First the pericardium and the adjacent N. phrenicus are exposed. The pericardium is opened ventrally. The heart can be dissected in situ or after separation from the great vessels. The removal of epicardial adipose tissue serves the purpose of tracing the branches of the coronary arteries. Using scissors, the ventricles are opened from the direction of the aorta and the pulmonary trunk, respectively, and the right atrium is opened from the direction of both Vv. cavae. After removal of the pericardium, the Oesophagus and the course of the Aorta thoracica, the Vv. azygos and hemiazygos, the N. vagus, and the Ductus thoracicus are presented in the posterior mediastinum. The parietal pleura is removed to facilitate the dissection of the sympathetic trunk with the corresponding Nn. splanchnici as well as intercostal neurovascular structures. Finally, the preparation of the superior mediastinum exposes the residual Thymus and the passageways to the neck are traced.

EXAM CHECK LIST

• Development: cardiac chambers and septation, foetal circulation, malformations • heart: situs with projections in radiology and auscultation of the valves, pericardial cavity and N. phrenicus, organisation (inner relief and valves, conducting system), Aa. coronariae including important branches and autonomic innervation • lungs: Cavitas pleuralis with recesses, projections of pulmonary borders, organisation in lobes and segments, Nodi lymphoidei • organisation and content of the mediastinum: branches of the aorta, Oesophagus with parts, constrictions and blood vessels, Trachea with bifurcation, Ductus thoracicus with dependent lymphatic drainage, organisation of the autonomic nervous system including the courses of the Truncus sympathicus and N. vagus [X]

5 Viscera of the Thorax

Heart → Lungs → Oesophagus →

Projection of the heart

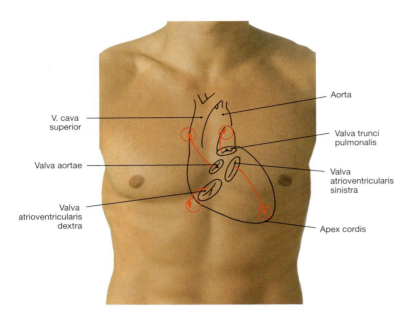

Fig. 5.1 Contours of the heart, cardiac valves and auscultation areas projected onto the ventral thoracic wall.
The **right heart contour** projects from the third to the sixth costal cartilage onto a line 2 cm lateral of the right sternal border.
The **contour of the left heart** projects onto a connecting line between the lower border of rib III (2–3 cm parasternal) and the left midclavicular line.
On each side, the heart contains an atrioventricular valve between the atrium and the ventricle and a semilunar valve between the ventricle and the respective artery.
The **projection of the four cardiac valves** forms a cross which is slightly deviating to the left side from the median axis.
The projection of the cardiac valves is of minor importance in clinical practice since the heart sounds and potential murmurs travel with the blood flow and are auscultated at the points of maximal intensity (circles).

	Surface Projection of Cardiac Valves	Auscultation Sites of Cardiac Valves
Pulmonary valve	left (!) sternal border, 3rd costal cartilage	parasternal left 2nd ICS
Aortic valve	left sternal border, 3rd ICS	parasternal right 2nd ICS
Mitral valve	left 4th to 5th costal cartilages	in the midclavicular line 5th ICS
Tricuspid valve	retrosternal 5th costal cartilage	parasternal right 5th ICS

ICS = intercostal space

Fig. 5.2 Projection of the heart onto the thorax; ventral view (according to [2])
We distinguish **four surfaces** of the heart: The ventrally oriented Facies sternocostalis predominantly represents the right ventricle. The Facies diaphragmatica points inferiorly and consists of parts of both ventricles. The Facies pulmonalis is formed by the right atrium on the right side and by the left ventricle on the left side. Thus, the right ventricle does not contribute to any of the cardiac borders.
The major part of the Facies sternocostalis is covered by the Pleura. These areas represent the **Recessus costomediastinales** of the pleural cavity. The pleural borders separate from each other inferior to rib IV and form the boundary of the **Trigonum pericardiacum** where the Pericardium is directly adjacent to the ventral wall of the Thorax.

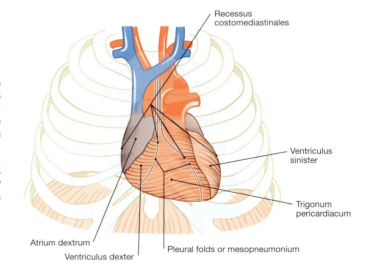

Clinical Remarks

During **auscultation** of the heart using a stethoscope **heart sounds** are detected at several locations. These sounds are the result of the normal heart action:
- The **first heart sound (S1)** is generated at the beginning of the systole due to ventricular contraction and closure of the atrioventricular valves.
- The **second heart sound (S2)** is generated at the beginning of the diastole due to the closure of the semilunar valves.

In contrast, **heart murmurs** are always pathological phenomena and are generated by malfunction of heart valves. Narrowing (stenosis) as well as insufficient closure (insufficiency) of the valves may cause heart murmurs. The time point and the location of the murmur provide information about the nature of the dysfunction of the affected valve. The **percussion** of the heart is used to assess its **size**.

The projection of the heart contours, which are covered by the Recessus costomediastinales, equals the **relative cardiac dullness** since the percussion sound is less absorbed. If this area extends to the left side beyond the midclavicular line, left ventricular hypertrophy is likely. The Trigonum pericardiacum is the area in which the heart is directly adjacent to the ventral thoracic wall. This is referred to as the area of the **absolute cardiac dullness** since the percussion sound is maximally absorbed. Although the Trigonum pericardiacum has only minor diagnostic value, it may be relevant to determine the position of the right ventricle for emergency **intracardiac injections**. Here, the risk of injuring the Pleura and thus inducing a pneumothorax is minimal. Intracardiac injections are performed in the fourth or fifth intercostal space approximately 2 cm left parasternal. However, this procedure is hazardous and not recommended anymore.

Thymus → Topography → Sections

Projection of the heart

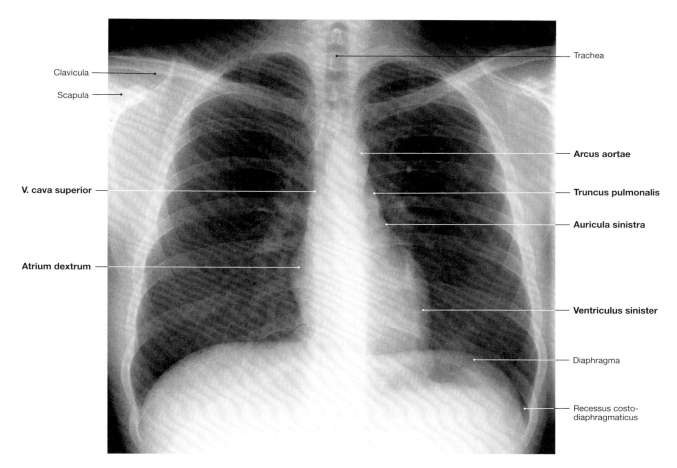

Fig. 5.3 Thoracic cage, Cavea thoracis, with thoracic viscera; radiograph in postero-anterior (PA) beam projection.

The radiograph can be used to assess the size of the heart. In addition to the absolute size, knowledge of the structures contributing to the heart contours is of importance.

Fig. 5.4 Schematic drawing of the heart contours in the radiograph.
From cranial to caudal, the **right border of the heart** is formed by the following structures:
- superior vena cava (V. cava superior)
- right atrium (Atrium dexter)

From cranial to caudal, the **left border of the heart** is formed by the following structures:
- aortic arch (Arcus aortae)
- Truncus pulmonalis
- left auricle (Auricula sinistra)
- left ventricle (Ventriculus sinister)

Thus, the right ventricle does not contribute to any of the cardiac borders!
M = Median axis of the body

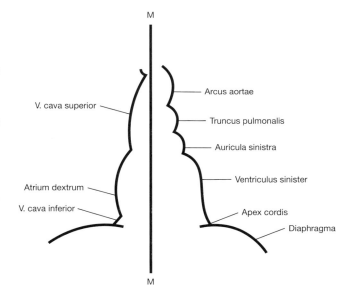

Clinical Remarks

The conventional radiograph of the Thorax provides information on the size of the heart. The transverse diameter of the heart shows individual differences. However, if it is larger than half of the diameter of the Thorax, an enlargement of the heart is present which may be caused by **hypertrophy** of the cardiac muscle or by **dilation** of the cardiac wall. Frequently, the heart is enlarged to the left side (Facies pulmonalis sinistra) indicative of left ventricular pathologies. **Arterial hypertension, stenosis,** or **insufficiency** of the **aortic** or **mitral valves,** respectively, may be causally involved. In contrast, an enlargement of the right ventricle, as in pulmonary hypertension, chronic obstructive pulmonary disease (COPD), or pulmonary emboli are not recognised with a sagittal radiograph of the Thorax. This is explained by the fact that the right ventricle does not contribute to any of the cardiac contours. In this case, lateral radiographic projections or tomographic methods such as computed tomography (CT) or magnetic resonance tomographic imaging (MRI) are required.

5 Viscera of the Thorax

Heart → Lungs → Oesophagus →

Development

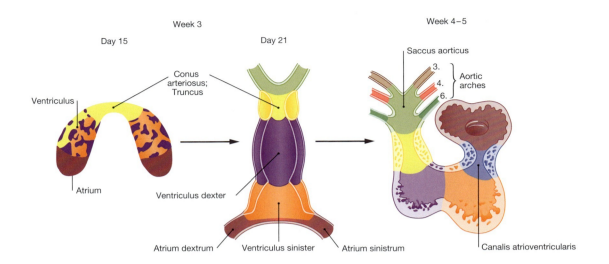

Fig. 5.5 Stages of cardiac development during weeks 3 to 5. (according to [2])
At **week 3,** the initially horseshoe-shaped **endocardial tube** develops from a vascular plexus in the cardiogenic mesoderm. Several gaps around the endocardial tube merge to establish the pericardial cavity which connects with the general body cavity. The inner layer of the pericardial cavity condenses to form the Myocardium. The Epicardium develops from cells which migrate from the Septum transversum and the liver primordium. The lateral crus of the endocardial tube fuse to build the **cardiac tube** which contracts rhythmically from the end of week 3 onwards. The cardiac tube initially comprises a paired atrium with the Sinus venosus collecting incoming blood, one ventricle, and the Conus arteriosus as the outflow segment. Caused by differential longitudinal growth and reorganisation of the respective segments, during weeks 4 – 5 the cardiac tube develops into the S-shaped **heart loop.** The transition between atrium and ventricle is constricted to form the unpaired atrioventricular canal. The latter originally opens into the left part of the ventricle, but is later shifted to the midline and partitioned into a right and left atrioventricular opening through endocardial cushions. These endocardial cushions later form the atrioventricular valves.

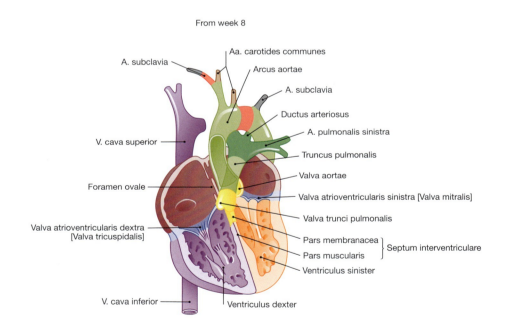

Fig. 5.6 Stages of cardiac development during weeks 5 to 7. (according to [2])
During weeks 5–7, the **interventricular septum** develops (Pars muscularis), which incompletely separates the two ventricles. The latter communicate until the end of week 7 when the formation of the Pars membranacea of the septum completes the ventricular separation. The Conus arteriosus of the outflow tract is separated spirally and, together with the adjacent Saccus aorticus, forms the **Truncus pulmonalis** and the **Aorta.**

The primitive **aortic arches** (arteries of the pharyngeal arches) derive from the Saccus aorticus. From the original six aortic aches, only the third, fourth and sixth contribute to the development of the great vessels. The A. carotis communis derives from the third aortic arch. Parts of the A. subclavia and the aortic arch develop from the fourth aortic arches on the right and left side, respectively. The proximal parts of the right and left pulmonary artery and the Ductus arteriosus develop from the right and left sixth aortic arches, respectively.

Development

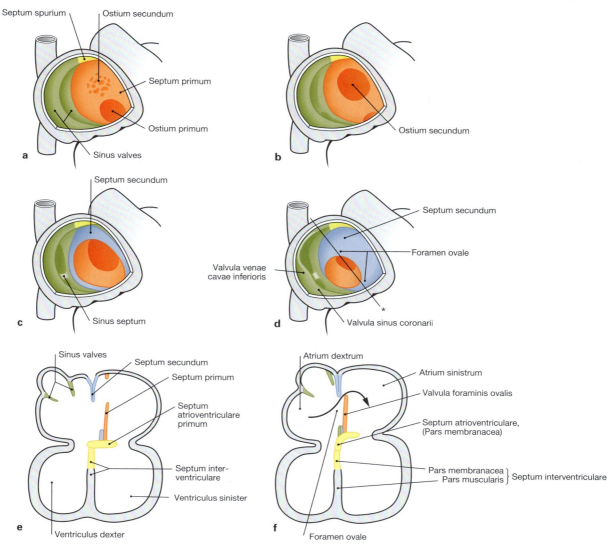

Figs. 5.7a to f Developmental steps in septum formation during weeks 5 (a, b), 6 (c, e), 7 and 8 (d, f); view from the opened right atrium (a–d) and in the four-chamber plane (e and f). (according to [2])

a Septum formation in the atria occurs during weeks 5–7 and begins with the growth of the **Septum primum** from dorsal and cranial until the **Ostium primum** is formed.

b Within the upper part of the Septum primum, the **Ostium secundum** is created through programmed cell death (apoptosis).

c, e On the right side of the Septum primum, the Septum secundum develops. Both septa lie adjacent to each other and outline the Foramen ovale.

d, f The Septum primum forms the **Valvula foraminis ovalis** which facilitates the directional blood flow from the right into the left atrium (→ Fig. 5.8). After birth, the Valvula foraminis ovalis closes the Foramen ovale due to the increased blood pressure in the left atrium (→ Fig. 5.10).

* sectional plane in e, f

Clinical remarks

Congenital cardiac defects are detected in 0.75% of all newborns and thus represent the most common developmental defects. Luckily, not all cardiac defects have functional relevance and require therapeutic intervention. To understand the cause and the symptoms of heart defects in children and adolescents, one has to be familiar with the basic steps in cardiac development. Because of their clinical significance and the relevance for exams in different disciplines, the most important developmental cardiac defects are briefly explained. They are divided in three pathophysiological groups:
- The most frequent defects are those with resulting **left-to-right shunt** (ventricular septal defect 25%, atrial septal defect 12%, patent ductus arteriosus [→ p. 9] 12%). Due to the higher blood pressure in the systemic circulation, the blood shunts from the left heart to the right heart and into the pulmonary circulation. If this shunt is not corrected surgically the developing pulmonary hypertension may cause a secondary right ventricular insufficiency.
- Defects with a **right-to-left shunt** (FALLOT's tetralogy 9%, transposition of the great vessels 5%) are characterised by a bluish tinge of the skin and mucous membranes (cyanosis) because deoxygenated blood enters the systemic circulation.
- Heart defects causing **obstruction** (pulmonary valve stenosis, aortic valve stenosis, aortic coarctation [→ p. 9] 6% each) result in the hypertrophy of the affected ventricle.

The **FALLOT's tetralogy** comprises a combination of a ventricular septal defect, pulmonary stenosis, right ventricular hypertrophy, and "overriding" aorta. Due to asymmetric septation of the Conus arteriosus, the pulmonary valve is too narrow and the aorta is too wide and shifted to the right side above the septum ("overriding"). Untreated, the pulmonary stenosis causes hypertrophy of the right ventricle with subsequent right-to-left shunt via the ventricular septal defect and cyanosis.

Viscera of the Thorax

Heart → Lungs → Oesophagus →

Prenatal circulation

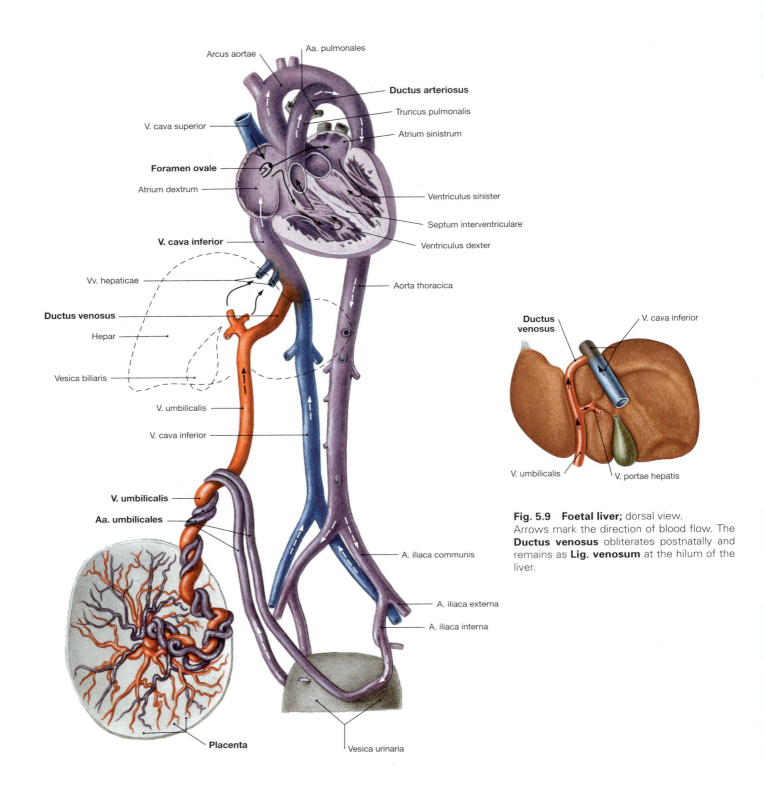

Fig. 5.8 Prenatal circulation (foetal circulation); schematic illustration.
This illustration distinguishes the different oxygen contents of the blood by colour codings: oxygenated blood (red), deoxygenated blood (blue), mixed blood (purple). The arrows mark the direction of blood flow.
The following aspects distinguish the foetal circulation from the postnatal circulation: umbilical blood vessels, Ductus venosus, Ductus arteriosus, Foramen ovale (→ Fig. 5.10).
Deoxygenated blood from the foetus is conveyed to the placenta by the **Aa. umbilicales** which derive from the Aa. iliacae internae. After oxygenation the blood from the placenta reaches the foetus via the **V. umbilicalis** and bypasses the liver through the **Ductus venosus** due to the high flow resistance of the foetal liver. A valve at the opening of the inferior vena cava (Valvula venae cavae inferioris) directs the incoming blood predominantly through the **Foramen ovale** to the left atrium. This way, the oxygenated blood takes the shortest way to reach the foetal organs. Blood from the superior vena cava enters the right atrium and right ventricle. From the right ventricle it reaches the Truncus pulmonalis and is shunted through the **Ductus arteriosus** directly into the Aorta, thus bypassing the non-functional lung circulation.

Fig. 5.9 Foetal liver; dorsal view.
Arrows mark the direction of blood flow. The **Ductus venosus** obliterates postnatally and remains as **Lig. venosum** at the hilum of the liver.

Thymus → Topography → Sections

Postnatal circulation

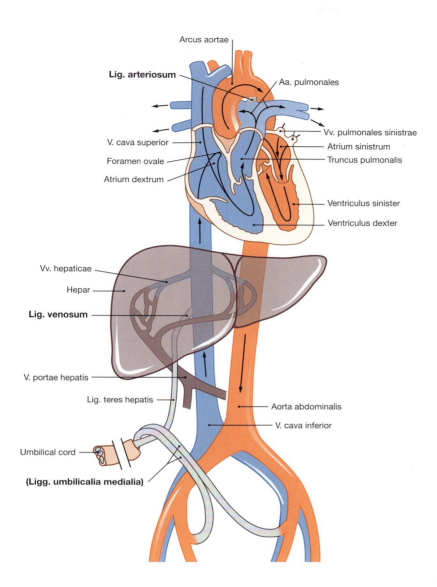

Fig. 5.10 Schematic illustration of the postnatal circulation.
After birth the placental circulation is interrupted. Inflation of the lungs due to breathing opens the pulmonary circulation and causes an increase in blood pressure in the left atrium. The switch from prenatal to postnatal circulation includes the following changes: The valve-like opening of the Foramen ovale between the right and left atrium is closed passively due to the increased blood pressure in the left atrium. Later, the Valvula foraminis ovalis fuses with the Septum secundum leaving the persistent **Fossa ovalis** in the right atrium.

The Ductus arteriosus functionally closes within a few days and later obliterates to the **Lig. arteriosum** (→ Fig. 5.13).
The Ductus venosus obliterates postnatally and remains as **Lig. venosum** at the hilum of the liver.
The umbilical vein obliterates and remains as **Lig. teres hepatis** between liver and ventral abdominal wall.
The distal parts of the umbilical arteries form the **Lig. umbilicale mediale** on the right and left side, which contribute to the formation of the respective Plica umbilicalis medialis at the internal relief of the ventral abdominal wall.

Clinical Remarks

Patent Ductus arteriosus: Since prostaglandin E_2 dilates the ductus, prostaglandin synthesis inhibitors may be successfully applied to close this vessel and prevent surgical intervention. However, their use as anti-inflammatory agents in pregnant women may result in premature closure of the Ductus arteriosus in the foetus.
Patent Foramen ovale: Approximately 20% of the adult population have a remaining opening in the area of the Foramen ovale. Usually, this has no functional relevance. In some cases, however, this opening may facilitate ascending emboli dislodged from crural thrombi to reach the systemic circulation and cause an organ infarction or stroke.

Aortic coarctation: If the closure of the Ductus arteriosus extends to the adjacent parts of the aortic arch this may cause an aortic coarctation. As a result, a left ventricular hypertrophy develops with concomitant arterial hypertension in the upper body and low arterial blood pressure in the lower body. Physical examination reveals a systolic heart murmur between both scapulae. Radiological findings may include notching of the ribs due to a strong collateral circulation from the A. thoracica interna via the intercostal arteries. The stenosis is treated surgically or with dilation to prevent heart failure or strokes which occur already at a young age.

Thoracic Viscera

Heart → Lungs → Oesophagus →

The heart in-situ

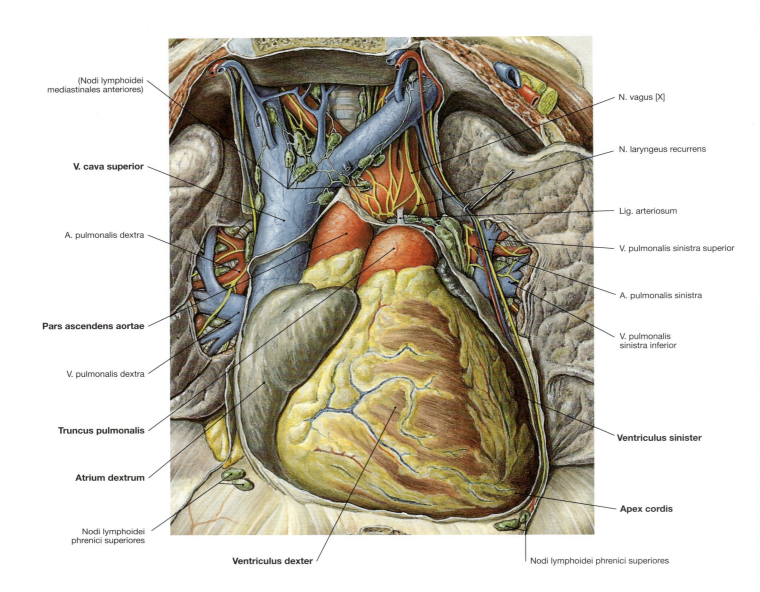

Fig. 5.11 Position of the heart, Cor, within the thorax, Situs cordis; ventral view; after opening of the Pericardium.

The heart is positioned within the pericardial cavity (Cavitas pericardiaca) in the inferior middle mediastinum. The broad base of the heart is oriented in an oblique direction towards the superior right side and corresponds to the valvular plane at the base of the great vessels. The apex of the heart (Apex cordis) points to the inferior left side and ventrally. Base and apex are connected by the **longitudinal axis** (12 cm) which shows an oblique course in the Thorax directed from the dorsal right side to the ventral left side. Thus, the longitudinal axis of the heart forms an **angle of 45° with all three anatominal planes.** The heart has four surfaces (→ Fig. 5.2). The anterior surface (Facies sternocostalis) is predominantly formed by the right ventricles. The inferior surface is adjacent to the diaphragm and consists of parts of the right and left ventricles. The inferior surface clinically represents the "posterior wall" in the diagnostic electrocardiogram (ECG) when referred to as posterior myocardial infarction. The Facies pulmonalis is determined by the right atrium on the right side and by the left ventricle on the left side.

Pericardium

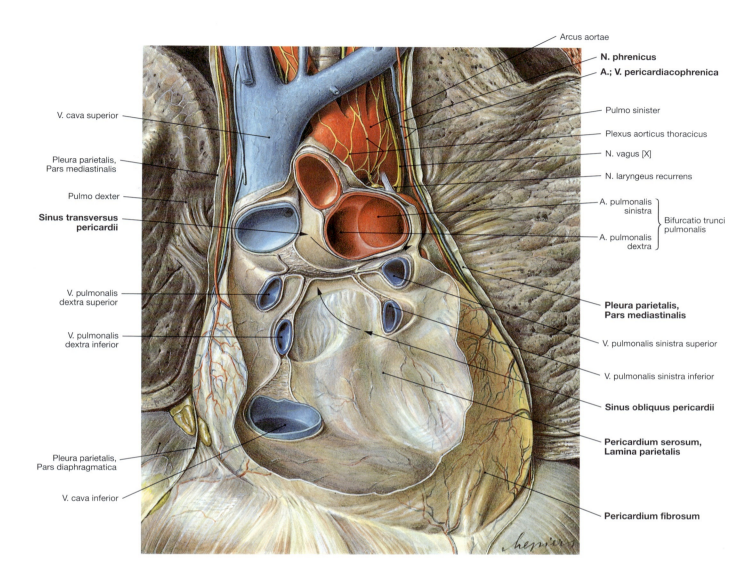

Fig. 5.12 Pericardium, Pericardium; ventral view; after removal of the anterior part of the Pericardium and the heart.
The Pericardium surrounds the heart, stabilises its position and enables the heart to contract without friction. The outer layer of dense connective tissue is the **Pericardium fibrosum**. Adjacent to the Pericardium fibrosum on the inner side is the Tunica serosa or **Pericardium serosum** which comprises the parietal layer (Lamina parietalis) of the Pericardium serosum. This Lamina parietalis is a continuation of the Lamina visceralis of the Pericardium (= **Epicardium**) folding back at the ventral side of the roots of the great cardiac vessels. At the posterior side of the atria, the reflection between the Epicardium and the parietal Pericardium forms a vertical fold between the V. cava inferior and superior and a horizontal fold between the upper pulmonary veins of the right and left side. These folds of the Pericardium create two sinuses of the pericardial cavity at the posterior side (Sinus pericardii, arrows):

- **Sinus transversus pericardii**: above the horizontal fold between the V. cava superior (posterior) and the Aorta and Truncus pulmonalis (anterior)
- **Sinus obliquus pericardii**: below the horizontal fold between the pulmonary veins on both sides

The Pericardium fibrosum is connected to:
- the Centrum tendineum of the diaphragm
- the posterior aspect of the Sternum (Ligg. sternopericardiaca)
- the tracheal bifurcation (Membrana bronchopericardiaca)

At the outer side, the fibrous Pericardium is covered by the **Pleura parietalis, Pars mediastinalis.** The N. phrenicus and the Vasa pericardiacophrenica course between these two layers.
The Epicardium is the visceral layer of the Pericardium serosum.

Clinical Remarks

The pericardial cavity usually contains 15 – 35 ml of serous fluid. The Pericardium has a total volume of 700 – 1100 ml, including the heart. With diseases accompanied by inflammatory reactions of the pericardium **(pericarditis)** or with insufficiency of the heart, additional fluid may accumulate **(pericardial effusion)** which may even impede the cardiac function.

Following rupture of the cardiac wall due to myocardial infarction or injury (stab wounds), blood may rapidly accumulate in the pericardial cavity and inhibit the cardiac functions resulting in death **(pericardial tamponade).**

Thoracic Viscera

Heart → Lungs → Oesophagus →

Heart

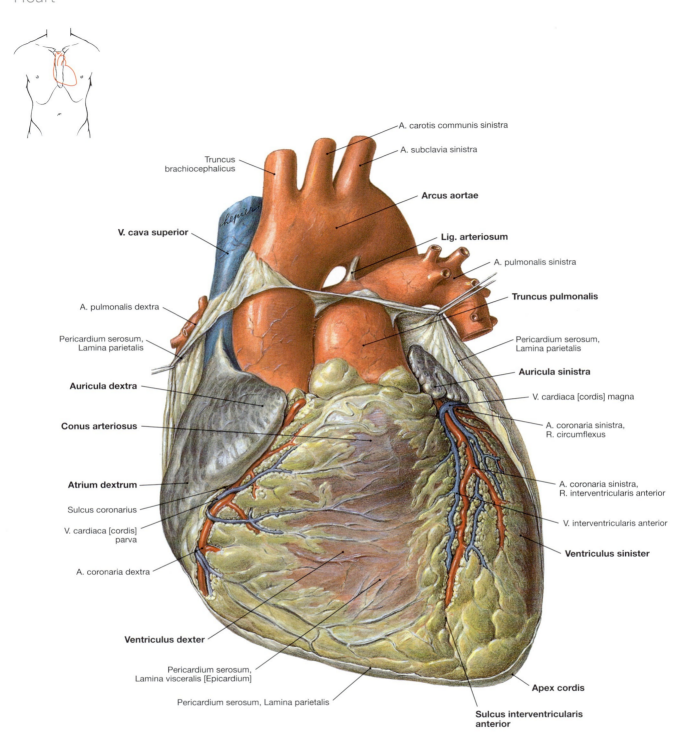

Fig. 5.13 Heart, Cor; ventral view.
The heart weighs 250–300 g and has approximately the size of the fist of the respective person. The apex of the heart (Apex cordis) is directed to the inferior left side. The base of the heart represents the position of the **Sulcus coronarius** which harbours, among other structures, the A. coronaria dextra. The heart consists of a ventricular chamber (ventricle) and an atrial chamber (atrium) on the right and left side, respectively. At the anterior surface (Facies sternocostalis), the **Sulcus interventricularis anterior** is visible. It depicts the position of the interventricular septum (Septum interventriculare) and contains the R. interventricularis anterior of the A. coronaria sinistra. At the inferior surface (Facies diaphragmatica), the border between the two ventricles is marked by the **Sulcus interventricularis posterior** (→ Fig. 5.14). Prior to the transition into the Truncus pulmonalis, the right ventricle is dilated as Conus arteriosus. The origin of the Aorta from the left ventricle is not visible from the outer surface due to the spiral course of the Aorta behind the Truncus pulmonalis. Therefore, the Aorta appears at the right side of the Truncus pulmonalis. The aortic arch is connected with the pulmonary trunk through the Lig. arteriosum, a developmental relict of the Ductus arteriosus of the foetal circulation (→ Fig. 5.8). Both atria have an anterior pouch which is referred to as auricle (Auriculae dextra and sinistra). The V. cava superior and inferior enter the right atrium, the four pulmonary veins enter the left atrium.

Heart

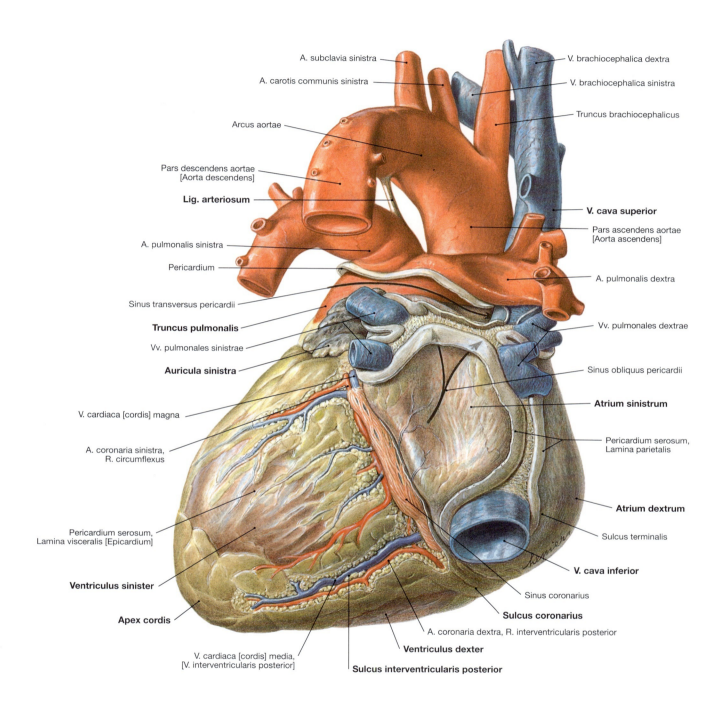

Fig. 5.14 Heart, Cor; dorsal view (explanation → Fig. 5.13).

Clinical Remarks

Most hearts seen in the gross anatomy dissection course are enlarged. This clearly shows how frequently diseases occur that present with either **hypertrophy** (e.g. arterial hypertension) or **dilation** (alcohol abuse, viral infections) of the heart.

The weight of the heart in professional athletes (training, anabolic substances) may reach 500 g. This is considered the **critical heart weight** since sufficient blood supply is not warranted above this weight with resulting risk of myocardial infarction. Some pathologic conditions may cause the heart to weigh up to 1100 g, a condition referred to a **cor bovinum** (bovine heart).

5 Thoracic Viscera

Heart → Lungs → Oesophagus →

Cardiac wall

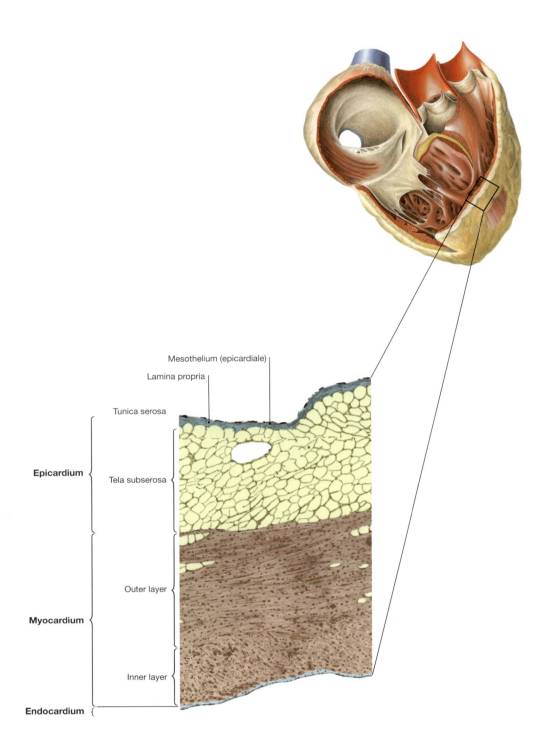

Fig. 5.15 Structure of the cardiac wall; microscopic detail from the right atrium. (according to [2])
The wall of the heart is composed of three layers:
- **Endocardium:** inner surface consisting of endothelium and connective tissue
- **Myocardium:** cardiac muscle with cardiomyocytes
- **Epicardium:** Tunica serosa and Tela subserosa at the outer surface of the heart, representing the visceral layer of the Pericardium serosum. In the human, the Tela subserosa contains plenty of white adipose tissue in which the coronary blood vessels and nerves are embedded.

Cardiac muscle

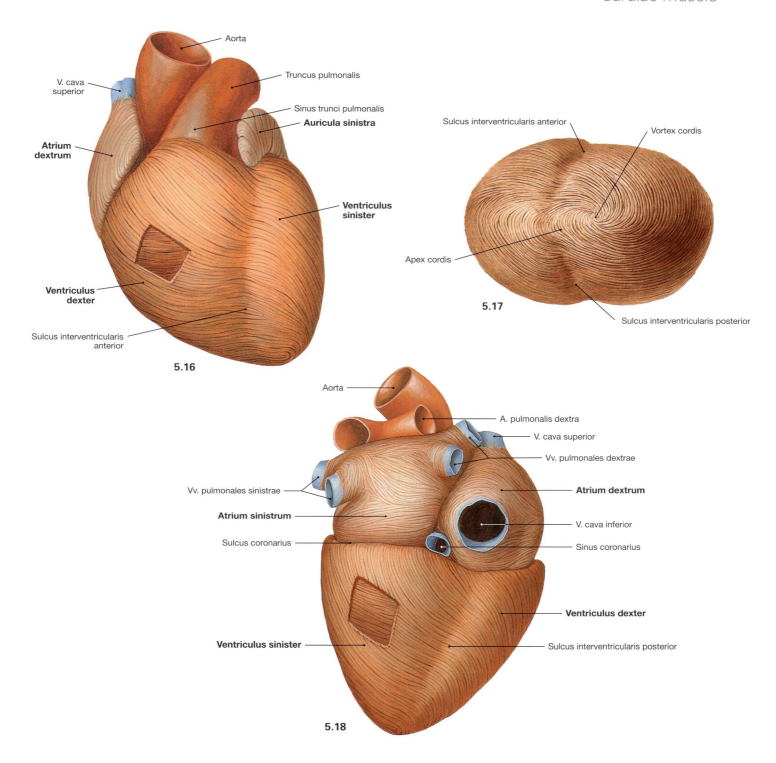

Fig. 5.16 to Fig. 5.18 Cardiac muscle, Myocardium; ventral view (→ Fig. 5.16), view from the apex (→ Fig. 5.17), and dorsocaudal view (→ Fig. 5.18).
The cardiac muscle fibres consist of cardiomyocytes and have a spiral arrangement within the cardiac wall. In the wall of the atria and the right ventricle they form two layers, in the wall of the left ventricle they even form three layers. Thus, the Myocardium and the cardiac wall are much thicker in the region of the left ventricle. In comparison to the right ventricle, this arrangement reflects the much higher pressure required in the left ventricle to pump the blood into the systemic circulation. The right ventricular wall is 3–5 cm thick, the left ventricular wall is 8–12 cm thick.

Clinical remarks

If the thickness of the **left ventricular wall exceeds 15 mm**, the term **hypertrophy** is used. A left ventricular hypertrophy may be caused for example by stenosis of the aortic valve or arterial hypertension. In the **right ventricle,** a hypertrophy is already diagnosed if the wall thickness **exceeds 5 mm.** This may be caused by a stenosis of the pulmonary valve or by pulmonary hypertension, resulting from chronic obstructive pulmonary diseases (COPD; e.g. asthma) or recurrent pulmonary emboli.

Thoracic Viscera

Heart → Lungs → Oesophagus →

Heart valves and skeleton of the heart

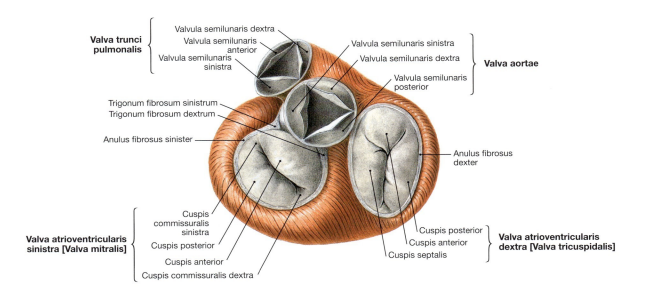

Fig. 5.19 Heart valves, Valvae cordis; cranial view; after removal of the atria, Aorta and pulmonary trunk.
The heart has two **atrioventricular valves** (Valvae cuspidales) between the atria and the ventricles of each side. The right atrioventricular valve (Valva atrioventricularis dextra) consists of three cusps **(tricuspid valve)**. The left atrioventricular valve (Valva atrioventricularis sinistra) has two cusps **(bicuspid valve, mitral valve)**. The cusps are anchored to the papillary muscles by tendinous cords (Chordae tendineae) to prevent a prolapse of the valves during ventricular contraction.

In addition, between the ventricles and the great arteries lie the **aortic valve** (Valva aortae) on the left side and the **pulmonary valve** (Valva pulmonalis) on the right side, both of which consist of three semilunar cusps (Valvulae semilunares). When blood is ejected from the ventricles into the great arteries during the **systole** the **semilunar valves are open** and the atrioventricular valves are closed. When the ventricles are filled with blood from the atria during the **diastole** the **atrioventricular valves are open** and the semilunar valves are closed.

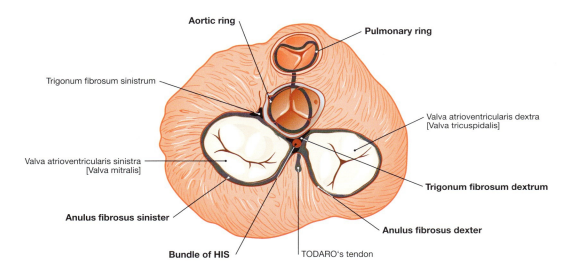

Fig. 5.20 Fibrous skeleton of the heart; cranial view, schematic illustration. (according to [2])
The valves are anchored to the cardiac skeleton. The latter consists of connective tissue forming a ring (Anuli fibrosi dexter and sinister) around the atrioventricular valves (Valvulae atrioventriculares) and a fibrous ring around the semilunar valves (Valvulae semilunares). Between the Anuli fibrosi lies the Trigonum fibrosum dextrum. Here, the bundle of HIS belonging to the conducting system of the heart passes over from the right atrium to the interventricular septum. In addition to the stabilisation of the valves, the fibrous skeleton of the heart serves as an electrical insulator between the atria and the ventricles because all cardiomyocytes are attached to the cardiac skeleton. Since there is no connection between atria and ventricles via cardiomyocytes, the electrical impulse reaches the ventricles exclusively through the bundle of HIS.

Clinical Remarks

If the valves are constricted (stenosis) or do not close properly (insufficiency), **heart murmurs** develop. These are most noticeable at the auscultation sites of the respective valves (→ Fig. 5.1). If a murmur is detected during **systole** (between the first and second heart sounds) in the area of one of the **atrioventricular (AV) valves**, an **insufficiency** of the respective valve is likely, since AV valves are normally closed during systole. If the murmur is detected in this area during **diastole, a stenosis** of the respective valve can be suspected since the AV valves are fully opened during diastole. The **opposite** is true for the **semilunar valves**. Valvular stenoses are either congenital or acquired (rheumatic diseases, bacterial endocarditis). Valvular insufficiencies are mostly acquired and may also be the result of a myocardial infarction if one or more of the papillary muscles are affected by the infarction.

Chambers of the heart

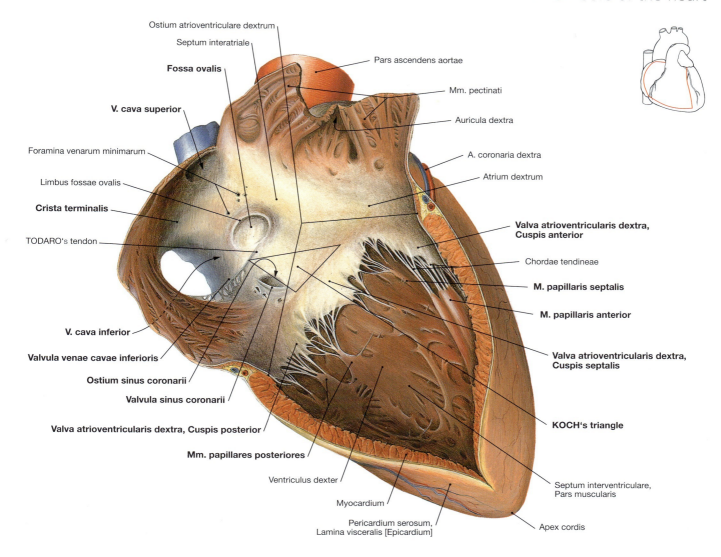

Fig. 5.21 Right atrium, Atrium dextrum, and right ventricle, Ventriculus dexter; ventral view.
The right atrium consists of a part with a smooth inner surface, the sinus of venae cavae (Sinus venarum cavarum), and of a muscular part with a rough inner surface consisting of the pectinate muscles (Mm. pectinati). Both parts are separated by the **Crista teminalis,** which serves as important landmark for the localisation of the sinu-atrial node (SA node) of the cardiac conducting system (→ pp. 20–22). The SA node is positioned at the outside (subepicardial) of this demarcation line between the entry of the V. cava superior and the right auricle (Auricula dextra). The interatrial septum (Septum interatriale) shows a remnant of the former Foramen ovale, the **Fossa ovalis** with its rim, the Limbus fossae ovalis. The opening of the **Sinus coronarius** (Ostium sinus coronarii), which represents the largest cardiac vein, has a valve (Valvula sinus coronarii) and the opening of the V. cava inferior is also demarcated by a valve (Valvula venae cavae inferioris). Both valves, however, are not able to close the respective lumen. Smaller cardiac veins enter the right atrium directly (Foramina venarum minimarum). An extension of the Valvula venae cavae inferioris is the TODARO's tendon (Tendo valvulae venae cavae inferioris). It serves as a landmark and, together with the opening of the Sinus coronarius and the tricuspid valve (Valva atrioventricularis dextra), it forms the **KOCH's triangle** which harbours the AV node (→ Figs. 5.25 to 5.27). In the right ventricle, the three cusps are attached via Chordae tendineae to the three **papillary muscles** (Mm. papillares anterior, posterior and septalis). Of the interventricular septum (Septum interventriculare) only the muscular part is visible in this illustration. Starting from the interventricular septum, specific fibres of the cardiac conducting system (moderator band described by LEONARDO DA VINCI, not visible here) course to the anterior papillary muscle **(M. papillaris anterior).** This connection is referred to as the **Trabecula septomarginalis** (→ Fig. 5.27).

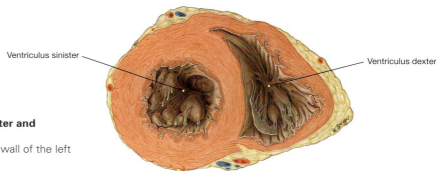

Fig. 5.22 Left and right ventricles, Ventriculus sinister and Ventriculus dexter; cross-section, cranial view.
Because of the substantially stronger muscle layer, the wall of the left ventricle is thicker than the wall of the right ventricle.

Thoracic Viscera

Heart → Lungs → Oesophagus →

Chambers of the heart

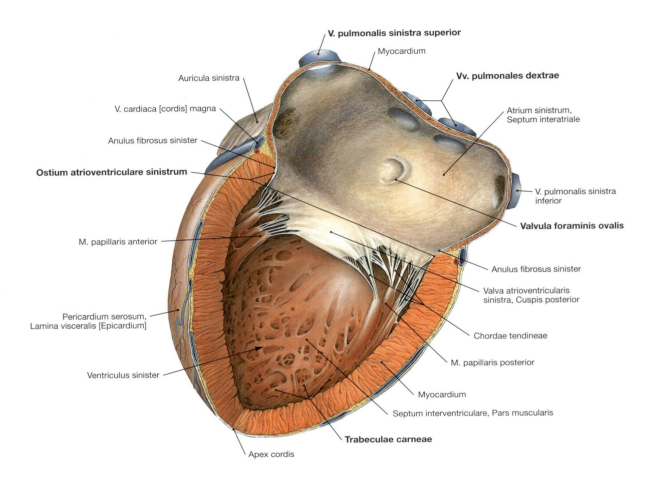

Fig. 5.23 Left atrium, Atrium sinister, and left ventricle, Ventriculus sinister; lateral view.
The auricle (Auricula sinistra) represents the muscular part of the left atrium. The four pulmonary veins (Vv. pulmonales) enter the smooth-walled part of the left atrium. The septal wall shows the crescent-shaped Valvula foraminis ovalis, a remnant of the Septum primum during the development of the heart (→ Fig. 5.7). The Ostium atrioventriculare sinistrum is the junction to the left ventricle and contains the Valva mitralis. The wall of the left ventricle is not smooth but structured by trabeculae of the ventricular Myocardium (Trabeculae carneae).

Thymus → Topography → Sections

Chambers of the heart

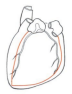

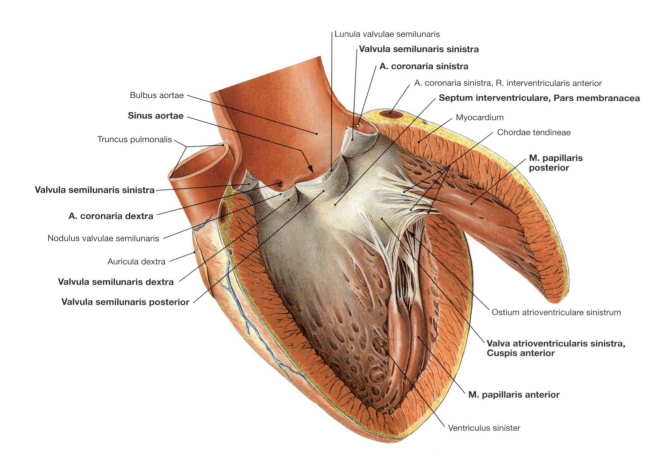

Fig. 5.24 Left ventricle, Ventriculus sinister; lateral view.
The mitral valve (Valva atrioventricularis sinistra) only consists of two cusps. Thus, only two **papillary muscles** are required (Mm. papillares anterior and posterior). Beneath the mitral valve, the approximately 1 cm² large area of the **Pars membranacea** of the interventricular septum is located. However, the major part of the interventricular septum consists of cardiac muscle fibres (Pars muscularis). Blood from the left ventricle is pumped through the aortic valve (Valva aortae) into the dilated part of the Aorta (Bulbus aortae). The **aortic valve** consists of three semilunar valves (Valvulae semilunares) which cover the Sinus aortae from which the right and left **coronary arteries** originate (Aa. coronariae dextra and sinistra).

19

Thoracic Viscera

Heart → Lungs → Oesophagus →

Electrical stimulation and conducting system of the heart

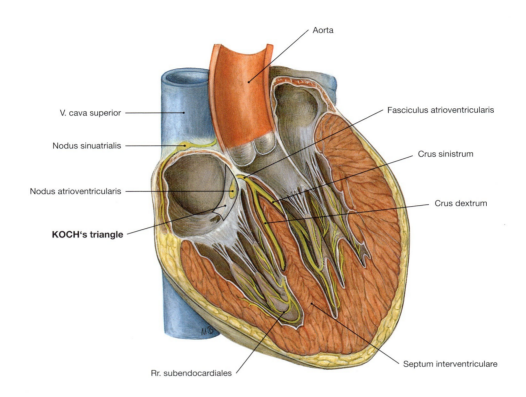

Fig. 5.25 Electrical stimulation and conducting system [Complexus stimulans et conducente cordis] along the axis of the sectioned heart.
The heart harbours an electrical stimulation and conducting system which consists of modified cardiomyocytes instead of nerve fibres. This system is divided into the following parts:
- **sinu-atrial node** (Nodus sinuatrialis, SA-node; node of KEITH-FLACK)
- **atrioventricular node** (Nodus atrioventricularis; AV-node, node of TAWARA)
- **atrioventricular bundle** (Fasciculus atrioventricularis, bundle of HIS)
- **right and left bundle branch** (Crus dextrum and sinistrum node of TAWARA)

The electrical stimulation is initiated independently within the **sinu-atrial node** by spontaneous depolarisation in the specialised myocardial cells and has a frequency of approximately 70/min. The SA-node has a size of approximately 3 × 10 mm and is located within the wall of the right atrium in a groove (Sulcus terminalis cordis) between the entry of the V. cava superior and the right auricle. This groove corresponds to the Crista terminalis at the inner surface of the right atrium. The SA node is occasionally covered by an area of subepicardial adipose tissue making it visible from outside. The SA node is supplied by the sinu-atrial nodal branch (R. nodi sinuatrialis) which derives from the A. coronaria dextra in most cases. The electrical signal spreads from the SA node through the Myocardium of both atria (myogenic conduction) and reaches the **AV node.** The latter slows down the frequency of the electrical signal to allow a sufficient filling of the ventricles.

The AV node, approximately 5 × 3 mm in size, is embedded within the Myocardium of the atrioventricular septum at KOCH's triangle. The KOCH's triangle is confined by the TODARO's tendon, the entry of the Sinus coronarius, and the septal cusp of the tricuspid valve (→ Fig. 5.21). The AV node is also supplied by a separate branch (R. nodi atrioventricularis) which usually derives from the dominant coronary artery (in most cases the A. coronaria dextra) near the branching of the R. interventricularis posterior.

From the AV node the electrical signal is conveyed by the **bundle of HIS** (approx. 4 × 20 mm) through the Trigonum fibrosum dextrum to the interventricular septum.

In the Pars membranacea of the interventricular septum the bundle of HIS divides into the **right and left bundle branch.** The left bundle branch splits into the anterior, septal and posterior subendocardial fasciculi to the respective parts of the Myocardium including the papillary muscles and the apex of the heart. The right bundle branch descends subendocardially in the septum to the apex of the heart and reaches the anterior papillary muscle via the Trabecula septomarginalis (→ Fig. 5.27).

Thymus → Topography → Sections

Electrical stimulation and conducting system of the heart

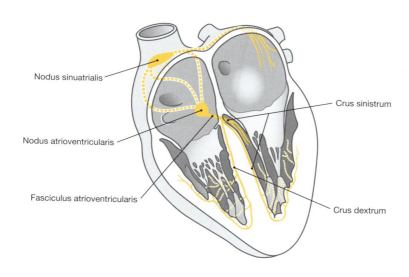

Fig. 5.26 Electrical stimulating and conducting system of the heart; schematic illustration.

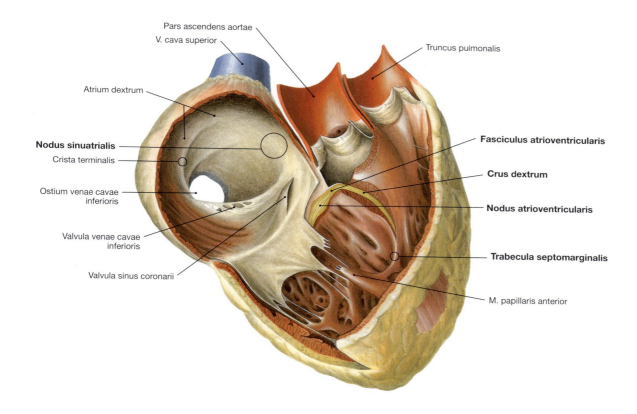

Fig. 5.27 Electrical stimulation and conducting system of the heart.
The electrical stimulation and conducting system is organised in **four parts** (→ Fig. 5.25).

The illustration demonstrates how a part of the right bundle branch (Crus dextrum) reaches the right anterior papillary muscle via the Trabecula septomarginalis.

Thoracic Viscera

Heart → Lungs → Oesophagus →

Electrical stimulation and conducting system of the heart

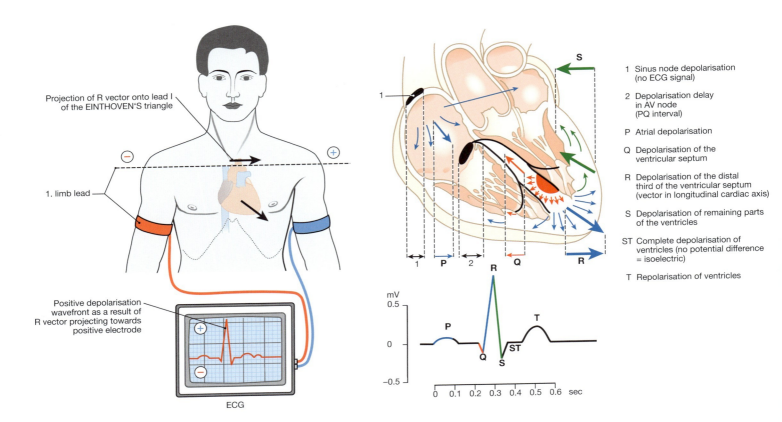

Fig. 5.28 Anatomical principles of the electrocardiogram (ECG). (according to [2])

The electrical signal spreads from the sinu-atrial node to the AV node which causes a delay in electrical conduction before reaching the interventricular septum via the bundle of HIS. The right and left bundle branches then divide and stimulate the ventricular Myocardium. This conduction of electrical impulses within the heart can be detected by electrodes on the surface of the body. If the electrical signal travels towards the electrode at the surface of the body, it results in a positive upward amplitude of the baseline voltage. Because of the small volume of the sinu-atrial node, the SA excitation is not detectable in the ECG. The depolarisation of the atria is represented by the **P wave**. The depolarisation delay by the AV node occurs during the PQ segment. The latter depicts the lack of polarisation changes during the depolarisation of the entire atrial Myocardium. The rapid retrograde direction of the depolarisation of the interventricular septum is illustrated by the **Q wave**. Depolarisation of the ventricular myocardium towards the apex of the heart is represented by the ascending limb of the **R wave**, whereas the propagation of the depolarisation away from the apex results in the descending limb of the R wave and in the short **S wave**. During the ST segment the entire ventricular Myocardium is depolarized. Since the repolarisation of the ventricular myocardium occurs in the same direction as the depolarisation, the **T wave** also shows a positive (upward) amplitude. Usually, three limb leads are recorded to determine the electrical axis of the heart according to the largest amplitude of the R wave. However, this electrical axis is influenced by the thickness of the Myocardium in both ventricles and by the excitability of the tissue and is therefore not identical with the anatomical axis of the heart.

Clinical Remarks

The ECG is used to detect **cardiac arrhythmias,** for example if the heart beats too fast **(tachycardia, > 100/ min),** too slow **(bradycardia, < 60/min),** or in an irregular way **(arrhythmia).** In addition, reduced arterial perfusion due to coronary artery disease (e.g. myocardial infarction), and other diseases such as myocardial inflammation result in alterations of the electrical conduction. The ECG is of particular importance for the identification of myocardial infarction.

If atrial fibres bypass the AV node and directly link to the bundle of HIS or the ventricular myocardium (KENT's bundles), cardiac arrhythmias are the result **(WOLFF-PARKINSON-WHITE syndrome).** If these arhythmias cause severe symptoms and resist pharmacological treatment, it may be necessary to interrupt the accessory bundles using a cardiac catheter device.

Innervation of the heart

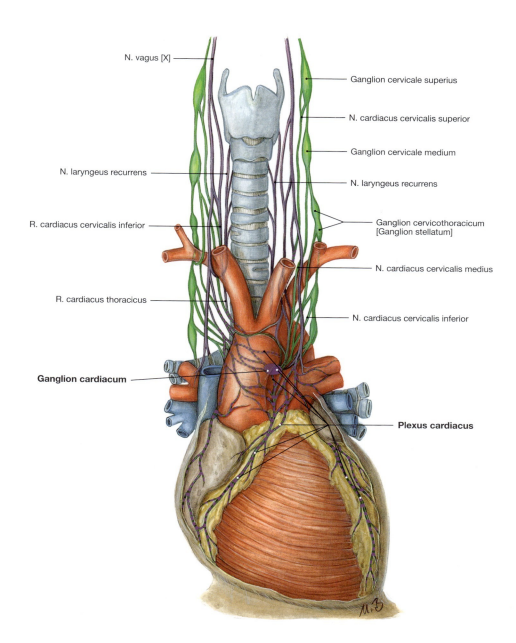

Fig. 5.29 Innervation of the heart: Plexus cardiacus with sympathetic (green) and parasympathetic (purple) nerve fibres; schematic illustration.
The function of the electrical conducting system and the Myocardium can be modified by autonomic innervation to adjust to the needs of the whole body. This is the purpose of the Plexus cardiacus as part of the autonomic nervous system. The Plexus cardiacus consists of sympathetic and parasympathetic nerve fibres. The cell bodies (Perikarya) of the postganglionic **sympathetic nerve fibres** reside within the cervical ganglia of the sympathetic trunk (Truncus sympathicus) and reach the Plexus cardiacus via three nerves (Nn. cardiaci cervicales superior, medius and inferior). **Sympathetic stimulation** increases the heart rate (positive chronotropic effect), the speed of conduction (positive dromotropic effect), and the excitability (positive bathmotropic effect) of the cardiomyocytes. In addition, sympathetic stimulation enhances the contractile force (positive inotropic effect) due to accelerated relaxation (positive lusitropic effect). **Parasympathetic stimulation** elicits negative chronotropic, dromotropic, and bathmotropic effects and, additionally, has negative inotropic effects on the atrial Myocardium. The **parasympathetic nerve fibres** derive as preganglionic nerve fibres from the N. vagus [X] and reach the Plexus cardiacus as Rr. cardiaci cervicales superior and inferior and as Rr. cardiaci thoracici. In the Plexus cardiacus, they are synapsed within numerous (up to 500) tiny ganglia (Ganglia cardiaca) onto postganglionic neurons.

Clinical Remarks

Increased sympathetic tonus, as in stress situations, is accompanied by increased heart rate **(tachycardia)** and elevated arterial blood pressure **(arterial hypertension)**. Injury to the parasympathetic fibres may also result in tachycardia. The increased activity of the heart also increases the oxygen consumption by the cardiomyocytes. This may cause an angina pectoris and myocardial infarction in the case of a pre-existing coronary artery stenosis (coronary artery disease).

Thoracic Viscera

Heart → Lungs → Oesophagus →

Coronary arteries

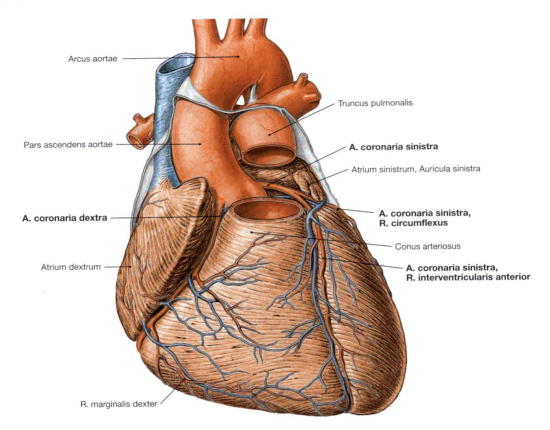

Fig. 5.30 Coronary arteries, Aa. coronariae; ventral view.
The **right coronary artery** (A. coronaria dextra) has its origin at the right aortic sinus and courses in the Sulcus coronarius to the inferior margin (Margo dexter). It continues to the Facies diaphragmatica where in most cases the **R. interventricularis posterior** branches off as a terminal branch.
The **left coronary artery** (A. coronaria sinistra) originates at the left aortic sinus and divides after 1 cm to form the **R. interventricularis anterior**, which courses to the apex of the heart, and the **R. circumflexus**. The latter courses in the Sulcus coronarius around the left cardiac margin to reach the posterior aspect of the heart.
Conventionally, the coronary dominance is determined by the artery that supplies the R. interventricularis posterior. In most cases the right coronary artery is dominant (in the "co-dominant" and the "right-dominant" perfusion type, together in 75% of all cases → pages 26 and 27).

Important Branches of the Right Coronary Artery (A. coronaria dextra)

- R. coni arteriosi
- R. nodi sinuatrialis (two-thirds of all cases): to the **SA node**
- R. marginalis dexter
- R. posterolateralis dexter
- R. nodi atrioventricularis: to the **AV node** (if "right dominant")
- R. interventricularis posterior (if "right dominant") with Rr. interventriculares septales, supplying the **bundle of HIS**

Important Branches of the Left Coronary Artery (A. coronaria sinistra)

R. interventricularis anterior:
- R. coni arteriosi
- R. lateralis (clinical term: R. diagonalis)
- Rr. interventriculares septales

R. circumflexus:
- R. nodi sinuatrialis (one-third of all cases): to the **SA node**
- R. marginalis sinister
- R. posterior ventriculi sinistri

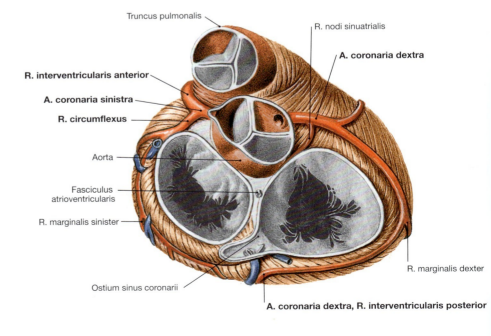

Fig. 5.31 Coronary arteries, Aa. coronariae; cranial view.

Veins of the heart

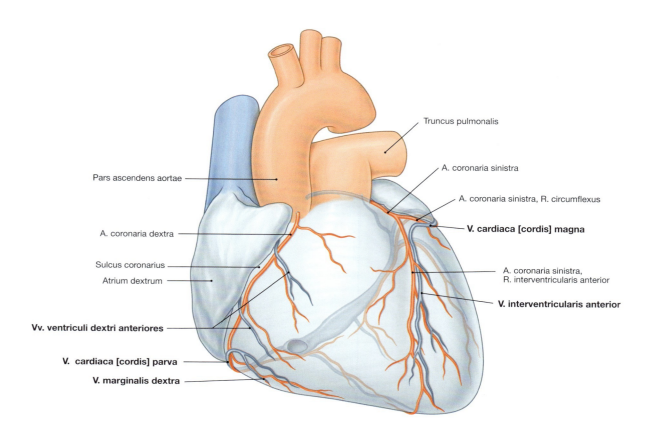

Fig. 5.32 Cardiac veins, Vv. cordis; ventral view. [8]
The venous blood from the heart is collected in **three major systems.** 75% of the venous blood are collected in the Sinus coronarius and drain into the right atrium. The remaining 25% of the venous blood drain into the atria and ventricles directly via the **transmural** and the **endomural system** (→ pages 17–19).

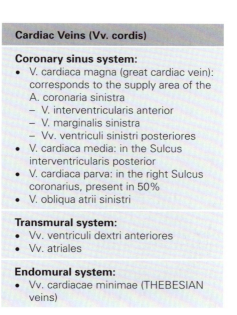

Cardiac Veins (Vv. cordis)

Coronary sinus system:
- V. cardiaca magna (great cardiac vein): corresponds to the supply area of the A. coronaria sinistra
  – V. interventricularis anterior
  – V. marginalis sinistra
  – Vv. ventriculi sinistri posteriores
- V. cardiaca media: in the Sulcus interventricularis posterior
- V. cardiaca parva: in the right Sulcus coronarius, present in 50%
- V. obliqua atrii sinistri

Transmural system:
- Vv. ventriculi dextri anteriores
- Vv. atriales

Endomural system:
- Vv. cardiacae minimae (THEBESIAN veins)

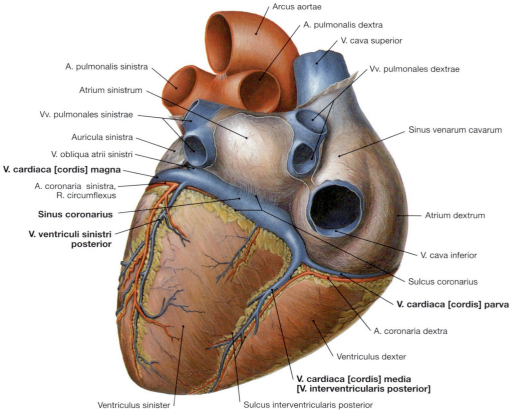

Fig. 5.33 Cardiac veins, Vv. cordis; dorsocaudal view.

Thoracic Viscera

Heart → Lungs → Oesophagus →

Coronary artery dominance

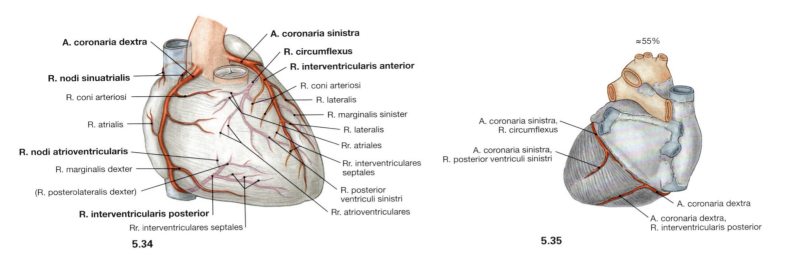

Fig. 5.34 and Fig. 5.35 "Balanced" or co-dominant coronary circulation between the coronary arteries, Aa. coronariae; ventral (→ Fig. 5.34) and dorsal (→ Fig. 5.35) views.

In 55% of all cases, the R. interventricularis posterior originates from the A. coronaria dextra but does not supply the posterior aspect of the left ventricle. This is referred to as a "balanced" or "co-dominant" perfusion type.

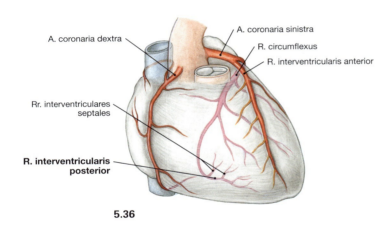
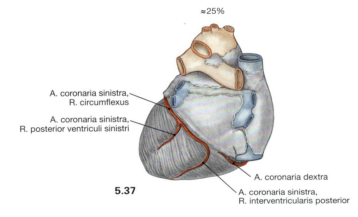

Fig. 5.36 and Fig. 5.37 "Left dominant" coronary circulation between the coronary arteries, Aa. coronariae; ventral (→ Fig. 5.36) and dorsal (→ Fig. 5.37) views.

In 25% of all cases, the R. interventricularis posterior originates from the A. coronaria sinistra.

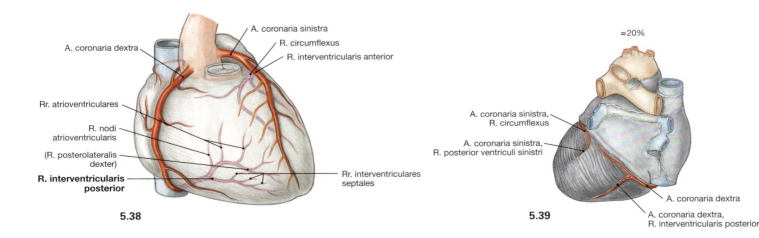

Fig. 5.38 and Fig. 5.39 "Right-dominant" coronary circulation between the coronary arteries, Aa. coronariae; ventral (→ Fig. 5.38) and dorsal (→ Fig. 5.39) views.

In 20% of all cases, the A. coronaria dextra not only branches off the R. interventricularis posterior but also supplies parts of the posterior aspect of the left ventricle.

Thymus → Topography → Sections

Coronary artery dominance

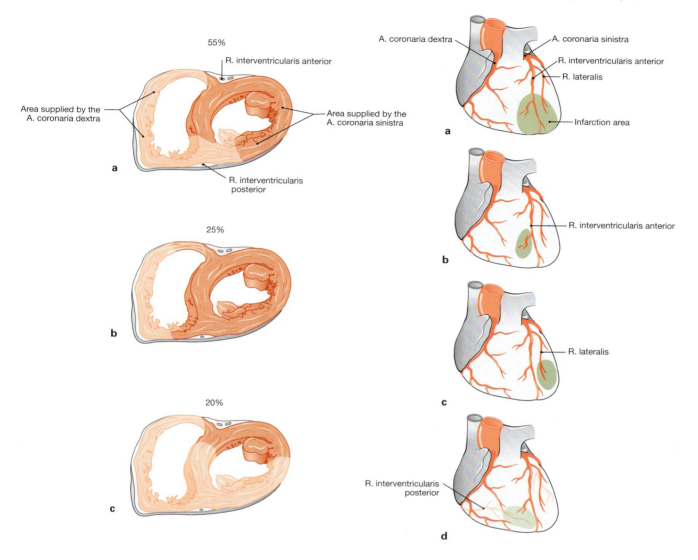

Figs. 5.40a to c Areas supplied by the A. coronaria dextra (light red) and sinistra (dark red) in the cross-section; caudal view. (according to [2])
a **Balanced or co-dominant perfusion type:** The left coronary artery supplies the anterior two-thirds of the septum via the Rr. interventriculares septales of the R. interventricularis anterior (left anterior descending [LAD] branch). Corresponding branches derived from the R. interventricularis posterior of the right coronary artery supply the posterior third of the septum.
b **Left-dominant perfusion type:** The left coronary artery supplies the entire septum and the AV node.
c **Right-dominant perfusion type:** Two thirds of the septum and large areas of the posterior aspect of the left ventricle are supplied by the A. coronaria dextra.
The perfusion type has effects on the severity of a myocardial infarction due to an occlusion of one of the coronary arteries.

Figs. 5.41a to d Infarction pattern owing to the occlusion of the coronary arteries.
a Isolated occlusion of the R. interventricularis anterior (left anterior descending [LAD] branch) results in an anterior myocardial infarction.
b Distal occlusion of the R. interventricularis anterior results in myocardial infarction of the apex of the heart, often referred to as apical infarction.
c If only the R. lateralis is occluded the myocardial infarction is restricted to the lateral wall of the ventricle.
d Occlusion of the R. interventricularis posterior results in a posterior myocardial infarction (PMI) of the Facies diaphragmatica.

Clinical Remarks

The **coronary artery disease** (CAD) is caused by a stenosis of the coronary arteries resulting from arteriosclerosis. Due to insufficient myocardial perfusion this may cause pain in the chest **(angina pectoris)** which may radiate into the arm (mostly the left arm) or into the neck. Total occlusion of an artery results in necrosis of the dependent Myocardium **(myocardial infarction, MI).** Functionally, coronary arteries are terminal arteries and a distinct infarction pattern results from the occlusion of the supplying arteries. These patterns may be detected in various leads in the ECG. The most definitive evidence is achieved through coronary catheterisation using a radiocontrast agents (coronary angiogram). The **posterior myocardial infarction** (PMI) is often accompanied by bradycardiac arrhythmias because the artery supplying the AV node originates near the outlet of the R. interventricularis posterior (→ Fig. 5.38). Mostly, the R. interventricularis posterior is the terminal branch of the A. coronaria dextra (in the balanced and the right-dominant perfusion types). Due to the low pressure system of the right heart, the Myocardium of the right ventricle requires less oxygen when compared to the left ventricle. Thus, even a proximal occlusion of the A. coronaria dextra may only result in an isolated posterior myocardial infarction. In this case, the bradycardia may be severe due to the insufficient perfusion of the SA node.

5 Thoracic Viscera

Heart → **Lungs** → Oesophagus →

Projection of trachea and bronchi

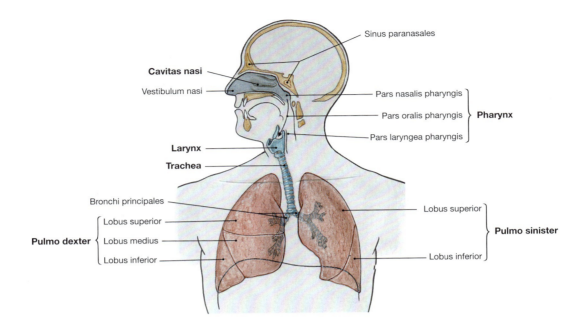

Fig. 5.42 Upper and lower respiratory tract; schematic illustration.
The respiratory system is devided in upper and lower parts.
The **upper** respiratory tract comprises:
- nasal cavity (Cavitas nasi)
- parts of the Pharynx

The **lower** respiratory tract comprises:
- Larynx
- wind pipe (Trachea)
- lungs (Pulmones)

The right lung (Pulmo dexter) has three lobes, the left lung (Pulmo sinister) has two lobes.

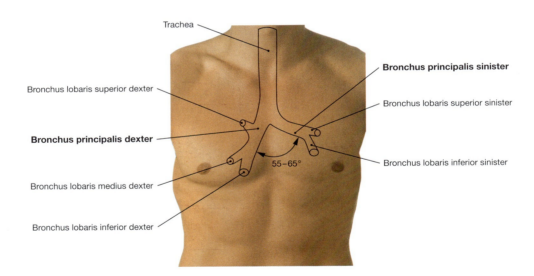

Fig. 5.43 Projection of the Trachea and main bronchi onto the anterior chest wall.
The Trachea is 10–13 cm long and elongates up to 5 cm during deep inspiration. The origin of the Trachea at the cricoid cartilage projects onto the 7th cervical vertebra; the bifurcation of the Trachea into the two main bronchi projects onto the 4th and 5th thoracic vertebrae (rib II to III). The angle between the main bronchi is 55° to 65°. The **right main bronchus** (Bronchus principalis dexter) is larger, 1–2.5 cm in length, and is positioned **nearly vertically.** The **left main bronchus** (Bronchus principalis sinister) is almost twice as long and located more horizontally.

Clinical Remarks

Because of the almost vertical position of the right main bronchus foreign bodies more frequently enter the **right lung** during inspiration **(aspiration).** This knowledge may provide the crucial time advantage when dealing with medical emergencies.

Thymus → Topography → Sections

Projection of the lungs

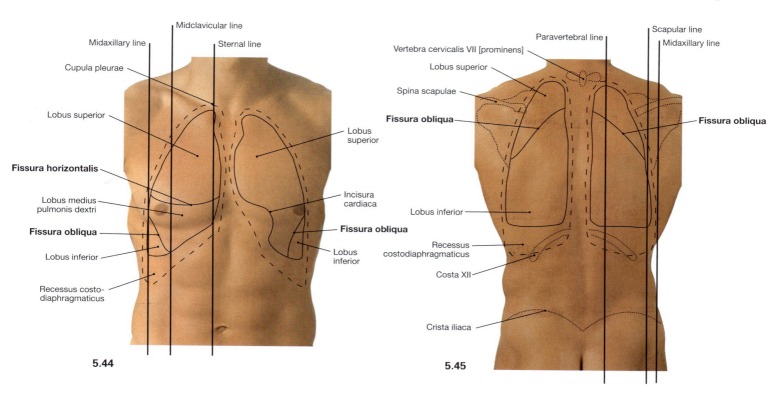

Fig. 5.44 and Fig. 5.45 Projection of the borders of the lungs and Pleura onto the anterior (→ Fig. 5.44) and posterior (→ Fig. 5.45) thoracic walls.
The **right lung** has three lobes which are separated by the **Fissura obliqua** and the **Fissura horizontalis**. On the dorsal side, the Fissura obliqua follows rib IV and, thus, separates the superior and the inferior lobes. From the midaxillary line onwards, the Fissura obliqua descends more steeply to reach rib VI at the midclavicular line. Anteriorly, the Fissura obliqua separates the middle and inferior lobes (→ Figs. 5.53 and 5.54). The Fissura horizontalis projects along rib IV on the anterior chest wall and separates the superior and the middle lobes.

The **left lung** only has two lobes which are separated by the **Fissura obliqua**. Because the heart enlarges the Mediastinum to the left side (Incisura cardiaca), the volume of the left lung is smaller and the position of the left lung differs in the sternal and midclavicular lines (see table).
Each **pleural cavity** (Cavitas pleuralis) is lined by the **parietal pleura** (Pleura parietalis). The Pleura parietalis is divided into Pars mediastinalis, Pars costalis, and Pars diaphragmatica (→ Fig. 5.65). The pleural cavities have four pleural recesses (Recessus pleurales). The largest recessus is the **Recessus costodiaphragmaticus** which expands laterally up to 5 cm in the midaxillary line.

	Borders of the Right Lung	Borders of the Left Lung
Sternal line	crosses rib VI	crosses rib IV
Midclavicular line	parallel to rib VI	crosses rib VI
Midaxillary line	crosses rib VIII	as right side
Scapular line	crosses rib X	as right side
Paravertebal line	crosses rib XI	as right side

pleural borders: one rib lower each

Clinical Remarks

Identifying lung and pleural borders is important during physical examination in order to determine the **size and mobility of the lungs during respiration**. In addition, these borders are invaluable for the **localisation of pathological changes** such as pulmonary infiltrations in pneumonia or increased fluid in the pleural cavity (pleural effusion). **Pleural effusions** are drained from the Recessus costodiaphragmaticus by thoracocentesis.

Nociceptive innervation and resulting **pain sensation** is restricted to the **Pleura parietalis**. Chest pain accompanying pneumonias or bronchial carcinomas therefore indicates an involvement of the Pleura parietalis.
If air enters the pleural cavity, the lung collapses completely or partially **(pneumothorax)**. This is detected by a loud (hypersonoric) sound during percussion.

5 Thoracic Viscera

Heart → Lungs → Oesophagus →

Development

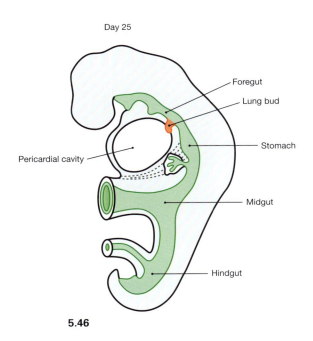

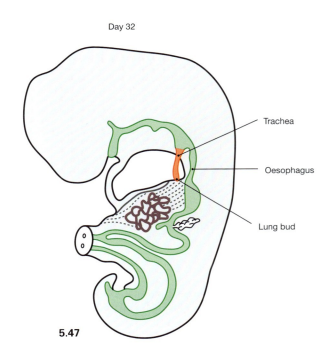

Fig. 5.46 and Fig. 5.47 Development of the lower respiratory tract on day 25 (→ Fig 5.46) and day 32 (→ Fig 5.47). (according to [3])

In week 4, the epithelial tissues of Larynx, Trachea, and lungs begin to develop from the endoderm of the foregut. Connective tissue, smooth muscles, and blood vessels derive from the surrounding mesoderm.

Clinical Remarks

Incomplete separation of the Oesophagus and the Trachea may result in the formation of pathological connections **(tracheo-oesophageal fistulas)** which are frequently associated with an oesophageal blind-ending pouch **(oesophageal atresia)**.

From **week 28** onwards, the alveoli produce and secrete **surfactant**, a lipoprotein mixture which reduces the surface tension of the alveoli. From week 35 on, surfactant production is usually sufficient to enable **spontaneous breathing**. Insufficient surfactant production results in a **respiratory distress syndrome** (RDS) which accounts for the most common cause of death in premature infants. Up to 60% of infants born before week 30 develop RDS.

It is only after birth with the first cry of the newborn, that the lungs inflate with air. Thus, in forensic medicine the **floating lung test** is used to differentiate whether a child was born alive (lung floats) or dead (lung sinks).

Thymus → Topography → Sections

Development

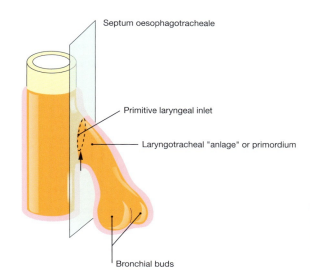

Fig. 5.48 Development of the Septum oesophagotracheale. [20]
During week 4 and 5, mesenchymal folds develop on both sides which fuse to the Septum oesophagotracheale and separate the primordium of the lower respiratory tract from the Oesophagus.

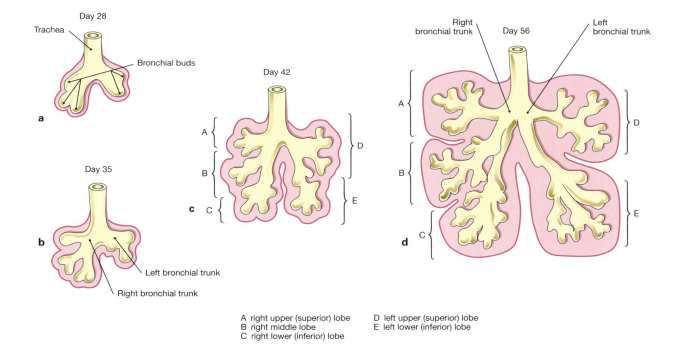

A right upper (superior) lobe
B right middle lobe
C right lower (inferior) lobe
D left upper (superior) lobe
E left lower (inferior) lobe

Figs. 5.49a to d Stages of the lung development. [20]
Three stages of the lung development are recognised which partly overlap:
- **pseudoglandular period** (weeks 7–17): development of the air conducting part of the respiratory tract
- **canalicular period** (weeks 13–26): early development of the respiratory part (gas exchange) of the respiratory tract
- **alveolar period** (week 23 to 8 years of life): development of alveoli

5 Thoracic Viscera

Heart → **Lungs** → Oesophagus →

Trachea and bronchi

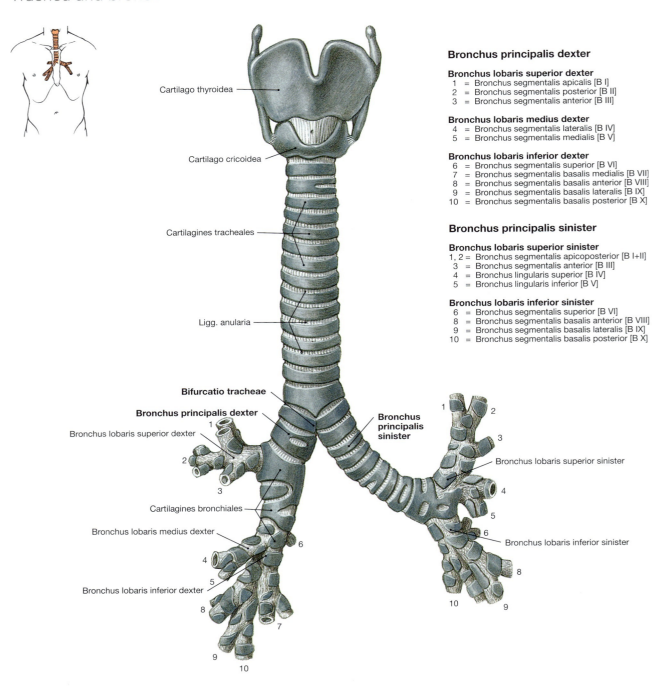

Fig. 5.50 Lower respiratory tract with larynx, Larynx, trachea, Trachea and bronchi, Bronchi; ventral view.
The Trachea is 10–13 cm long and extends from the cricoid cartilage of the Larynx to its division (Bifurcatio tracheae) into the two main (primary) bronchi **(Bronchi principales)**. The Trachea is organised in a cervical part (Pars cervicalis) and a thoracic part (Pars thoracica). Projection and topography are described in → Fig 5.43. The main bronchi further divide in three and two lobar bronchi **(Bronchi lobares)** on the right and left sides, respectively. The lobar bronchi give rise to the segmental bronchi **(Bronchi segmentales)**. The right lung has 10 segments and, thus, 10 segmental bronchi. In the left lung, however, segment 7 and the respective Bronchus are missing.

The more detailed systematic description of the bronchial tree is not illustrated here. The bronchi further divide six- to twelvetimes before continuing as bronchioles. **Bronchioles** have a diameter smaller than 1 mm and lack cartilage and glands within their walls. Each bronchiole is associated with a pulmonary lobule (Lobulus pulmonis) and further divides three- to fourtimes before continuing as terminal bronchioles **(Bronchioli terminales)**. These represent the last segment of the **air conducting part** of the respiratory system which has a volume of 150–170 ml. Each Bronchiolus terminalis opens into a pulmonary acinus **(Acinus pulmonis)** which generates 10 additional generations of Bronchioli respiratorii with Ductus and Sacculi alveolares. All parts of the acinus contain alveoli and, thus, the acinus belongs to the gas-exchanging part of the respiratory system.

Clinical Remarks

The volume of the air conducting part of the respiratory system **(150–170 ml)** is equivalent to the **anatomical dead-space** and has an important practical relevance for **resuscitation**. During ventilation the volume of oxygenated air needs to exceed 170 ml to effectively reach the alveoli and avoid just moving the air column within the conducting part. Thus, artificial ventilation is more effective when performed slower with larger volume than with high frequency and smaller volume.

Thymus → Topography → Sections

Structure of trachea and bronchi

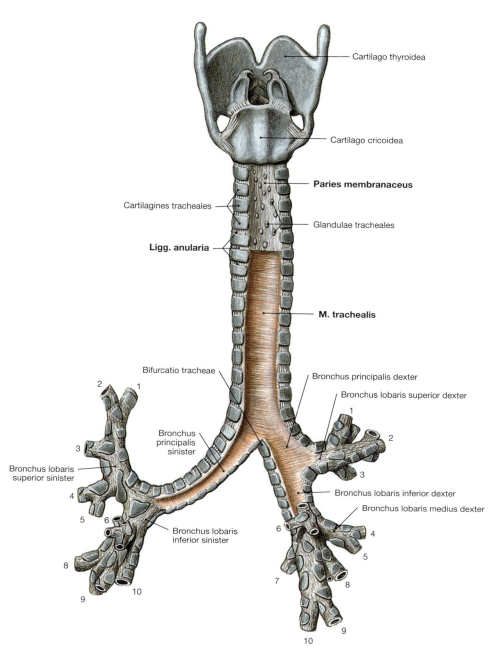

Fig. 5.51 Lower respiratory tract with larynx, Larynx, trachea, Trachea, and bronchi, Bronchi; dorsal view.
The systematic composition of the bronchial tree is described in → Figure 5.50. The dorsal view clearly shows that the dorsal walls of the Trachea and the main bronchi do not consist of cartilage (Paries membranaceus) but predominantly of smooth muscles (M. trachealis). The incomplete tracheal cartilages are connected by Ligg. anularia. These comprise elastic connective tissue and enable the elongation of the trachea for up to 5 cm during deep inspiration.

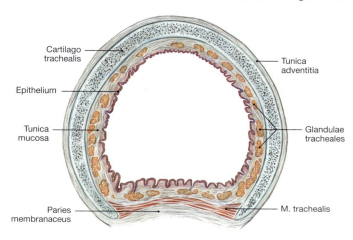

Fig. 5.52 Trachea, Trachea; cross-section, microscopic view.
The walls of the trachea and the main bronchi comprise a mucous membrane (Tunica mucosa) on the luminal side followed by the Tunica fibromusculocartilaginea and the Tunica adventitia. The Tunica fibromusculocartilaginea consists of 16 to 20 horseshoe-shaped incomplete tracheal cartilages of hyaline cartilage, which are bridged posteriorly by a smooth muscle (M. trachealis).

Thoracic Viscera

Heart → **Lungs** → Oesophagus →

Lungs

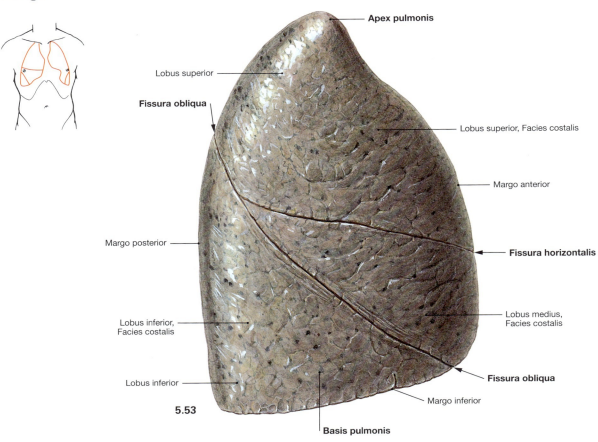

5.53

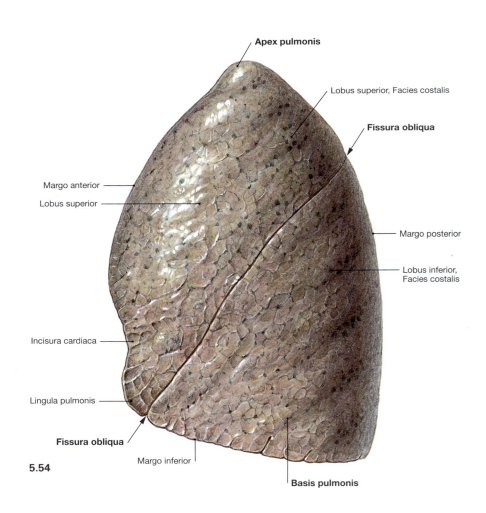

5.54

Fig. 5.53 and Fig. 5.54   Right lung, Pulmo dexter (→ Fig. 5.53), **and left lung, Pulmo sinister** (→ Fig. 5.54); lateral view.

The right lung has three lobes (Lobi superior, medius and inferior) which are separated by the Fissura obliqua and the Fissura horizontalis. The left lung has only two lobes (Lobi superior and inferior) separated by the Fissura obliqua. The Lingula pulmonis of the superior lobe is equivalent to the middle lobe of the right lung and forms a tongue-like extension inferior to the Incisura cardiaca.

The volume of the right lung encompasses 2–3 l, during maximal inspiration even 5–8 l. This volume is equivalent to a gas exchange area of 70–140 m^2. Due to the left-shifted position of the heart the volume of the left lung is smaller by 10–20%.

The apex of the lung (Apex pulmonis) is cranial part, the broad base of the lung (Basis pulmonis) is the caudal part of the lung. The surface of the lung is covered by the Pleura visceralis and has three surface alignments. The Facies costalis is located laterally and continues at the Margo inferior as the Facies diaphragmatica (→ Figs. 5.55 and 5.56). At the Margo anterior and the blunt Margo posterior it continues as the Facies mediastinalis towards the Mediastinum.

Lungs

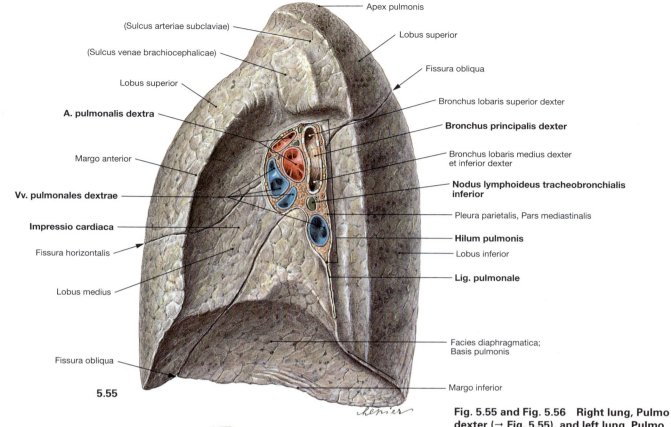

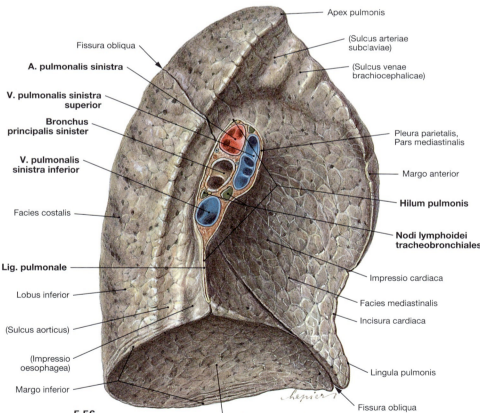

Fig. 5.55 and Fig. 5.56 Right lung, Pulmo dexter (→ Fig. 5.55), and left lung, Pulmo sinister (→ Fig. 5.56); medial view.

The Hilum pulmonis is the medially positioned entry for the main bronchi and the neurovascular structures to the lungs, which together are referred to as the root of the lung (Radix pulmonis). At the hilum, the Pleura visceralis is blends into the Pleura parietalis and both parts line the pleural cavity. This pleural fold extends inferiorly into the Lig. pulmonale.

The topographical orientation of the main bronchi in relation to the great blood vessels at the hilum of the lung is different for both lungs. At the **right lung,** the **Bronchus principalis** is the **most superior** structure and the Vv. pulmonales are positioned anteriorly. In contrast, the main bronchus of the left lung is positioned below the A. pulmonalis. When dissecting the root of the lung, the hilum frequently shows several lymph nodes (Nodi lymphoidei tracheobronchiales), which are normally black due to deposits of carbon dust. The Facies mediastinalis is concave-shaped (more pronounced at the left side) by the heart (Impressio cardiaca). Both lungs show impressions which are caused by adjacent blood vessels or, on the left side, the oesophagus. These impressions nicely demonstrate the topographical relations of the lungs to neighbouring organs but they are, similar to the margins of the lungs, only apparent in the fixed lungs (fixation artefacts).

Clinical Remarks

The apex of the lung extends up to 5 cm above the level of the superior thoracic aperture. Thus, with placement of a **central venous catheter** (CVC) via the V. subclavia, injury to the lung may occur and accidental injury of the cervical pleura may cause a **pneumothorax** with resulting collapse of the lung. But in catheterisation of the V. jugularis interna at the neck there is also a risk of pneumothorax since during this procedure the catheter is directed towards the sternoclavicular joint near the apex of the lung. But this risk is much higher when using the V. subclavia for a CVC since the latter directly contacts the Pleura (→ Fig. 5.99) before continuing as V. brachiocephalica.

Thoracic Viscera

Heart → **Lungs** → Oesophagus →

Bronchopulmonary segments

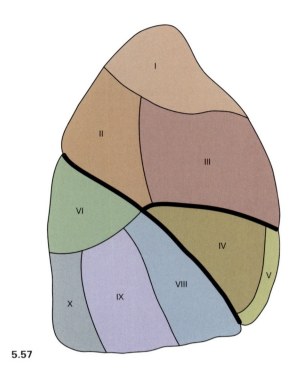

5.57

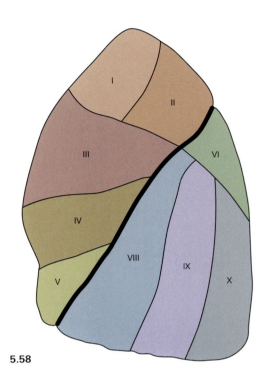

5.58

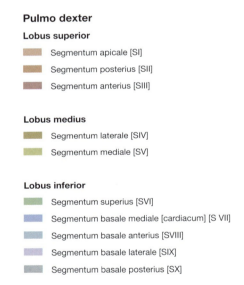

Pulmo dexter

Lobus superior
- Segmentum apicale [SI]
- Segmentum posterius [SII]
- Segmentum anterius [SIII]

Lobus medius
- Segmentum laterale [SIV]
- Segmentum mediale [SV]

Lobus inferior
- Segmentum superius [SVI]
- Segmentum basale mediale [cardiacum] [S VII]
- Segmentum basale anterius [SVIII]
- Segmentum basale laterale [SIX]
- Segmentum basale posterius [SX]

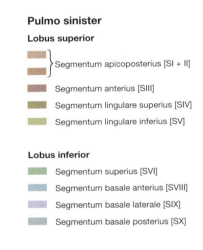

Pulmo sinister

Lobus superior
- Segmentum apicoposterius [SI + II]
- Segmentum anterius [SIII]
- Segmentum lingulare superius [SIV]
- Segmentum lingulare inferius [SV]

Lobus inferior
- Segmentum superius [SVI]
- Segmentum basale anterius [SVIII]
- Segmentum basale laterale [SIX]
- Segmentum basale posterius [SX]

Fig. 5.57 and Fig. 5.58 Bronchopulmonary segments, Segmenta bronchopulmonalia, of the right lung (→ Fig. 5.57) and the left (→ Fig. 5.58) lung; lateral view.
The lobes of the lung are organised in cone-shaped lung (bronchopulmonary) segments which are incompletely divided by septations of connective tissue. The segmental borders are not visible on the surface of the lung. The lung segments are associated with **segmental bronchi** and segmental branches of the pulmonary artery. The **right lung** has **ten segments,** three in the superior, two in the middle, and five in the inferior lobe. The **left lung** only has **nine segments** since segment VII (Segmentum basale mediale → Fig. 5.59) on the left side is missing or drastically reduced and fused with segment VIII due to the larger extension of the Mediastinum. The organisation of the other lung segments is similar on both sides since the segments of the middle lobe of the right lung are equivalent to the two segments of the Lingula pulmonis in the left lung.

Thymus → Topography → Sections

Bronchopulmonary segments

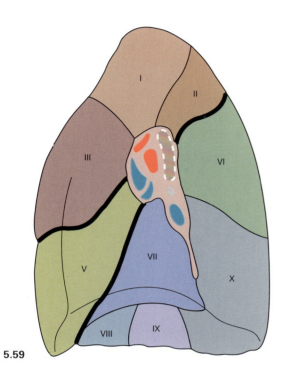

5.59

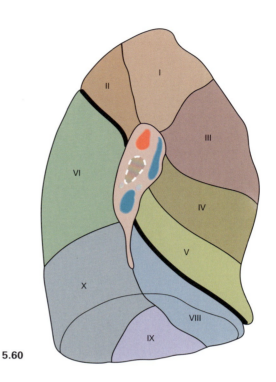

5.60

Fig. 5.59 and Fig. 5.60 Bronchopulmonary segments, Segmenta bronchopulmonalia, of the right lung (→ Fig. 5.59) and the left (→ Fig. 5.60) lung; medial view.

The right lung has ten segments. The left lung only has nine segments; segment VII (Segmentum basale mediale) is missing.

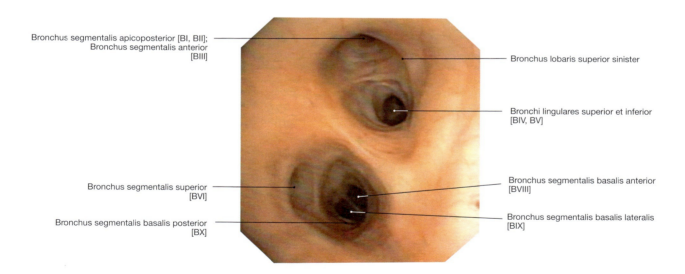

Fig. 5.61 Bronchi, Bronchi; bronchoscopy showing the segmental bronchi of the left side. It is apparent that the segmental bronchus VII is missing on the left side (→ Fig. 5.60).

Clinical Remarks

The knowledge of the lung segments is crucial for orientation during **bronchoscopy.** A bronchoscopy is performed if radiological imaging revealed a suspicious nodule and biopsies are needed to rule out or diagnose a tumour. Another indication for bronchoscopy is to acquire material for pathogen identification in cases of drug resistent pneumonia.

Thoracic Viscera

Heart → Lungs → Oesophagus →

Blood vessels of the Lungs

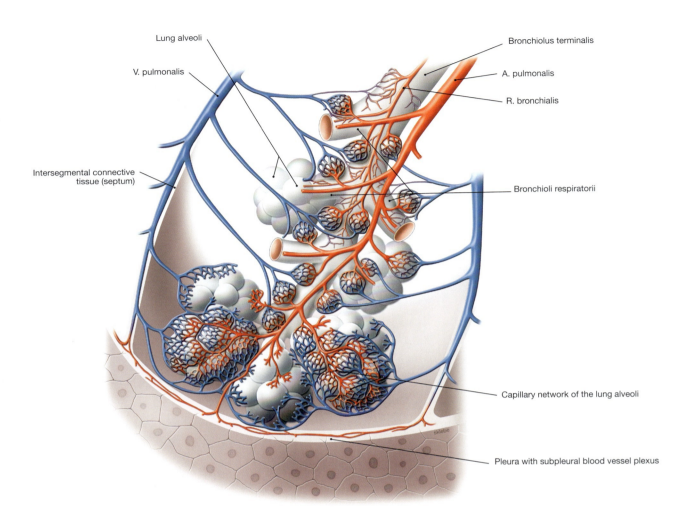

Fig. 5.62 Acinus of the lung, Acinus pulmonis, with blood vessels.
The lung has two blood vessel systems which communicate through their terminal branches in the wall of the alveoli (alveolar septa). The Aa. pulmonales and Vv. pulmonales of the pulmonary circulation constitute the **Vasa publica** which serve for the gas exchange of the blood. Branches of the Aa. pulmonales course in the peribronchial and subpleural connective tissue and transport the deoxygenated blood from the right heart to the alveoli. The Vv. pulmonales are located in the intersegmental connective tissue and transport the oxygenated blood to the left atrium.

The **Vasa privata** of the lung supply the lung tissue itself. The arterial Rr. bronchiales and the Vv. bronchiales course together with the bronchi.

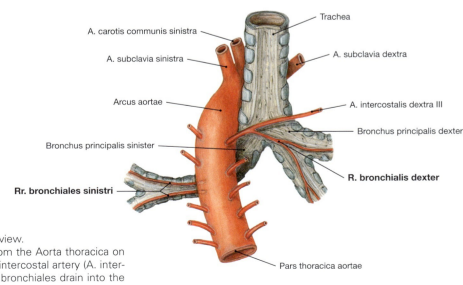

Fig. 5.63 Vasa privata of the lung; dorsal view.
The arterial Rr. bronchiales derive directly from the Aorta thoracica on the left side, but usually branch off the third intercostal artery (A. intercostalis dextra III) on the right side. The Vv. bronchiales drain into the azygos system (not shown here).

Lymph vessels and lymph nodes of the lung

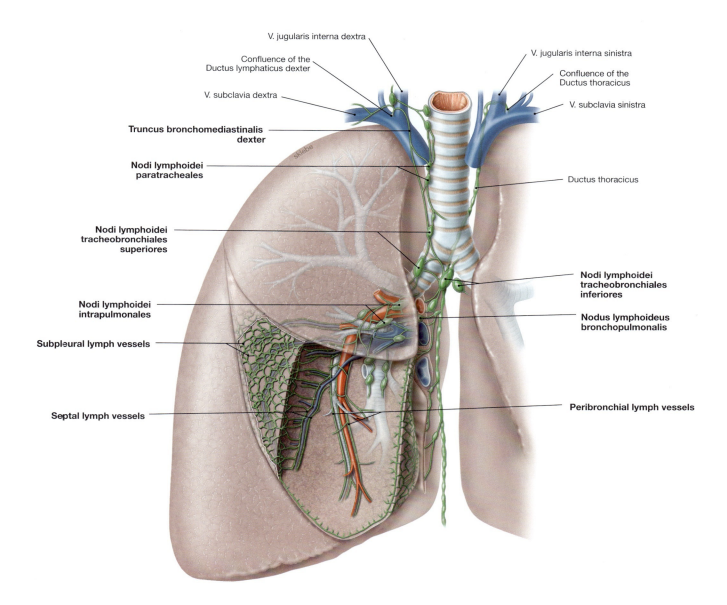

Fig. 5.64 Lymph vessels, Vasa lymphatica, and lymph nodes, Nodi lymphoidei, of the lung; ventral view; schematic illustration.
The lung has two lymph vessel systems which converge at the hilum. The **peribronchial system** follows the bronchi and feeds into several lymph node stations. The first station are the Nodi lymphoidei intrapulmonales at the transition from lobar to segmental bronchi. The second station comprises the Nodi lymphoidei bronchopulmonales at the hilum of the lung. The subsequent Nodi lymphoidei tracheobronchiales are located already at the root of the lung. Nodi lymphoidei tracheobronchiales superiores and inferiores are distinguished according to their location above and below the tracheal bifurcation. From here the lymph passes on to the Nodi lymphoidei paratracheales or to the Trunci bronchomediastinales on both sides. Thus, there is no strict separation of the lymph drainage from the different sides.

The **subpleural** and the **septal lymph system** drain into the Nodi lymphoidei tracheobronchiales as the first station. Their delicate lymph vessels form a polygonal network at the surface of the lung. This network represents the boundaries of distinct pulmonary lobules. Due to carbon dust deposits (exhaust fumes and cigarette smoke) these lymph vessels and the boundaries of the pulmonary lobules are clearly visible.

Clinical Remarks

Clinicians usually summarise all lymph nodes of the lung with the term **hilar lymph nodes.** However, this disregards the fact that the Nodi lymphoidei intrapulmonales are located deep within the lung parenchyma. This linguistic blurring may entail the misinterpretation of parenchymal processes as separate disease entities and neglect the association with lymph node enlargement which may initiate unnecessary diagnostic procedures.

Viscera of the Thorax

Heart → Lungs → Oesophagus →

Lungs and pleural cavities

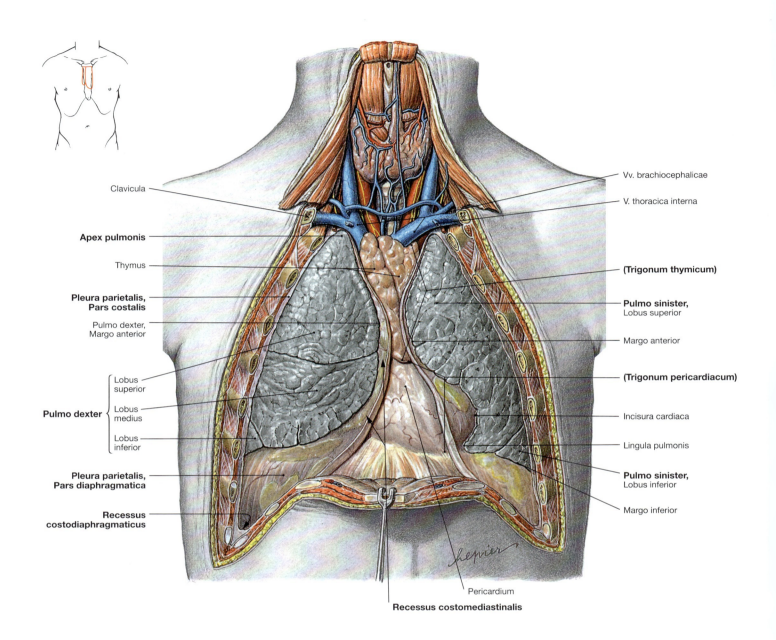

Fig. 5.65 Lungs, Pulmones, and pleural cavities, Cavitates pleurales, of an adolescent; ventral view; after removal of the anterior thoracic wall.

The pleural cavity **(Cavitas pleuralis)** is covered by the parietal Pleura (Pleura parietalis). The parietal Pleura is divided into Pars mediastinalis, Pars costalis, and Pars diaphragmatica. The visceral Pleura **(Pleura visceralis)** covers the outer surface of the lungs. The capillary space between both pleural layers contains 5 ml of a serous fluid which lubricates the pleural surfaces and reduces friction during breathing. The pleural cupula **(Cupula pleurae)** extends up to 5 cm above the superior thoracic aperture. The superior and inferior medial borders of the Pleura form the boundaries of the Trigonum thymicum and the Trigonum pericardiacum, respectively. The pleural cavities possesses four pleural recesses (Recessus pleurales) into which the lungs can expand during deep inspiration:

- **Recessus costodiaphragmaticus:**
  lateral, in the midaxillary line up to 5 cm deep
- **Recessus costomediastinalis:**
  ventral, to both sides of the Mediastinum and chest wall
- **Recessus phrenicomediastinalis:**
  caudal, between diaphragm and Mediastinum
- **Recessus vertebromediastinalis:**
  dorsal, adjacent to the vertebral column (→ Fig. 5.104)

Clinical Remarks

Increased fluid in the pleural cavity **(pleural effusion)** may be caused by inflammatory reactions in pneumonia (pleuritis), by congestion in the pulmonary circulation due to a (left) ventricular insufficiency, or by tumours of the lung or the Pleura. In addition, there are chylous pleural effusions if lymph from the Ductus thoracicus enters the pleural cavity. Pleural effusions cause a dull percussion sound. Diagnostic puncture of a pleural effusion from the Recessus costodiaphragmaticus is performed to sample fluid for diagnosis and to improve breathing.

Thymus → Topography → Sections

Thoracic viscera, radiography

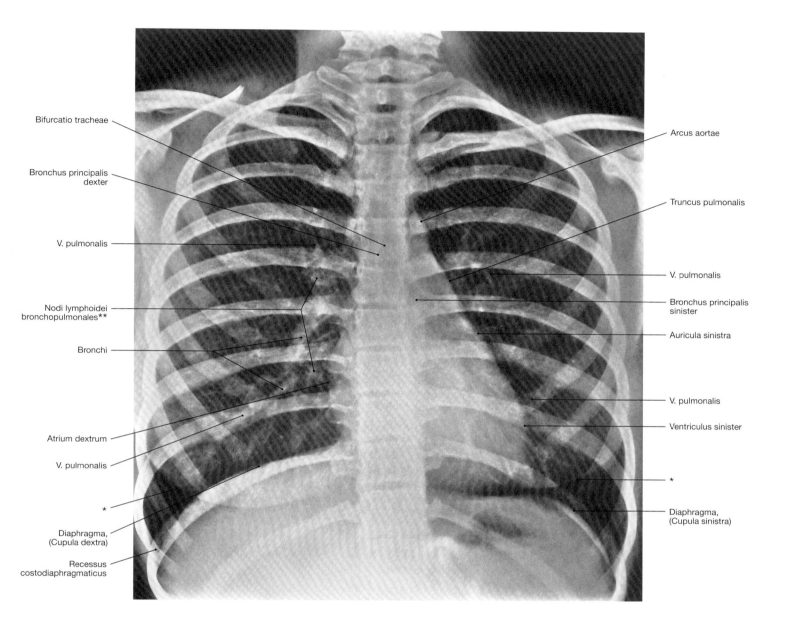

Fig. 5.66 Thoracic cage, Cavea thoracis, with thoracic viscera; radiograph in postero-anterior (PA) beam projection. [27]

The course of the bronchi is partly visible. On the right side, clusters of lymph nodes in the area of the hilum of the lung are visible.

* contour of the breast (mamma)
** clinical term: hilar lymph nodes

Clinical Remarks

Chest radiographs are frequently taken if **pathological processes** of the lungs or the pleura are suspected, such as inflammations (pneumonia, pleuritis) or tumours (bronchial carcinoma). Parenchymal alterations are often present as "shadows" because they absorb more of the radiation than the intact lung tissue. In the upright position, a pleural effusion blunts the Recessus costodiaphragmaticus and forms a horizontal fluid level.

5 Thoracic Viscera

Heart → Lungs → **Oesophagus** →

Projection of the oesophagus

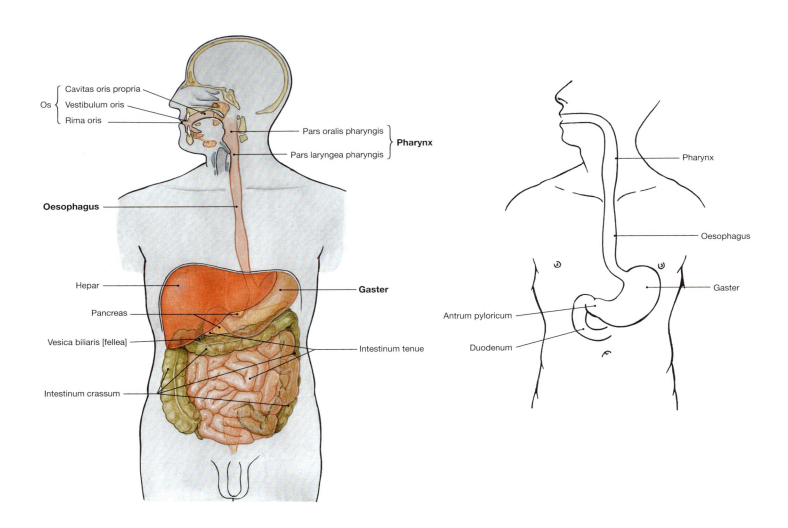

Fig. 5.67 Overview of the digestive tract.
The Oesophagus is a muscular tube connecting the Pharynx with the stomach (Gaster). It transports the ingested food.

Fig. 5.68 Projection of the Oesophagus onto the ventral thoracic wall.
The Oesophagus is 25 cm long and originates at the cricoid cartilage which projects onto the 6th cervical vertebra. It ends at the Cardia of the stomach at the level of the 10th thoracic vertebra (beneath the Proc. xiphoideus of the Sternum).

Clinical Remarks

The projection of the Oesophagus explains why an inflammation of the oesophageal mucosa by gastric acid reflux **(gastro-(o)esophageal reflux disease, GERD)** causes a retrosternal burning sensation and pain at a similar location as a myocardial infarction. Afferent nerve fibres from both organs and the ventral chest wall converge at the same spinal cord segments. The brain cannot differentiate whether the pain originates from internal organs or the body surface. These organ-associated dermatomes are referred to as HEAD's zones, the phenomenon is called "referred pain".

Thymus → Topography → Sections

Oesophagus

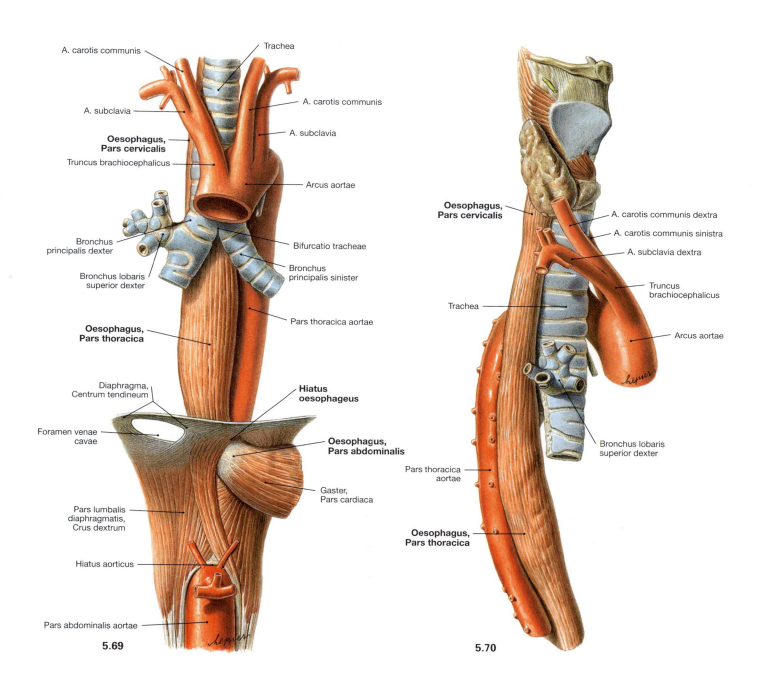

Fig. 5.69 and Fig. 5.70   Oesophagus, Oesophagus, trachea, Trachea, and thoracic aorta, Pars thoracica aortae; ventral view (→ Fig. 5.69) and view from the right side (→ Fig. 5.70).
The Oesophagus is 25 cm long and is organised in three parts:
- Pars cervicalis (5–8 cm)
- Pars thoracica (16 cm)
- Pars abdominalis (1–4 cm)

The **Pars cervicalis** is adjacent to the vertebral column. The **Pars thoracica** crosses the aortic arch which is adjacent on the dorsal left side. This part runs along the left main bronchus and descends ventrally with increasing distance to the vertebral column. The dorsal view shows the close proximity of the Pars thoracica to the Pericardium and to the left atrium (→ Fig. 5.71). After traversing the Hiatus oesophageus of the diaphragm, the short intraperitoneally located **Pars abdominalis** begins.

5 Thoracic Viscera

Heart → Lungs → Oesophagus →

Structure of the oesophagus

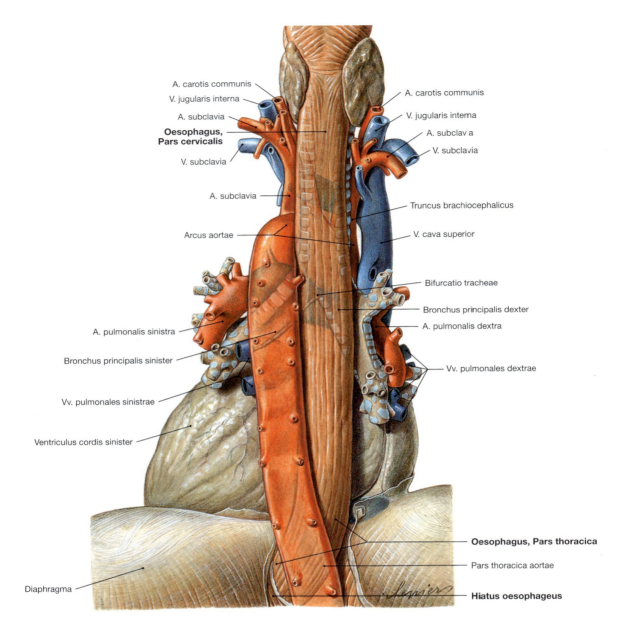

Fig. 5.71 Oesophagus, Oesophagus, pericardium, Pericardium, and thoracic aorta, Pars thoracica aortae; dorsal view.

The caudal part of the Pars thoracica of the Oesophagus is separated from the left atrium only by the pericardium.

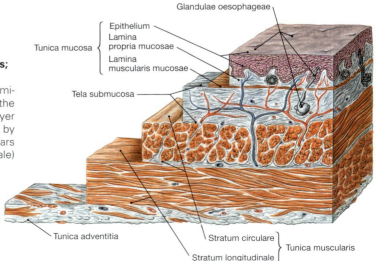

Fig. 5.72 Structure of the wall of the oesophagus, Oesophagus; microscopic view.

Similar to the entire gut, the wall of the Oesophagus consists of a luminal mucous membrane (**Tunica mucosa**) which is separated from the muscular layer (**Tunica muscularis**) by a loose connective tissue layer (**Tela submucosa**). The Partes cervicalis and thoracica are covered by the **Tunica adventitia**. The outer surface of the intraperitoneal Pars abdominalis is covered by visceral peritoneum (Peritoneum viscerale) which constitutes the **Tunica serosa**.

Constrictions and diverticula of the oesophagus

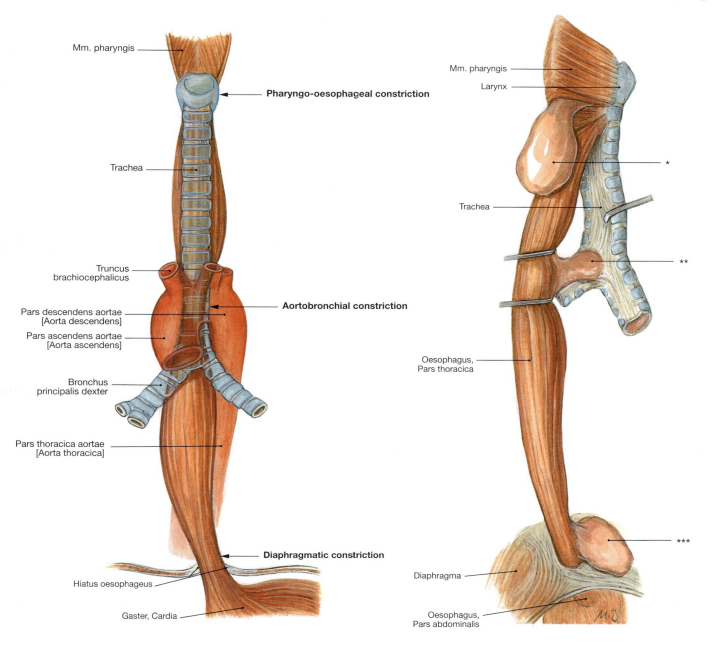

Fig. 5.73 Constrictions, Angustiae, of the Oesophagus; ventral view.
The Oesophagus has three constrictions:
- cervical constriction at the cricoid cartilage (Angustia cricoidea; pharyngo-oesophageal constriction)
- thoracic constriction at the Aorta (Angustia aortica; aortobronchial constriction)
- diaphragmatic constriction (Angustia diaphragmatica)

The **cervical constriction** has the smallest lumen and is located at the level of the upper oesophageal sphincter and the 6th cervical vertebra.
The **thoracic constriction** is created by the direct proximity of the aortic arch from the left and dorsal side (level of the 4th thoracic vertebra).
The **diaphragmatic constriction** lies in the Hiatus oesophageus (level

Fig. 5.74 Diverticula of the Oesophagus; view from the right dorsal side.

- * clinical term: ZENKER's diverticulum
- ** clinical term: traction diverticulum
- *** clinical term: epiphrenic diverticulum

of the 10th thoracic vertebra). There is no true sphincter muscle but an angiomuscular mechanism that acts like a valve under extension (lower oesophageal sphincter, LES). Elastic connective tissue (Lig. phrenicooesophageale) attaches the outside of the Oesophagus to the Hiatus oesophageus.

Clinical Remarks

Swallowed **foreign bodies** (e.g. fish bones) may get stuck at the oesophageal constrictions. True diverticula (outpouchings) of the entire oesophageal wall may occur at several locations. **ZENKER's diverticula** (70%) are most common. These diverticula bulge through the KILLIAN's triangle of the hypopharyngeal muscles and are wrongly categorised as oesophageal diverticula. Responsible for these diverticula is a defective relaxation of the inferior pharyngeal constrictor (Pars cricopharyngea). **Traction diverticula** (22%) are "true" diverticula and involve the entire oesophageal wall. They are either caused by incomplete separation between Oesophagus and Trachea during development (→ Fig. 5.48) or they result from inflammatory reactions involving adjacent structures. **Epiphrenic diverticula** (8%) are believed to be evoked by a disturbed function of the angiomuscular lower oesophageal sphincter.

5 Thoracic Viscera

Heart → Lungs → Oesophagus →

Blood vessels of the oesophagus

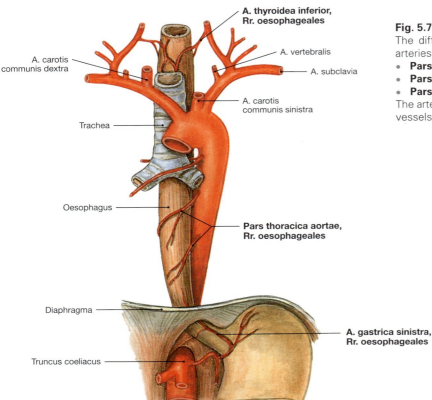

Fig. 5.75 Arteries of the Oesophagus; ventral view.
The different parts of the Oesophagus are supplied by surrounding arteries:
- **Pars cervicalis:** A. thyroidea inferior
- **Pars thoracica:** Rr. oesophageales of the Aorta
- **Pars abdominalis:** A. gastrica sinistra and A. phrenica inferior

The arterial and venous supply of the Trachea is equivalent to the blood vessels of the cervical and thoracic parts of the Oesophagus.

Fig. 5.76 Veins of the oesophagus, Vv. oesophageae; ventral view.
The complex venous network of the Tunica adventitia drains into different veins:
- **Pars cervicalis:** V. thyroidea inferior
- **Pars thoracica** and **Pars abdominalis:** via V. azygos and V. hemiazygos into the V. cava superior

The inferior parts gain **access to the portal venous system** via the gastric veins (V. gastrica sinistra). These veins may be utilised as **portocaval anastomoses** with increased pressure in the portal vein (portal hypertension) (→ Fig. 5.77).

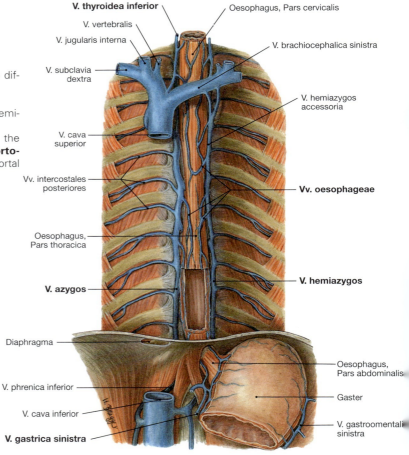

Clinical Remarks

In contrast to other organs of the gastrointestinal tract, the **Oesophagus** has **no dedicated arteries** but is supplied by blood vessels from the surrounding organs. This has implications for surgical procedures and poses challenges to oesophageal surgery.

Veins of the oesophagus

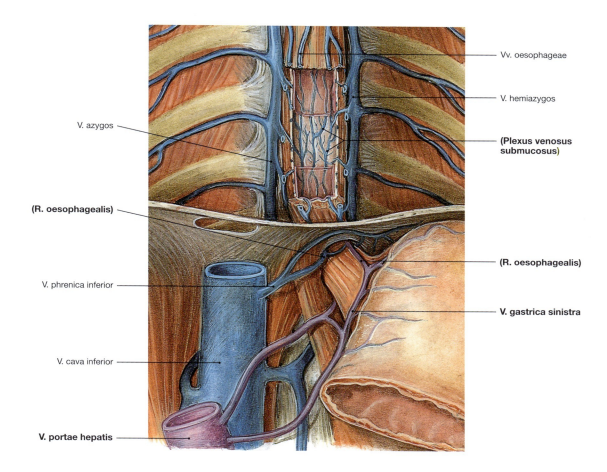

Fig. 5.77 Veins of the oesophagus, Vv. oesophageae, with illustration of the portocaval anastomoses between portal vein, V. portae hepatis, and V. cava superior; ventral view.
The extensive venous network in the Tunica adventitia is connected to the submucosal veins (Plexus venosus submucosus). The blood drains via V. azygos (right side) and V. hemiazygos (left side) upwards to the V. cava superior. The lower parts of the Oesophagus also connect to the V. portae hepatis via the veins at the lesser curvature of the stomach (V. gastrica sinistra).

Clinical Remarks

If pressure in the portal venous system increases **(portal hypertension)**, e.g. due to increased liver parenchymal resistance (cirrhosis of the liver), the venous blood is redirected to the Vv. cavae superior and inferior via **portocaval anastomoses.** Clinically, the most important portocaval anastomoses are the connections of the Oesophagus to the gastric veins. This may result in dilations of the oesophageal submucosal veins **(oesophageal varices → Fig. 5.81).** Rupture of these varices is associated with a mortality of approximately 50% and is, thus, the most frequent cause of death in patients with liver cirrhosis. Rupture into the lumen leads to the accumulation of darkened blood in the stomach, the rare external rupture results in bleeding into the peritoneal cavity.

Thoracic Viscera

Heart → Lungs → Oesophagus →

Lymph vessels of the oesophagus

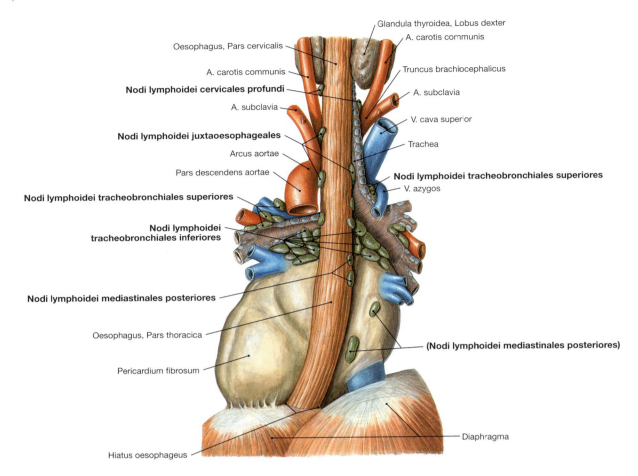

Fig. 5.78 Lymph nodes, Nodi lymphoidei, of the posterior mediastinum; dorsal view.
The lymph of the Oesophagus drains into the lymph nodes directly adjacent to the Oesophagus (Nodi lymphoidei juxtaoesophageales):
- **Pars cervicalis:** Nodi lymphoidei cervicales profundi

- **Pars thoracica** and **Pars abdominalis:** lymph nodes of the Mediastinum (Nodi lymphoidei mediastinales posteriores, Nodi lymphoidei tracheobronchiales and paratracheales) and of the peritoneal cavity (Nodi lymphoidei phrenici inferiores on the abdominal side of the diaphragm and Nodi lymphoidei gastrici on the lesser curvature of the stomach)

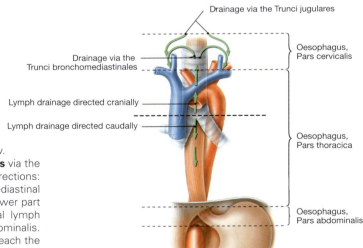

Fig. 5.79 Lymph drainage of the Oesophagus; ventral view.
The lymph of the Pars cervicalis reaches the **Truncus jugularis** via the deep cervical lymph nodes. The Pars thoracica drains in two directions: the upper part above the tracheal bifurcation drains via the mediastinal lymph nodes into the **Truncus bronchomediastinalis;** the lower part beneath the tracheal bifurcation connects to the abdominal lymph nodes which are the regional lymph nodes for the Pars abdominalis. From here the lymph passes the Nodi lymphoidei coeliaci to reach the **Truncus intestinalis.**

Clinical Remarks

The direction of lymphatic drainage influences the location of metastases in **oesophageal and gastric carcinomas.** Metastases of carcinomas of the lower oesophagus are likely to occur in the abdominal lymph nodes. Similar drainage ways appear to exist for the venous blood since oesophageal carcinomas below the tracheal bifurcation frequently cause liver metastases, whereas carcinomas above the tracheal bifurcation ususally metastasise into the lungs.

Oesophagus, oesophagoscopy

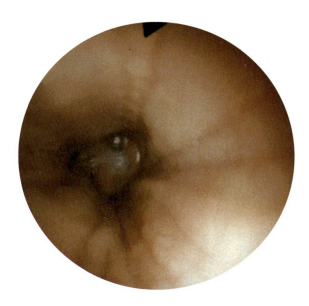

Fig. 5.80 **Oesophagus, Oesophagus;** oesophagoscopy, normal finding. [12]

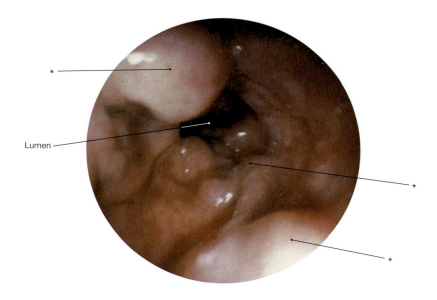

Fig. 5.81 **Oesophagus, Oesophagus;** oesophagoscopy, oesophageal varices in liver cirrhosis. [12]

* clinical term: varicose vein

Clinical Remarks

In **portal hypertension,** the dilation of **portocaval anastomoses** involving the veins of the Oesophagus may develop into **oesophageal varices.** The rupture of these varices frequently results in **life-threatening bleedings.** Therefore, prophylactic treatment is performed in oesophageal varices including banding ligation (endoscopic band ligation) or the endoscopic injection of sclerosing agents (sclerotherapy).

5 Thoracic Viscera

Heart → Lungs → Oesophagus →

Thymus

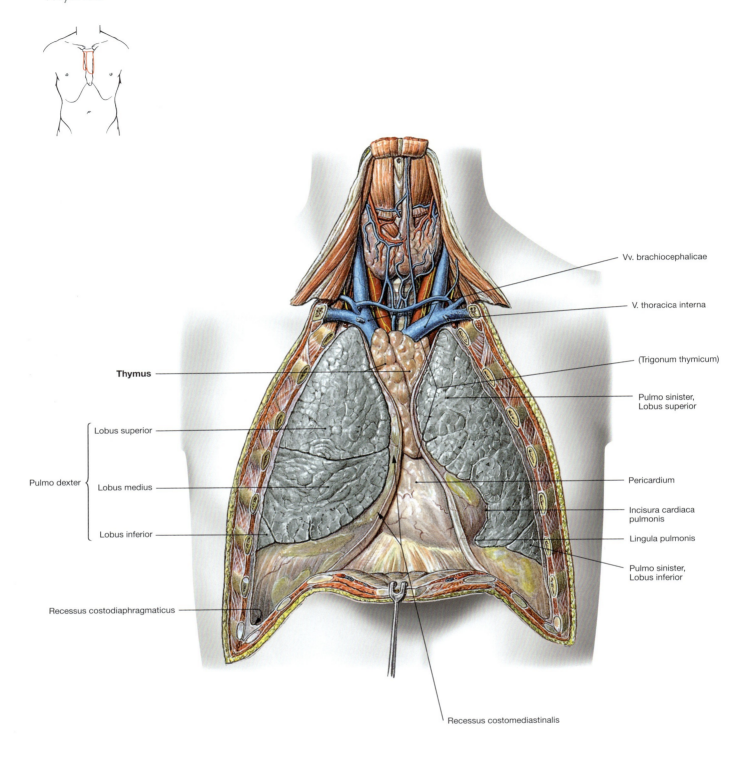

Fig. 5.82 Thymus, Thymus, mediastinum and pleural cavities, Cavitates pleurales, of an adolescent; ventral view; after removal of the anterior thoracic wall.
The Thymus is located in the Trigonum thymicum between the mediastinal borders of the pleural cavities. The Thymus is relatively large in a young adult. In an older individual it is almost completely replaced with adipose tissue. Thus, in the dissection of anatomical specimens only residual thymic tissue is found which is identified only due to smaller arterial branches derived from the A. thoracica interna or venous connections to the Vv. brachiocephalicae.

Thymus → Topography → Sections

Thymus

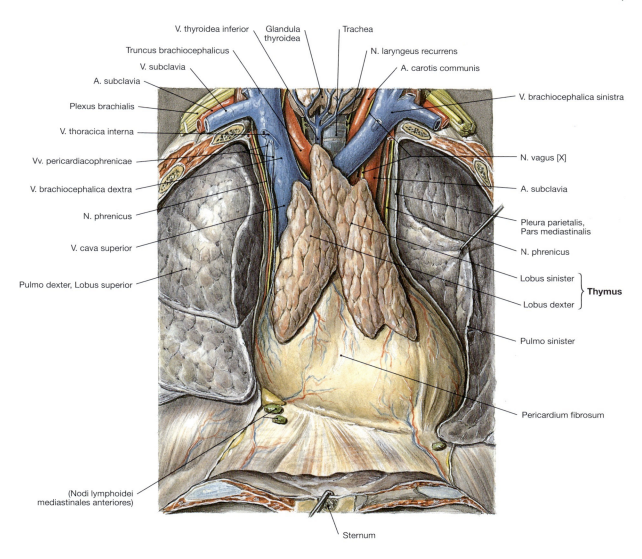

Fig. 5.83 Thymus, Thymus, of an adolescent; ventral view.
The Thymus is a primary lymphatic organ. It serves for the proliferation and selection of T-lymphocytes which then leave the Thymus to settle in secondary lymphatic organs to function in the adaptive immune responses.

The Thymus develops from the endoderm of the third pharyngeal pouch and the ectoderm of the third pharyngeal cleft. It consists of two lobes (Lobi dexter and sinister) which cover the great vessels of the superior Mediastinum. Microscopically, these lobes are subdivided into smaller lobules.

The composition of the thymic tissue changes continuously during life. Since its volume remains almost the same, its relative size is larger in the newborn than in the adult (→ Fig. 5.84). After puberty, the specific thymic parenchyma is gradually substituted by adipose tissue and the residual thymus is hardly visible in elder persons. However, functional thymic tissue remains present at all times to warrant adequate immune reactions.

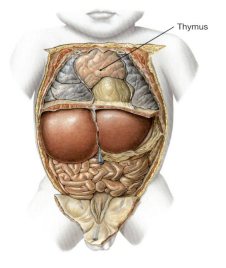

Fig. 5.84 Position of the thymus, Thymus, in a newborn; ventral view; after removal of the ventral thoracic wall.

Thoracic Viscera

Heart → Lungs → Oesophagus →

Mediastinum

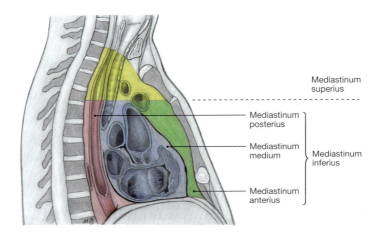

Fig. 5.85 Organisation of the Mediastinum.
The mediastinum is divided into a Mediastinum inferius which contains the heart, and a Mediastinum superius. The Mediastinum inferius is further divided into the Mediastinum anterius in front of the heart, the Mediastinum medium, containing the Pericardium, and the Mediastinum posterius behind the Pericardium.

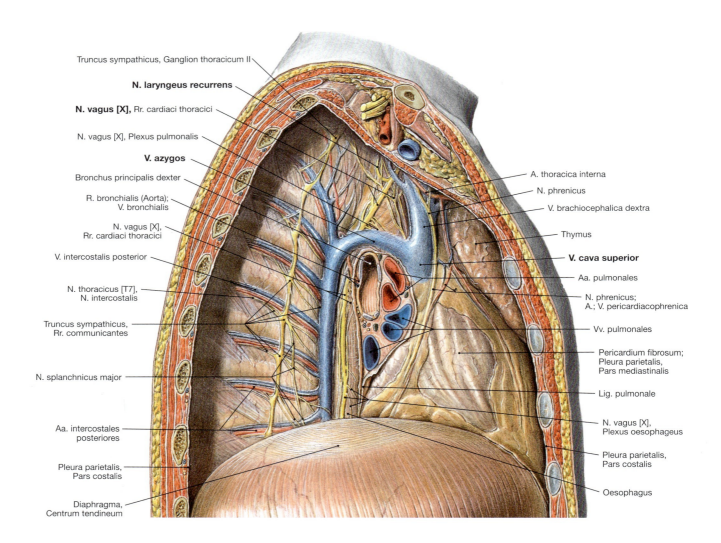

Fig. 5.86 Mediastinum and pleural cavity, Cavitas pleuralis, of an adolescent; view from the right side; after removal of the lateral thoracic wall and the right lung.
The view from the right side demonstrates clearly the **V. azygos** which ascends next to the vertebral column in the Mediastinum posterius. The V. azygos crosses the root of the right lung superiorly and enters the V. cava superior from dorsal at the level of the 4th / 5th thoracic vertebrae. After branching off the N. vagus [X], the N. laryngeus recurrens winds around the A. subclavia on the right side.

52 → dissection link

Thymus → **Topography** → Sections

Mediastinum

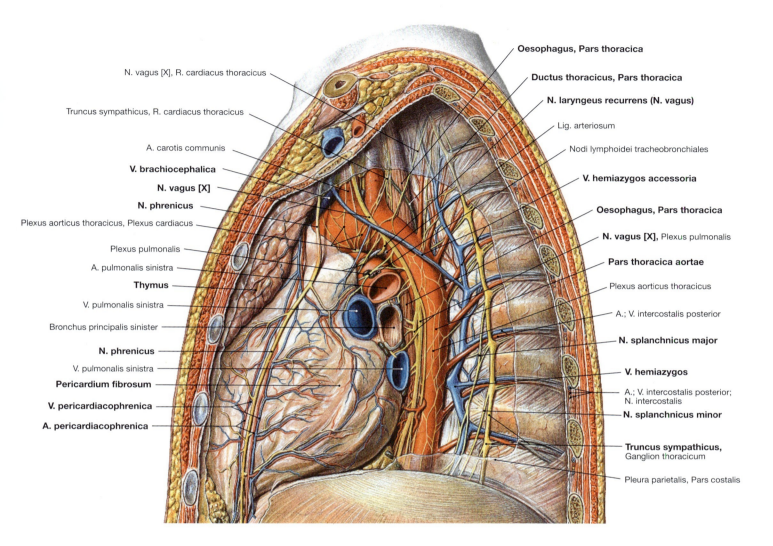

Fig. 5.87 Mediastinum and pleural cavity, Cavitas pleuralis, of an adolescent; view from the left side; after removal of the lateral thoracic wall and the left lung.
The view from the left side demonstrates clearly the Aorta thoracica which descends on the left side of the vertebral column in the Mediastinum posterius. The V. hemiazygos ascends on the lateral aspect of the vertebral bodies and drains ino the V. azygos at the level of the thoracic vertebrae 10th to 7th. Frequently, the V. hemiazygos communicates with the V. hemiazygos accessoria which collects the blood from the superior intercostal veins.

Further lateral, next to the heads of the ribs, the ganglia of the Truncus sympathicus are positioned which branch off the N. splanchnicus major and the N. splanchnicus minor. The N. vagus [X] descends behind the root of the lung next to the Oesophagus after releasing the N. laryngeus recurrens. On the left side, the N. laryngeus recurrens winds around the aortic arch. The Mediastinum medium harbours the Pericardium and the adjacent N. phrenicus accompanied by the Vasa pericardiacophrenica. In the Mediastinum superius the Thymus covers the great vessels ventrally.

Contents of the Mediastinum superius	Contents of the Mediastinum inferius
• Thymus • Trachea • Oesophagus • Aorta and Truncus pulmonalis • Vv. brachiocephalicae and V. cava superior • Lymph vessels: lymphatic trunks (Ductus thoracicus, Trunci bronchiomediastinales) and mediastinal lymph nodes • Autonomic nervous system (Truncus sympathicus, N. vagus [X] with N. laryngeus recurrens) • N. phrenicus	• **Mediastinum anterius:** retrosternal lymph drainage of the mammary gland • **Mediastinum medium:** pericardium with great vessels, N. phrenicus and Vasa pericardiacophrenica • **Mediastinum posterius:** Aorta, Oesophagus with Plexus oesophageus from the N. vagus, Ductus thoracicus, Truncus sympathicus with Nn. splanchnici, V. azygos and V. hemiazygos and intercostal neurovascular structures

Thoracic Viscera

Heart → Lungs → Oesophagus →

N. phrenicus

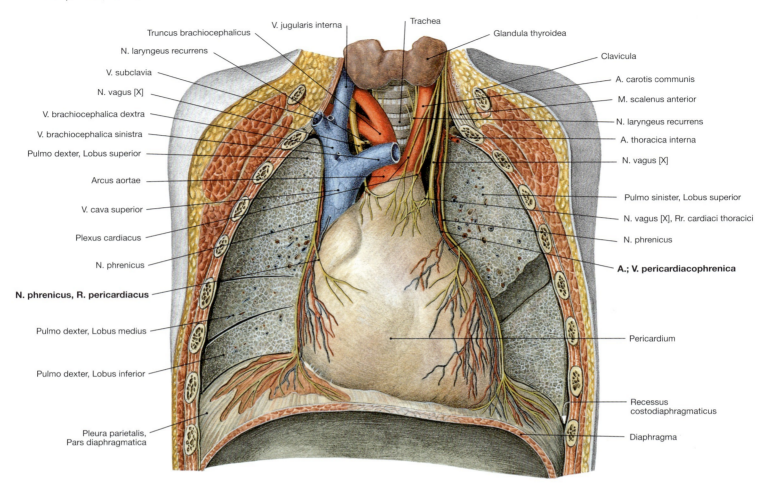

Fig. 5.88 Middle mediastinum; ventral view; after removal of the ventral thoracic wall, the lungs were dissected in the frontal plane.

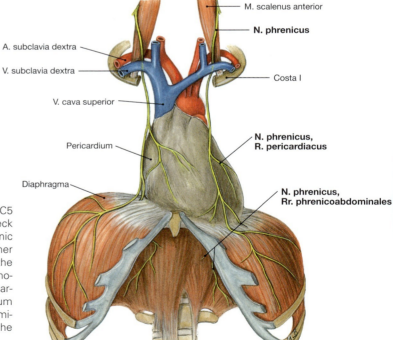

Fig. 5.89 Course of the N. phrenicus.
The N. phrenicus originates from the spinal cord segments C3 to C5 (predominantly C4) of the Plexus cervicalis and descends on the neck anterior to the M. scalenus anterior (guiding muscle!). Next the phrenic nerve courses anterior to the root of the lung and descends together with the Vasa pericardiacophrenica between the Pericardium and the Pleura mediastinalis to the diaphragm. The N. phrenicus provides motor innervation to the diaphragm and sensory innervation to the Pericardium (R. pericardiacus), the Pleura diaphragmatica, and the Peritoneum parietale at the abdominal side of the diaphragm (Rr. phrenicoabdominales). The Rr. phrenicoabdominales also convey sensory fibres to the Peritoneum viscerale on liver and gallbladder.

Clinical Remarks

The developmentally based course of the N. phrenicus has important clinical implications in cervical **spinal cord injuries** (tetraplegia). Injuries of the spinal cord below C4 do not compromise breathing, whereas injuries involving segment C4 bear the risk of suffocation and may require assisted ventilation.

Sensory innervation of the **liver** and **gallbladder** by the Rr. phrenicoabdominales may cause **referred pain in the right shoulder** (e.g. in liver biopsies, inflammation of the gallbladder). Similarly, ruptures of the spleen may cause referred pain in the left shoulder.

Thymus → Topography → Sections

Aortic arch

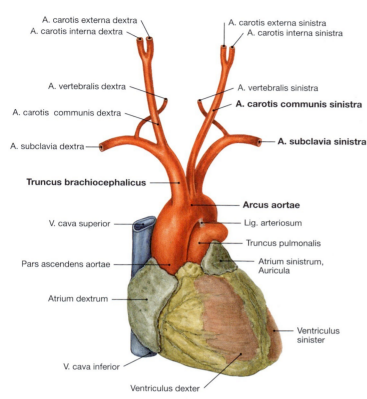

Fig. 5.90 Heart, Cor, and aortic arch, Arcus aortae, with branching of the great vessels; ventral view.
The Pars ascendens aortae continues as the aortic arch which is connected to the Truncus pulmonalis via the Lig. arteriosum. The aortic arch continues with the descending part (Pars descendens) of the Aorta thoracica (→ Fig. 5.92). The aortic arch has the following branches:
- Truncus brachiocephalicus (right side) which divides into the A. subclavia dextra and A. carotis communis dextra
- A. carotis communis sinistra
- A. subclavia sinistra

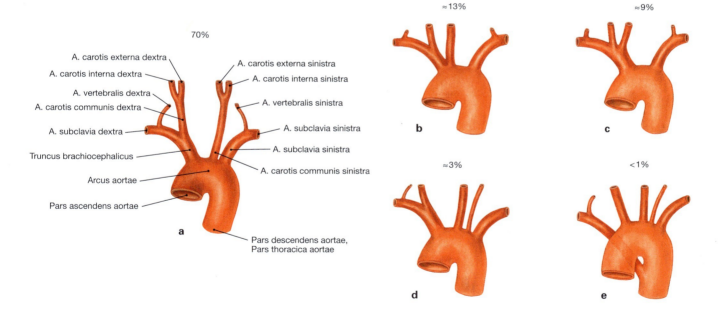

Figs. 5.91a to e Branching variations of the great vessels from the aortic arch.
a "textbook case"
b common origin of Truncus brachiocephalicus and A. carotis communis sinistra
c common stem for Truncus brachiocephalicus and A. carotis communis sinistra
d independent branching of the A. vertebralis sinistra off the Arcus aortae
e branching of the A. subclavia dextra as the last branch of the Arcus aortae. This unusual artery mostly courses behind the Oesophagus to the right side and may cause problems with swallowing (dysphagia lusoria).

The existence of an independent **A. thyroidea ima** coursing to the thyroid gland is uncommon. When existent, it either derives from the Truncus brachiocephalicus or as a second branch from the aortic arch.

5 Thoracic Viscera

Heart → Lungs → Oesophagus →

Arteries of the posterior mediastinum

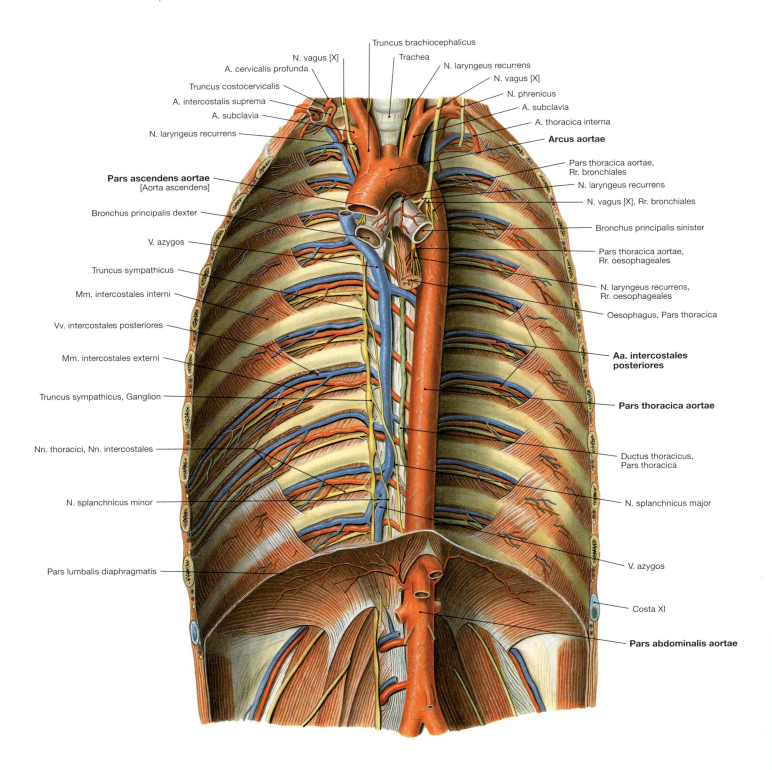

Fig. 5.92 Aorta and its branches; ventral view onto the posterior wall of the trunk. The Pars descendens of the Aorta descends in the Mediastinum posterius (Pars thoracica) and traverses the diaphragm (Pars abdominalis).

Branches of the Pars thoracica aortae	
Parietal branches to the wall of the trunk	• Aa. intercostales posteriores: 9 pairs (the first two are branches of the Truncus costocervicalis from the A. subclavia) • A. subcostalis: the last pair below rib XII • A. phrenica superior: to the upper side of the diaphragm
Visceral branches to the thoracic viscera	• Rr. bronchiales: Vasa privata of the lung (on the right side mostly from the A. intercostalis posterior dextra III) • Rr. oesophageales: 3–6 branches to the Oesophagus • Rr. mediastinales: small branches to Mediastinum and Pericardium

Veins of the posterior mediastinum

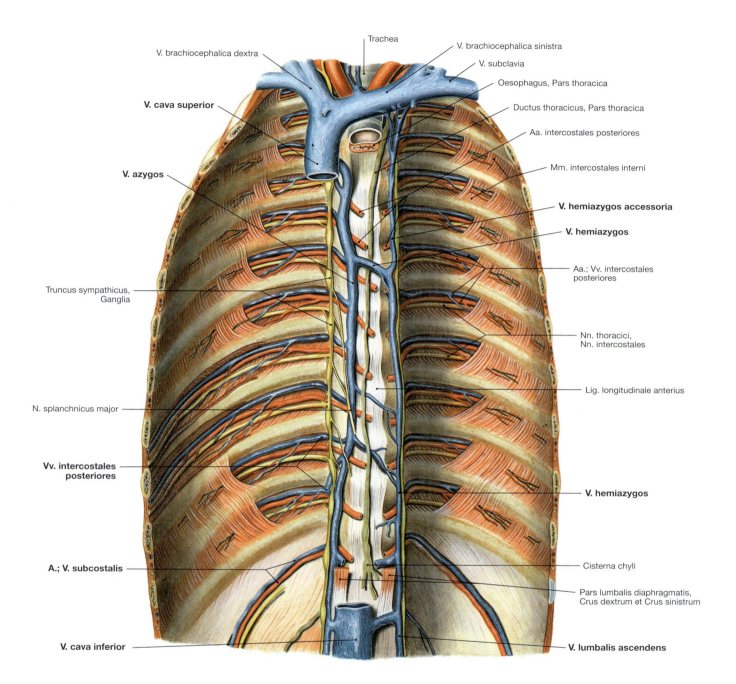

Fig. 5.93 Veins of the azygos system; ventral view onto the posterior wall of the trunk; after removal of the diaphragm.
The azygos system connects the Vv. cavae superior and inferior and its tributaries are equivalent to the branches of the Aorta. The **V. azygos** ascends on the **right side** of the vertebral column and drains into the V. cava superior from dorsal on the level of the 4th/5th thoracic vertebrae. The equivalent blood vessel on the **left side** is the **V. hemiazygos** which merges with the V. azygos at the level of the thoracic vertebrae 7th to 10th. Blood from the upper intercostal veins drains into the **V. hemiazygos accessoria**. Beneath the diaphragm, the V. lumbalis ascendens on each side continues the course of the azygos vein and connects to the V. cava inferior.

Tributaries:
- Vv. mediastinales: from the mediastinal organs (Vv. oesophageales, Vv. bronchiales, Vv. pericardiacae)
- Vv. intercostales posteriores and V. subcostalis: from the posterior wall of the trunk

Thoracic Viscera

Heart → Lungs → Oesophagus →

Nerves of the posterior mediastinum

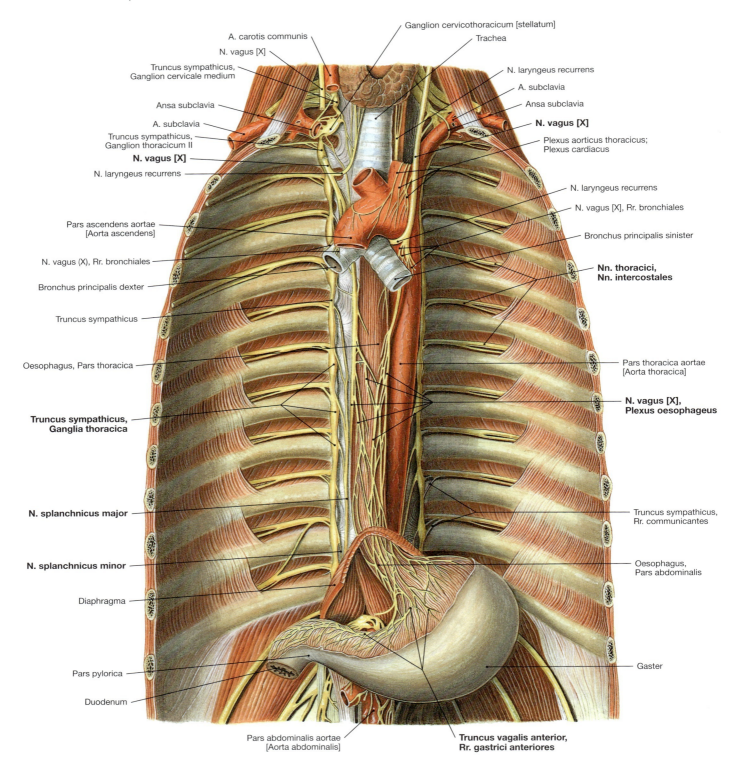

Fig. 5.94 Nerves of the posterior mediastinum; ventral view onto the posterior wall of the trunk; after removal of the diaphragm.
The posterior mediastinum contains the intercostal nerves (Nn. intercostales) of the **somatic nervous system** and parts of the sympathetic (Truncus sympathicus) and parasympathetic systems (Nn. vagi) as components of the **autonomic nervous system**. The **sympathetic trunk** (Truncus sympathicus) forms a paravertebral chain of twelve thoracic ganglia which are connected via Rr. interganglionares. The preganglionic sympathetic neurons are located in the lateral horns (C8 – L3) of the spinal cord and exit the vertebral canal with the spinal nerves. The Rr. communicantes albi guide the preganglionic fibres to the ganglia of the Truncus sympathicus where they are synapsed to postganglionic neurons. Axons of the postganglionic neurons join the spinal nerves and their branches again via the Rr. communicantes grisei. Some pregan-glionic fibres are not synapsed in the ganglia of the sympathetic trunk but continue as Nn. splanchnici major and minor to the nerve plexus around the Aorta abdominalis where they eventually synapse. The preganglionic fibres of the **Nn. vagi** course behind the root of the lung adjacent to the Oesophagus and form the Plexus oesophageus. The latter is the origin for the two vagal trunks (Trunci vagales anterior and posterior) which traverse the diaphragm together with the Oesophagus to reach the autonomic nerve plexus of the Aorta abdominalis. However, synapses to the postganglionic parasympathetic neurons mostly occur in closer proximity to the respective target organs.

Lymph vessels and lymph nodes of the mediastinum

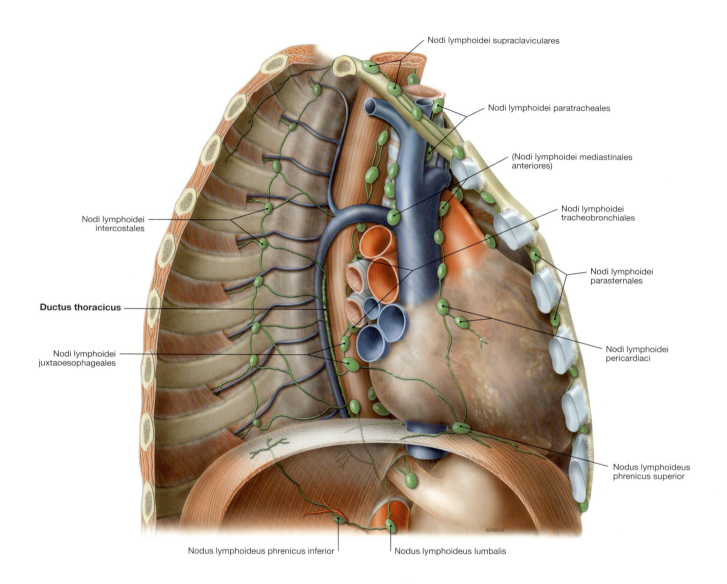

Fig. 5.95 Lymph vessels and lymph nodes of the mediastinum; view from the right ventrolateral side after removal of the lateral chest wall. (according to [2])
The Mediastinum harbours several different groups of lymph nodes which are categorised into parietal lymph nodes (drainage of the wall of the trunk) and visceral lymph nodes (drainage of the thoracic viscera). These drain into the large lymphatic trunks.

Parietal lymph nodes:
- Nodi lymphoidei parasternales: on both sides of the Sternum. They drain lymph from the anterior chest wall, the mammary glands and the diaphragm into the Truncus subclavius.
- Nodi lymphoidei intercostales: between the heads of the ribs. They drain lymph from the posterior chest wall. Their efferent lymph vessels drain directly into the Ductus thoracicus.

Visceral lymph nodes with connection to the Trunci bronchomediastinales:
- Nodi lymphoidei mediastinales anteriores: on both sides of the great vessels, tributaries from lungs and Pleura, diaphragm (Nodi lymphoidei phrenici superiores), heart and Pericardium (Nodi lymphoidei pericardiaci), and Thymus.
- Nodi lymphoidei mediastinales posteriores: at bronchi and Trachea (Nodi lymphoidei tracheobronchiales and paratracheales) and Oesophagus (Nodi lymphoidei juxtaoesophageales)

Lymphatic trunks:
The Ductus thoracicus traverses the diaphragm anterior to the vertebral column (→ Fig. 5.93) and ascends in the Mediastinum posterius, first behind the Aorta then behind the Oesophagus, to reach the 7th cervical vertebra. Next, the ductus crosses the left pleural cupula and opens into the left jugular-subclavian junction of veins from dorsal (between V. subclavia and V. jugularis interna). Shortly before draining into the jugular-subclavian junction, it collects the lymph of the Truncus bronchoMediastinalis sinister, which courses independently in the Mediastinum, the Truncus subclavius sinister (from the arm), and the Truncus jugularis sinister (from the neck). On the right side, a short (1 cm) Ductus lymphaticus dexter connects the respective lymphatic trunks and enters the right jugular-subclavian junction of veins.

5 Thoracic Viscera

Heart → Lungs → Oesophagus →

Superior thoracic aperture

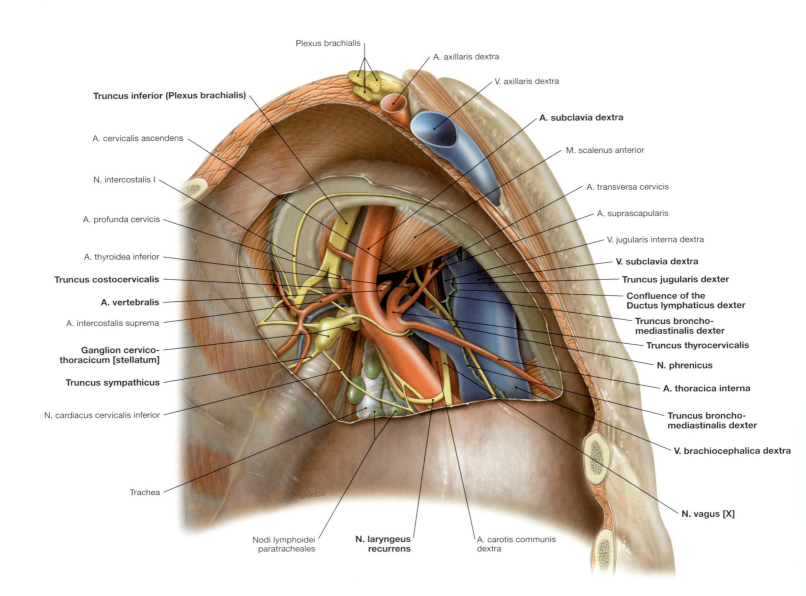

Fig. 5.96 Neurovascular structures of the superior thoracic aperture, right side; caudal view; after removal of the cervical pleural cupula.
The V. subclavia crosses the pleural cupula anterior to the M. scalenus, whereas the A. subclavia and the Plexus brachialis course posterior to the M. scalenus **(scalene gap)**. Branches of the A. subclavia are the A. thoracica interna descending to the lateral aspect of the Sternum, the A. vertebralis, and the Truncus thyreocervicalis with its branches. The Truncus costocervicalis branches off dorsal of the M. scalenus anterior and divides into the A. profunda cervicis and the A. intercostalis suprema. The N. phrenicus is located ventral to the V. brachiocephalica. The N. vagus courses dorsal to the V. brachiocephalica and releases the N. laryngeus recurrens which winds around the A. subclavia to ascend to the neck. Posterior to the A. subclavia, the Truncus sympathicus with its Ganglion cervicothoracicum (stellatum) is found. Most difficult to identify is the short Ductus lymphaticus dexter which drains into the right venous angle (between V. subclavia and V. jugularis interna) after merging the Truncus bronchomediastinalis and the Truncus subclavius.

Superior thoracic aperture

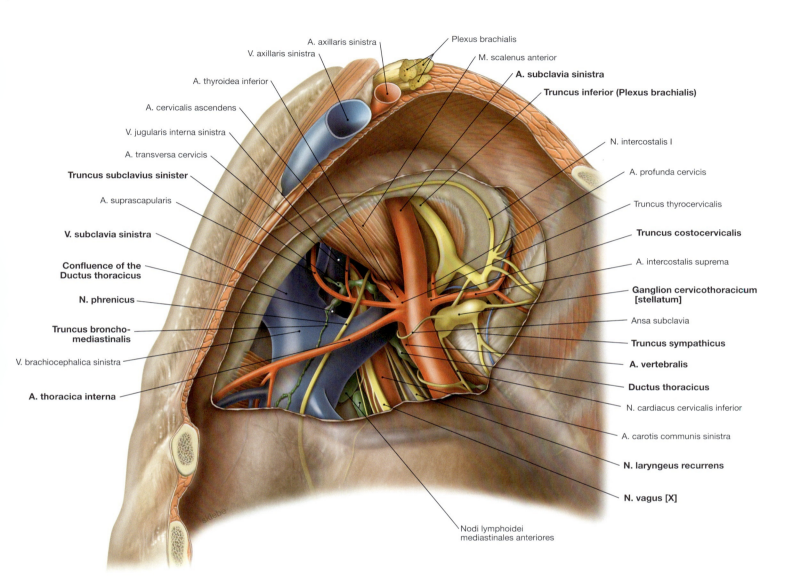

Fig. 5.97 Neurovascular structures of the superior thoracic aperture, left side; caudal view; after removal of the pleural cupula. Here, only structures are described which differ in their course from the neurovascular structures of the right side (→ Fig. 5.96).
On the left side, the **N. vagus [X]** descends further before releasing the N. laryngeus recurrens which then winds around the aortic arch (not visible here) and ascends to the neck. Particular attention must be paid to the **Ductus thoracicus** which is often injured during dissection in this region. The Ductus thoracicus ascends in the Mediastinum posterius and crosses the left pleural cupula before entering the left jugular-subclavian junction of veins (junction between V. subclavia and V. jugularis interna) from dorsal. Just before reaching the jugular-subclavian junction, it joins with the Truncus bronchomediastinalis, the Truncus subclavius, and the Truncus jugularis (not visible here).

5 Thoracic Viscera

Heart → Lungs → Oesophagus →

Thoracic cavity, midsagittal section

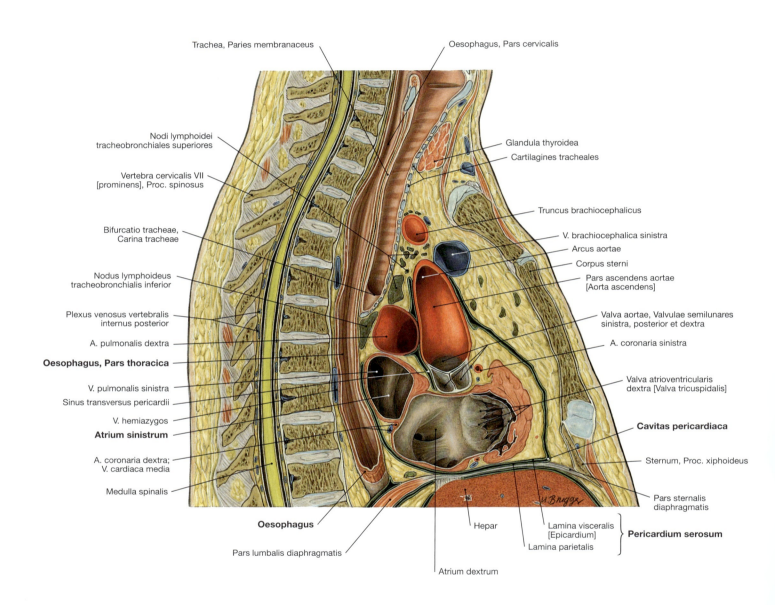

Fig. 5.98 Thoracic cavity, Cavitas thoracis; midsagittal section; lateral view from the right side.

In this section, the close proximity of the Oesophagus to the left atrium of the heart (Atrium sinistrum) in the Mediastinum posterius is obvious. Both structures are only separated by the pericardial cavity (Cavitas pericardiaca).

Clinical Remarks

The spatial proximity of the Oesophagus to the heart is useful when performing a **transoesophageal echocardiography.** With the ultrasound transducer in the Oesophagus, more detailed images of the heart and in particular, the heart valves, can be acquired than from outside of the chest wall.

Thymus → Topography → **Sections**

Thoracic cavity, transverse sections

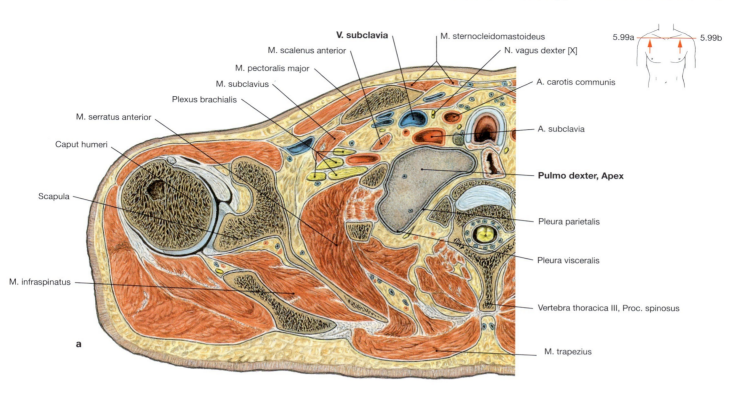

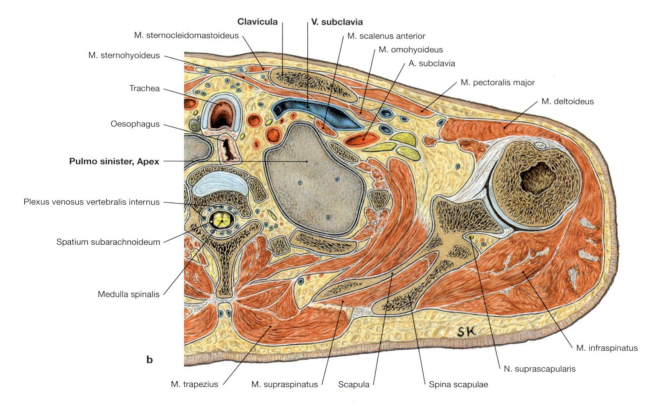

Figs. 5.99a and b Pleural cupula, Cupula pleurae; transverse sections; at the level of the shoulder joint; caudal view.

These sections demonstrate that the pleural cupula extends behind the neurovascular bundle of the arm above the superior thoracic aperture. Thus, the apex of the lung is positioned immediately posterior to the V. and A. subclavia.

Clinical Remarks

The extension of the pleural cupula needs to be considered when placing a **central venous catheter** (central line, CVC) in the **V. subclavia**. For this procedure the cannula is placed just below the anterior convexity of the clavicle in the direction towards the sternoclavicular joint. If the cannula is positioned too steep the pleural cavity may be injured which leads to an intrusion of air into the pleural cavity and results in collapsing of the lung **(pneumothorax)**.

5 Thoracic Viscera

Heart → Lungs → Oesophagus →

Thoracic cavity, transverse sections

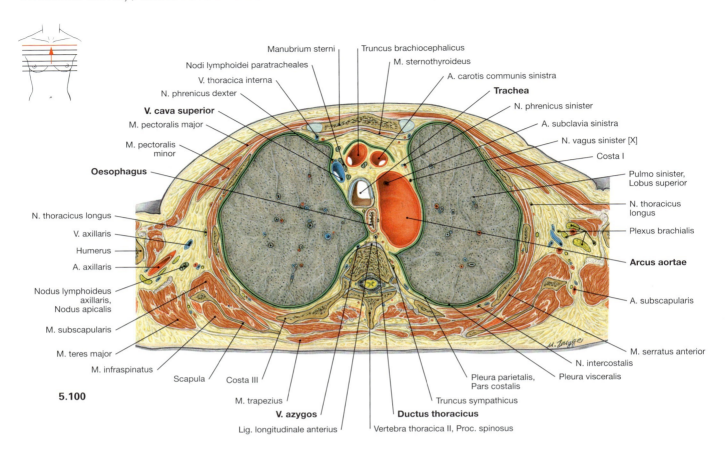

5.100

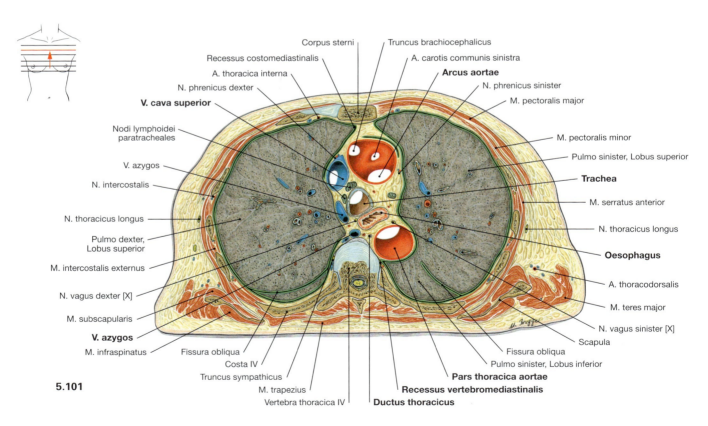

5.101

Fig. 5.100 and Fig. 5.101 Thoracic cavity, Cavitas thoracis; transverse sections at the level of the aortic arch; caudal view.
In the Mediastinum superius, the aortic arch is located ventrally and the V. cava superior is located at the right side of the aortic arch. Positioned dorsal to these blood vessels are the Trachea and, to the left side, the Oesophagus and the thoracic aorta. Posteriorly, the Aorta borders at the Recessus vertebromediastinalis of the pleural cavity. Positioned directly on the vertebral column are the V. azygos on the right side and the Ductus thoracicus on the left side.

Thymus → Topography → **Sections**

Thoracic cavity, transverse sections

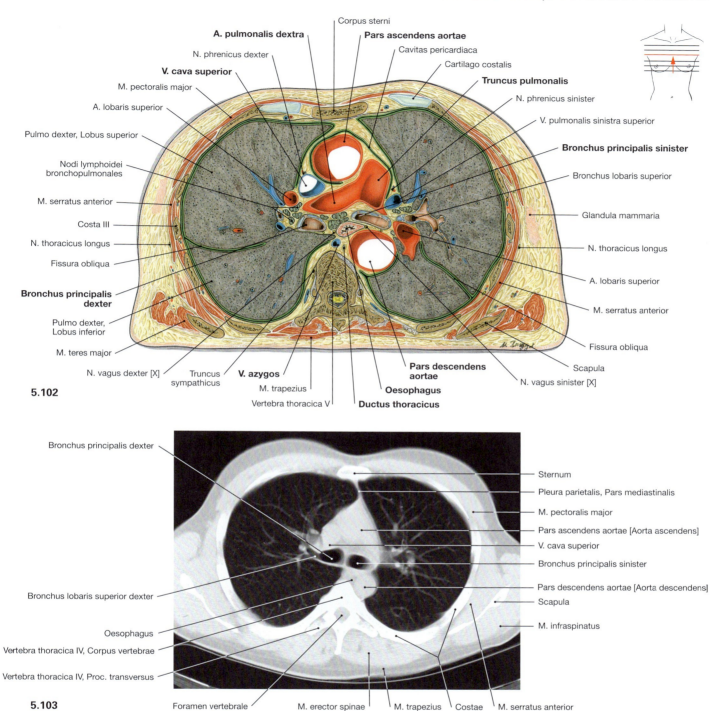

Fig. 5.102 and Fig. 5.103   Thoracic cavity, Cavitas thoracis; transverse section at the level of the Aorta descendens (→ Fig. 5.102) and computed tomographic cross-section (CT; → Fig. 5.103); caudal view.

In the Mediastinum superius, the Aorta ascendens is positioned most ventrally followed posteriorly and to the left side by the Truncus pulmonalis which branches into the pulmonary arteries. The V. cava superior is located at the right side of the Aorta. Behind the pulmonary arteries (Aa. pulmonales) are the main bronchi (Bronchi principales) and the Oesophagus. The Aorta descendens is visible on the left side of the vertebral column, the V. azygos on the right side.

Clinical Remarks

Cross sectional imaging with **computed tomography** (CT; → Fig. 5.103) or **magnetic resonance tomographic imaging** (MRI) is of high relevance in medical diagnostics. It is the general convention that these images are always displayed with a view from caudal. The advantage in **computed tomography (CT)** is based on the fact that all structures with their spatial distribution are imaged in a stack of sections with a thickness of a few millimeters. In contrast, in conventional radiography the structures are projected on top of each other. In tomography, the density of pathological structures already provides information regarding the tissue composition. Using **CT-controlled punctures,** biopsies can be obtained from individual enlarged lymph nodes which enables microbiological and pathological diagnosis.

Thoracic Viscera

Heart → Lungs → Oesophagus →

Thoracic cavity, transverse section

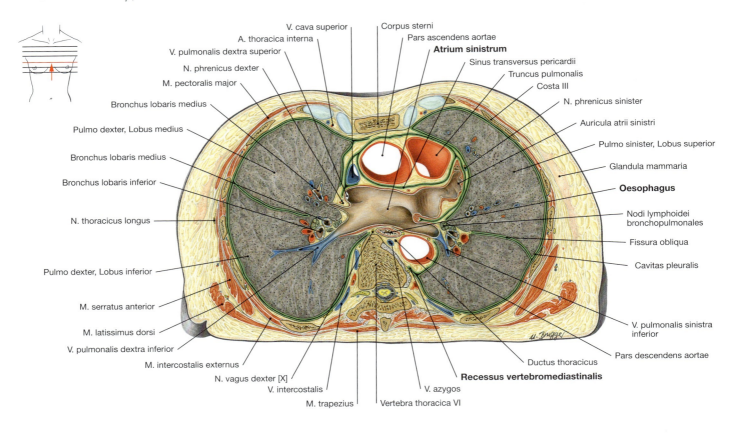

Fig. 5.104 Thoracic cavity, Cavitas thoracis; transverse section at the level of the left atrium; caudal view.

The left atrium of the heart (Atrium sinistrum) reaches further cranial than the right atrium and is positioned behind the great vessels. The Oesophagus is directly adjacent to the dorsal aspect of the left atrium.

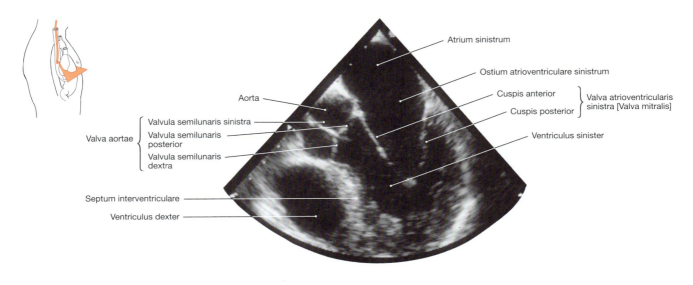

Fig. 5.105 Heart, Cor; ultrasound image taken from within the Oesophagus (transoesophageal echocardiography).

Clinical Remarks

The spatial proximity of the Oesophagus to the heart is useful when performing a **transoesophageal echocardiography** (→ Fig. 5.98). With the ultrasound transducer in the Oesophagus, more detailed images of the heart and particularly the heart valves, can be taken than from outside of the chest wall.

Thoracic cavity, transverse sections

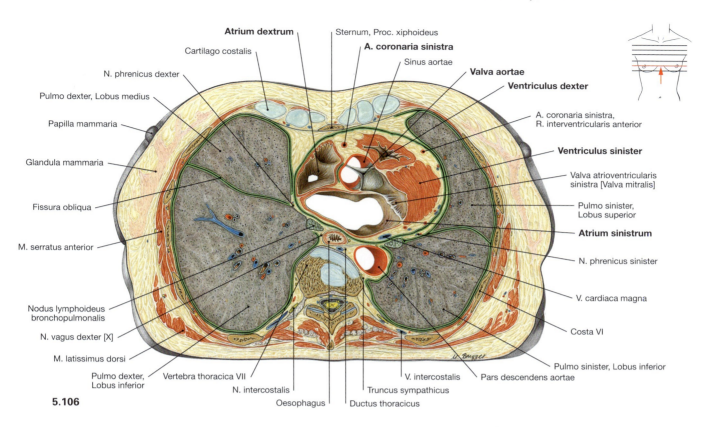

5.106

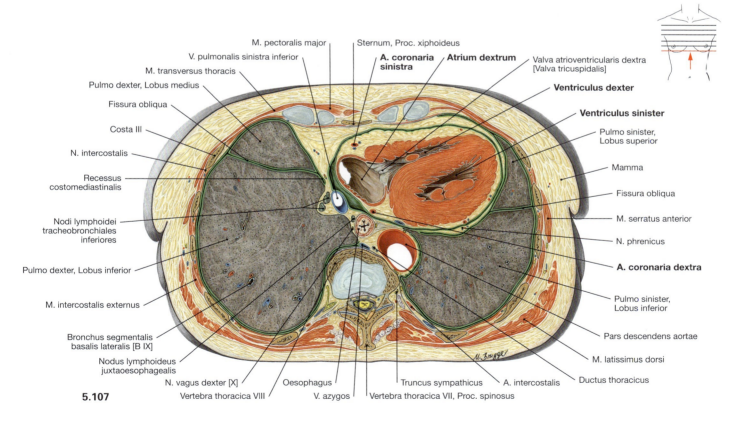

5.107

Fig. 5.106 and Fig. 5.107 Thoracic cavity, Cavitas thoracis; transverse sections at the level of the aortic valve (→ Fig. 5.106) and beneath the aortic valve (→ Fig. 5.107); caudal view.
These sections show that the Mediastinum medium, which contains the heart and the pericardium, extends further to the left side than to the right side. This results in a smaller volume of the left lung.

In the Pericardium, a thick layer of subepicardial adipose tissue is evident in which the coronary arteries are embedded. The lateral aspect of the heart (Facies pulmonalis of the heart) at this sectional level is confined by the right atrium on the right side and the left ventricle on the left side. The right ventricle does not participate in the borders of the heart but, instead, forms the anterior aspect of the heart (Facies sternocostalis).

Thoracic Viscera

Heart → ... → Sections

Thoracic cavity, frontal sections

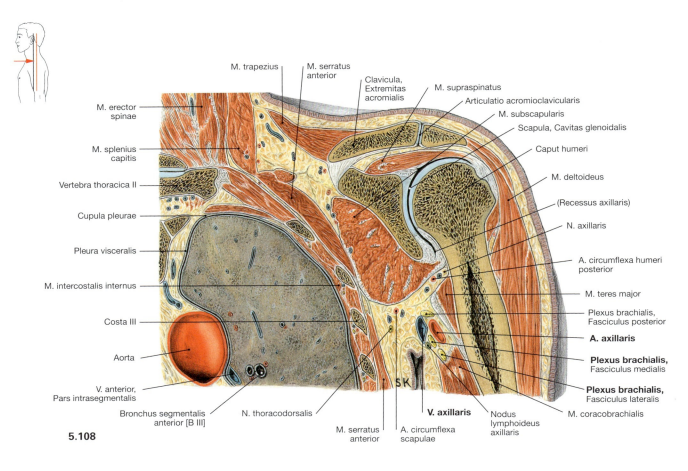

5.108

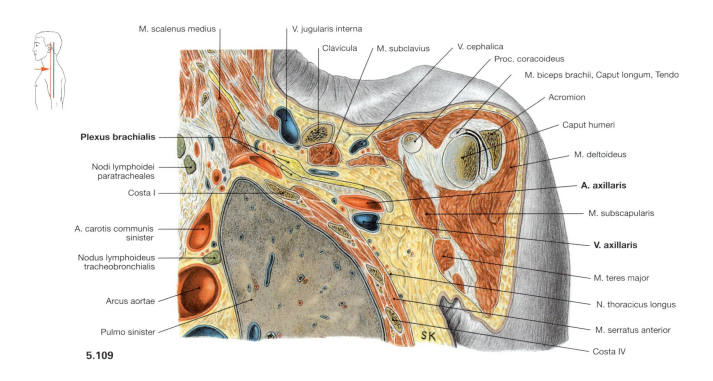

5.109

Fig. 5.108 and Fig. 5.109 Thoracic cavity, Cavitas thoracis, axillary fossa, Axilla, and shoulder joint, Articulatio humeri; frontal sections at the level of the shoulder joint (→ Fig. 5.108) and anterior to the shoulder joint (→ Fig. 5.109); ventral view.

These illustrations show that the neurovascular structures supplying the arm, A. and V. axillaris and the Plexus brachialis, course ventral to the shoulder joint in close topographical relation to the apex of the lung.

Viscera of the Abdomen

Development 72
Stomach 74
Intestines 86
Liver and Gallbladder 102
Pancreas 120
Spleen 128
Topography 130
Sections 148

6

The Abdomen – Concealed Organs

The origin of the terms abdomen and abdominal for the organs that lie in its cavity (Cavitas abdominalis), are derived from the Latin verb "abdo" – "I hide". In fact, the abdomen does not only hide many organs, but even more causes for diseases.

At a First Glance

Once opened, one looks into an abdominal cavity which is tightly filled with soft and solid organs (Viscera). This is called the situs, "the positioning" of the organs in relation to one another. The inside of the abdominal wall as well as the surfaces of the abdominal organs are covered with soft, moist, and shiny linings, known as the **Peritoneum**. The wall-covering Peritoneum is the parietal layer; the organ-covering Peritoneum is the visceral layer. The smooth peritoneum enables for example the peristaltic movements of stomach and intestines, allowing intestinal loops to slide against each other.

Upper Abdominal Situs

The organs of the upper abdomen lie beneath and between the arches of the rib cage, beneath the dome of the diaphragm, in the Regiones hypochondriacae and the Regio epigastrica. This region contains the **liver** (Hepar) and the **Pancreas,** the largest glands in the human body. The liver occupies the entire Regio hypochondriaca dextra and parts of the Regio epigastrica, where its surface clings closely to the diaphragm. At its inferior surface it bears the reservoir for its secretion, the **gallbladder** (Vesica biliaris). The **stomach** (Gaster) is just below the ribs of the Regio hypochondriaca sinistra. At the right Regio epigastrica, the stomach transitions into the **Duodenum** (the first part of the small intestine) at the Pylorus (M. sphincter pyloricus). Between the Duodenum and stomach on one side and the inferior surface of the liver on the other spans a peritoneal duplication, called the **Omentum minus**. The **Pancreas** and a greater part of the **Duodenum** are located dorsal and slightly caudal to the stomach at the dorsal wall of the abdominal cavity. Lateral and posterior to the stomach, in the "outer left corner" of the Regio hypochondriaca sinistra, the **spleen** (Splen) is located in its "niche". It is also not visible at first, but easily palpable when one glides the hand over the stomach towards the spleen.

Lower Abdominal Situs

In the remaining larger part of the abdomen, in the Regiones abdominales laterales, inguinales, umbilicalis, and pubica, the **intestines** (Intestinum) are located – hardly visible at first. Hanging down from the lower margin of the stomach, the **Omentum majus** resembles an apron containing adipose tissue. Lifting it, one observes the convolution of the intestines. The lower segments of the **small intestine** (Intestinum tenue), Jejunum and Ileum, are strongly wound and several meters long. If the small intestines are slightly moved back and forth, one notices that they are framed by the **Colon** (Intestinum crassum) like an inverted "U": the Colon ascendens on the right hand side, the Colon transversum (where the Omentum majus is attached to in a similar way as to the stomach) marks the border to the Epigastrium, and the Colon descendens on the left hand side. Then, with an elegant swing, the Colon sigmoideum disappears in the lower pelvis where it transitions into the Rectum.

"Mesos" and Peritoneal Relationships

Some of the organs of the Situs viscerum (e.g. Intestinum tenue) are attached to planar, adipose-rich duplications of the Peritoneum (**"Mesos"**) which project into the lumen of the body cavity. The Mesos carry blood vessels and nerves for the particular Viscera. Depending on the organ associated with the Meso, it is referred to as the Mesocolon (of the Colon transversum), the mesentery (of the small intestine) or the Mesogastrium (of the stomach). The "Mesos" can be pictured as so-called "planar stems" that serve to suspend the respective organs from the abdominal wall. As a result, the entire organs are covered by Peritoneum, except on the "seam-line" to the Meso. They are therefore called **intraperitoneal.**

Other organs (such as the Colon ascendens, the Colon descendens or the Pancreas) are located at the dorsal wall of the abdomen and fixed in place by connective tissue; hence they have no "stalks". Therefore these organs are less mobile, they are covered by Peritoneum only on their ventral surfaces facing the abdominal cavity, and are referred to as **retroperitoneal.** In contrast to the organs of the retroperitoneal situs (see below), these organs shifted to the dorsal body wall during development and are, therefore, called secondary retroperitoneal.

The position of these two groups of organs is not only of academic interest, but essential for all surgical disciplines: in contrast to the organs of the retroperitoneal situs, intraperitoneal organs can only be reached once the abdominal cavity is opened and this increases the risk of infection and complications.

Retroperitoneal Situs

If the space occupied by the gastro-intestinal tract, including its accessory glands, were "cleared", the organs behind the Peritoneum parietale would become visible on the dorsal wall of the Cavitas abdominalis, which resembles the retroperitoneal space (→ p. 158). The kidneys (Renes) are located ventral to the lowest ribs. The V. cava inferior ascends just to the right side of the vertebral column. It arises at the level of the lowest lumbar vertebra from the confluence of the two Vv. iliacae communes. Nota bene, the V. cava inferior receives no direct venous inflow from the abdominal viscera. Instead their venous blood is collected in the hepatic portal vein, the V. portae hepatis, and flows through the capillary bed of the liver before it enters the V. cava inferior. The **Aorta abdominalis** descends in the median plane along the vertebral bodies, and divides into the Aa. iliacae communes ventral to the fourth lumbar vertebra. Three large, unpaired arterial trunks, which leave the Aorta ventrally, supply the organs of the upper abdomen (Truncus coeliacus) and the intestines (Aa. mesentericae superior and inferior).

Abdominal Pain

Abdominal pain has several causes which range from innocuous situations to imminent disasters. The abdominal wall can be soft and hardly tender to palpation, but also show board-like rigidity and rebound tenderness. It takes a skilled internist or surgeon to accurately diagnose the causal pathology of an "acute abdomen", which per se is only a symptom, to provide appropriate therapeutic options. This will only be successful, if one has a clear picture of the composition of the abdomen.

Clinical Remarks

Relevance for the Physician
Diseases of abdominal organs are of high importance not only for the general practitioner, but also for the specialist in internal medicine, among them gastroenterologists and hepatologists. Inflammatory diseases of the stomach (**gastritis**) or **gastric ulcers** are common. Peptic ulcers may perforate and erode the blood vessels of the stomach causing potentially life-threatening complications. Bile stones with inflammation of the gallbladder (**cholecystitis**) and Pancreas (**pancreatitis**) are in the Western world as common as liver diseases, from the fatty degeneration to fibrous destruction (liver cirrhosis), due to alcohol abuse and excessive nutrition. Liver cirrhosis may cause hypertension in the portal venous system (portal hypertension) potentially resulting in portocaval anastomoses and subsequently in life-threatening **bleeding from oesophageal varices**. Organs such as the stomach or the Colon are common sites for malignant **tumours**. In these cases, the anatomical knowledge of the supplying blood vessels and the lymphatic drainage pathways is of clinical importance for diagnostic staging as well as surgical therapy. Other organs such as the spleen are at risk of rupturing due to a blunt abdominal trauma and may be the source of life-threatening internal bleedings.

→ *Dissection Link*
After opening the abdominal cavity, initially the undissected situs with the Bursa omentalis and the Omenta majus and minus should be demonstrated, as dissection significantly changes the relative positions of the structures. Alternatively, only the organs of the lower abdomen or all organs of the peritoneal cavity as a block should be removed to dissect the retroperitoneum and pelvic situs. Prior to resection, the three unpaired blood vessels of the abdominal aorta (Truncus coeliacus, Aa. mesentericae superior and inferior) must first be identified and cut, if needed. After transection and ligation of the Oesophagus or Duodenum proximally, and of the terminal ileum and the Rectum distally, the intraperitoneal and secondary retroperitoneal organs are mobilised bluntly. In addition, the liver should be separated from the V. cava inferior. Afterwards, neurovascular structures of the organs remaining in situ and the removed organs must be traced. At stomach, spleen, and intestines, primarily the blood vessels are to be dissected and displayed. The extrahepatic bile ducts are dissected in the region of the hilum of the liver and the gallbladder.

EXAM CHECK LIST

• Development: abdominal situs, Pancreas with malformations • topography: positions of the organs with ligaments, recessus of the peritoneal cavity with Bursa omentalis, CT sectional diagnostics • organs: all organs including neurovascular structures and lymphatic drainage pathways (particularly Gaster and Intestinum crassum), liver segments and structures of the liver hilum • portal venous system • portocaval anastomoses with clinical relevance • Vesica biliaris with CALOT's triangle • course and junctions of the extrahepatic bile ducts • secretory ducts of the Pancreas

6 Viscera of the Abdomen   Development → Stomach → Intestines → Liver and gallbladder →

Development of the upper abdominal situs

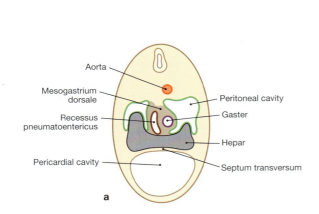
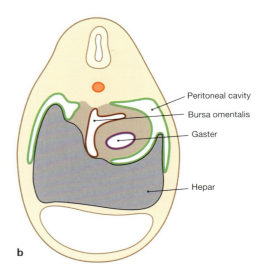
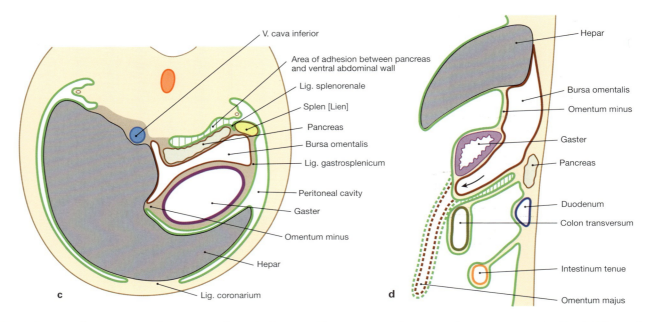

Figs. 6.1a to d   Development of the upper abdominal situs at the end of week 4 (a), at the beginning of week 5 (b), and at the beginning of week 7 (c); transverse sections (a to c) and paramedian section (d) of the upper abdomen. Peritoneum (green); Peritoneum of the Recessus pneumatoentericus and the Bursa omentalis (dark red), respectively. (according to [1])

The **primordial gut** predominantly derives from the endoderm and parts of the yolk sac. In the surrounding mesoderm, developing gaps fuse to form the body cavity. The mesoderm covering the primordial gut later forms the Peritoneum viscerale and, as Peritoneum parietale, lines the abdominal cavity. The Peritoneum viscerale also forms the mesenteries which contain the supplying neurovascular structures and serve as attachments. The dorsal mesentery connects the primordial gut with the dorsal wall of the trunk. The upper abdomen also contains a ventral mesentery.

At the beginning of **week 4,** an endodermal outgrowth develops ventral to the primordial gut at the level of the later Duodenum and gives rise to the epithelial tissues of liver, gallbladder, bile ducts and Pancreas. Subsequently, the following restructuring occurs:

1. The liver expands into the Mesogastrium ventrale and, thus, creates a division into the Mesohepaticum ventrale (between ventral wall of the trunk and liver) and the Mesohepaticum dorsale (between liver and stomach) (**a** and **b**). The Mesohepaticum ventrale later forms the **Lig. coronarium** cranially and the **Lig. falciforme hepatis** caudally. The **Lig. teres hepatis** at the caudal margin is a remnant of the umbilical vein. The Mesohepaticum dorsale becomes the Omentum minus.
2. In the Mesogastrium dorsale a gap appears at the right side (Recessus pneumatoentericus) which later forms the **Bursa omentalis** (a and b).
3. The stomach rotates **90°** in a **clockwise** direction (cranial view) and thus is located in a frontal position at the left side of the body **(c)**. The Omentum minus connects the liver and lesser curvature of the stomach also in a frontal plane and forms the ventral border of the Bursa omentalis which has reached a position on the left side behind the stomach.
4. In the Mesogastrium dorsale, the **Pancreas** and the **spleen** develop. The Pancreas subsequently acquires a retroperitoneal position, and the spleen remains intraperitoneal.
5. The Mesogastrium dorsale eventually separates into the **Lig. gastrosplenicum** (from the greater curvature of the stomach to the spleen) and the **Lig. splenorenale** (from the splenic hilum to the dorsal abdominal wall) and forms the other portions of the Omentum majus (apron-like at the greater curvature of the stomach; **d**). Therefore, due to its development and the neurovascular supply, the **Omentum majus** is associated with the upper abdominal situs.

Pancreas → Spleen → Topography → Sections

Development of the lower abdominal situs

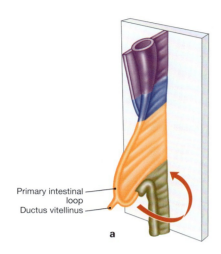
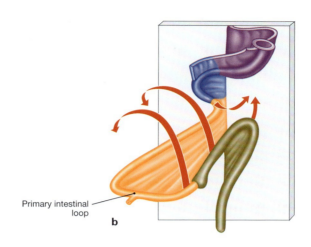
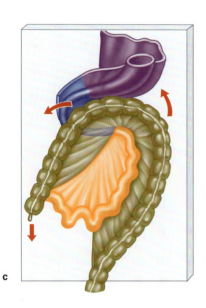
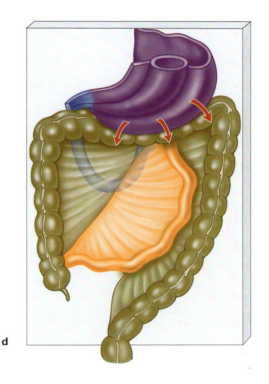

Figs. 6.2a to d Schematic illustrations of the intestinal rotation. Intestinal segments and their mesenteries are highlighted in different colours: Gaster and Mesogastrium (purple), Duodenum and Mesoduodenum (blue), Jejunum and Ileum with associated mesenteries (orange), Colon and Mesocolon (ochre). (according to [1])

1. Caused by the longitudinal growth of the primordial gut, a ventrally oriented loop forms **(primary intestinal loop)**. The proximal (upper) limb of this loop develops into the major part of the small intestine, the distal (lower) limb develops into the colon including the Colon transversum. The distal large intestine develops from the hindgut and, thus, differs in its neurovascular supply.
2. Due to a lack of space, the primary intestinal loop is temporarily located outside of the embryo in the umbilical cord **(physiological umbilical hernia)** and remains connected to the yolk sac via the Ductus vitellinus. If the intestines fail to relocate entirely into the embryo, a congenital umbilical hernia **(omphalocele)** remains which contains portions of the intestinal segments and their mesenteries. Because this congenital hernia traverses through the later umbilical ring, it is covered by amnion only but not by muscles of the abdominal wall.
3. Remnants of the Ductus vitellinus may remain as **MECKEL's diverticulum** located at the small intestine.
4. The elongation of the intestines initiates a **270° counter-clockwise** rotation, resulting in the colon to surround the small intestine like a frame.
5. Colon ascendens and Colon descendens are secondarily relocated in a retroperitoneal position.

Clinical Remarks

MECKEL's diverticula are common (3% of the population) and are usually located in the part of the small intestine that is located approximately 100 cm cranial of the iliocaecal valve. Due to the fact that these diverticula frequently contain disseminated gastric mucosa, inflammation and subsequent bleeding thereof may mimic symptoms of an appendicitis. Disturbances of the intestinal rotation can cause a **malrotation** (hypo- and hyperrotation). These may result in intestinal obstruction (ileus) or an abnormal positioning of the respective intestinal segments, a condition that may impede the diagnosis of an appendicitis. A **Situs inversus** describes a condition where all organs are positioned mirror-inverted.

6 Viscera of the Abdomen Development → Stomach → Intestines → Liver and gallbladder →

Projection of the stomach

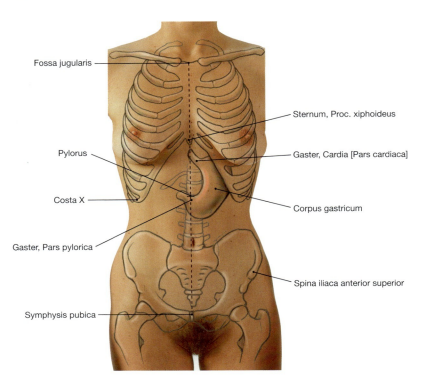

Fig. 6.3 Projection of the stomach, Gaster, onto the ventral wall of the trunk.
The cardiac orifice (Cardia) projects onto the level of the 10th thoracic vertebra, thus, ventrally below the Proc. xiphoideus of the sternum. The position of the caudal part of the stomach is relatively variable at the level of the 2nd to 3rd lumbar vertebra. The Pylorus, on the other hand, regularly locates halfway along a virtual line connecting the pubic symphysis (Symphysis pubica) and the jugular fossa (Fossa jugularis), projecting onto the 1st lumbar vertebra.

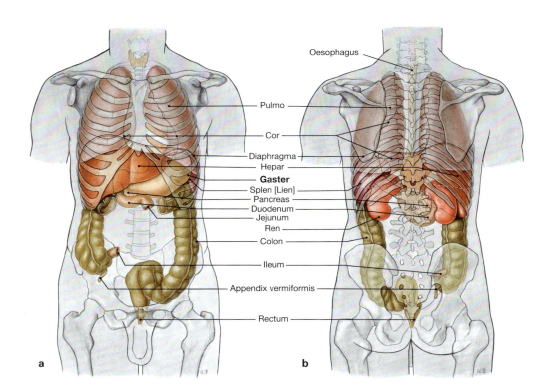

Figs. 6.4a and b Projection of the internal organs onto the body surface; ventral (**a**) and dorsal (**b**) views.
The stomach is positioned **intraperitoneally** in the left Epigastrium between the left lobe of the liver and the spleen. The stomach is mostly covered by the left costal arch but a small area is directly adjacent to the ventral abdominal wall. This area is clinically relevant since PEG-tubes (**p**ercutaneous **e**ndoscopic **g**astrostomy) can be placed here for parenteral nutrition.

Pancreas → Spleen → Topography → Sections

Divisions of the stomach

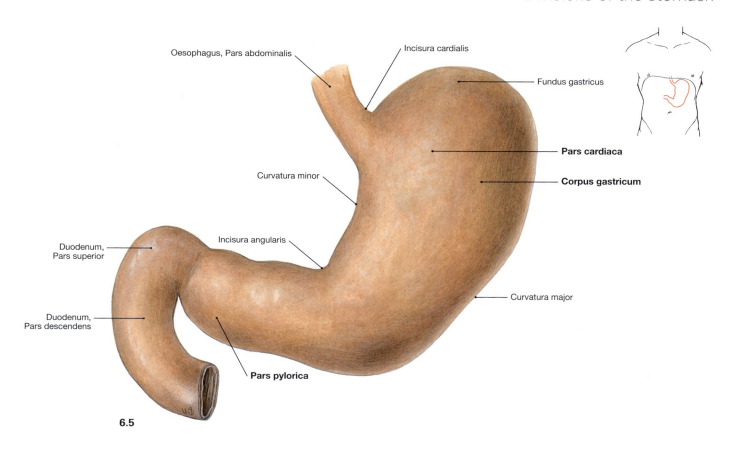

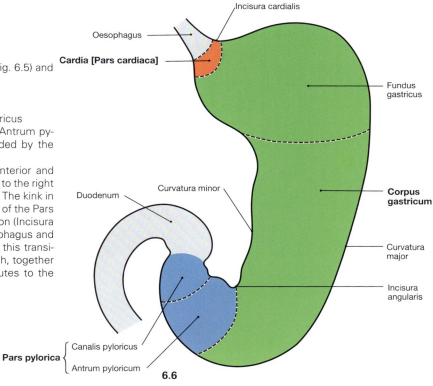

Fig. 6.5 and Fig. 6.6 Stomach, Gaster; ventral view (→ Fig. 6.5) and schematic illustration (→ Fig. 6.6). (Fig. 6.6 according to [1])
The stomach has three parts:
- **Pars cardiaca:** entrance to the stomach
- **Corpus gastricum:** main part with superior Fundus gastricus
- **Pars pylorica:** exit of the stomach which continues as Antrum pyloricum and Canalis pyloricus, the latter being surrounded by the sphincter muscle (M. sphincter pyloricus).

The stomach has an anterior and posterior wall (Paries anterior and posterior). The lesser curvature (Curvatura minor) is directed to the right side, the greater curvature (Curvatura major) to the left side. The kink in the lesser curvature (Incisura angularis) marks the beginning of the Pars pylorica. The greater curvature also begins with an indentation (Incisura cardialis) which marks the angle of HIS between the Oesophagus and the stomach (cardiac notch). At the inside of the stomach, this transition between both organs is marked by a mucosal fold which, together with the angiomuscular gastro-oesophageal valve, contributes to the closure of the stomach.

Clinical Remarks

If the cardiac notch is straightened and the angle of HIS is lost, such as in sliding hiatal hernias, the resulting reflux of gastric juice into the Oesophagus may cause **gastro-(o)esophageal reflux disease (GERD)** with inflammation of the oesophageal mucosa. If therapeutic approaches with proton pump inhibitors (antacids) to reduce the gastric acid production are not successful, surgical procedures, such as fixing the fundus around the Oesophagus (NISSEN fundoplication) are performed, to restore the gastro-oesophageal valve mechanism.

6 Viscera of the Abdomen → Development → Stomach → Intestines → Liver and gallbladder →

Muscles of the stomach

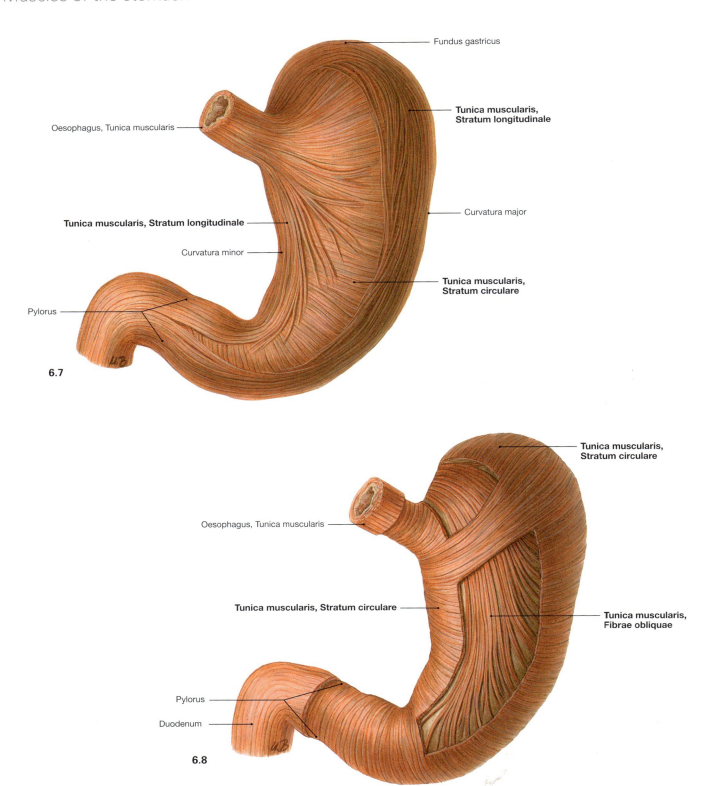

Fig. 6.7 and Fig. 6.8 Outer (→ Fig. 6.7) and inner (→ Fig. 6.8) muscular layers of the stomach, Gaster; ventral view.
The wall of the stomach comprises three muscular layers (Tunica muscularis) not consistently found in all regions of the stomach. The external longitudinal layer (Stratum longitudinale) is adjacent to the circular layer (Stratum circulare). The innermost layer consists of the oblique muscle fibres (Fibrae obliquae) which are missing at the lesser curvature.

Pancreas → Spleen → Topography → Sections

Inner relief of the stomach

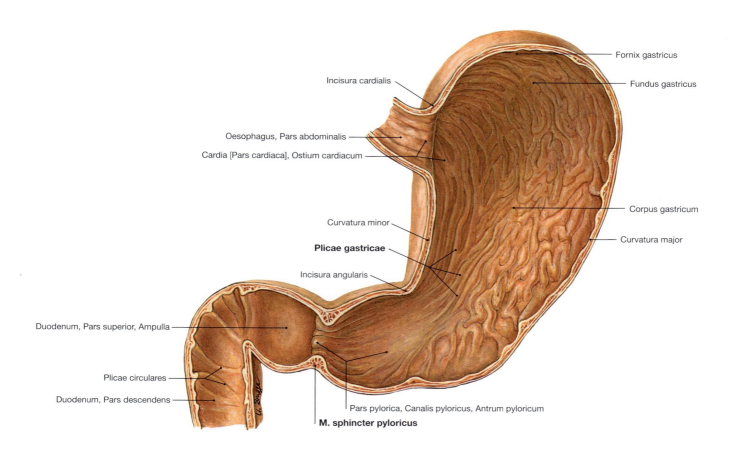

Fig. 6.9 Stomach, Gaster, and duodenum, Duodenum; ventral view.
The gastric mucosa has a characteristic relief serving the enlargement of the inner surface. The macroscopically recognisable gastric folds (Plicae gastricae) are longitudinally oriented and form the functional canal along the lesser curvature (gastric canal). The mucosal folds reveal small microscopic areas (Areae gastricae; → Fig. 6.10). At the exit of the stomach (Pylorus), the circular muscle layer is thickened to form the pyloric sphincter muscle (M. sphincter pyloricus).

6 Viscera of the Abdomen Development → Stomach → Intestines → Liver and Gallbladder →

Structure of the wall of the stomach

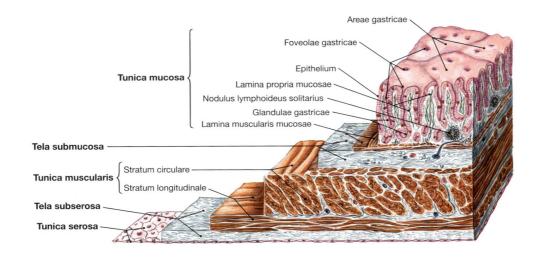

Fig. 6.10 Wall of the stomach, Gaster; microscopic view.
Similar to the whole intestines, the wall of the stomach comprises an inner mucosal layer (Tunica mucosa) which is separated from the muscular layer (Tunica muscularis, → Figs. 6.7 and 6.8) by a layer of loose connective tissue (Tela submucosa). As an intraperitoneal organ the outer surface of the stomach is covered by visceral peritoneum (Peritoneum viscerale) which forms the Tunica serosa.

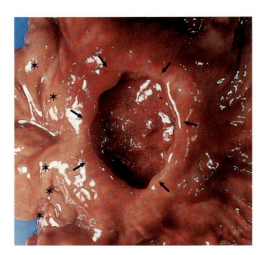

Fig. 6.11 Gastric ulcer (Ulcus ventriculi). [5]
Gastric ulcers are peptic defects which affect the entire wall of the stomach. Asterisks mark the pyloric ring, arrows mark the rim of the ulcer.

Clinical Remarks

More than 80% of all **gastric and duodenal ulcers** are caused by the bacterium Helicobacter pylori. In addition, an increased production of gastric acid or a reduced production of mucus, e.g. caused by pain treatment with acetylsalicylic acid, may promote the formation of peptic ulcers. Thus, therapeutic approaches include antibiotic treatment and antacids. Complications may include a perforation into adjacent organs or the abdominal cavity with resulting life-threatening peritonitis, or the erosion of a gastric artery (→ p. 80) with subsequent severe bleeding. These complications require surgical intervention.

Pancreas → Spleen → Topography → Sections

Topographical relations of the stomach

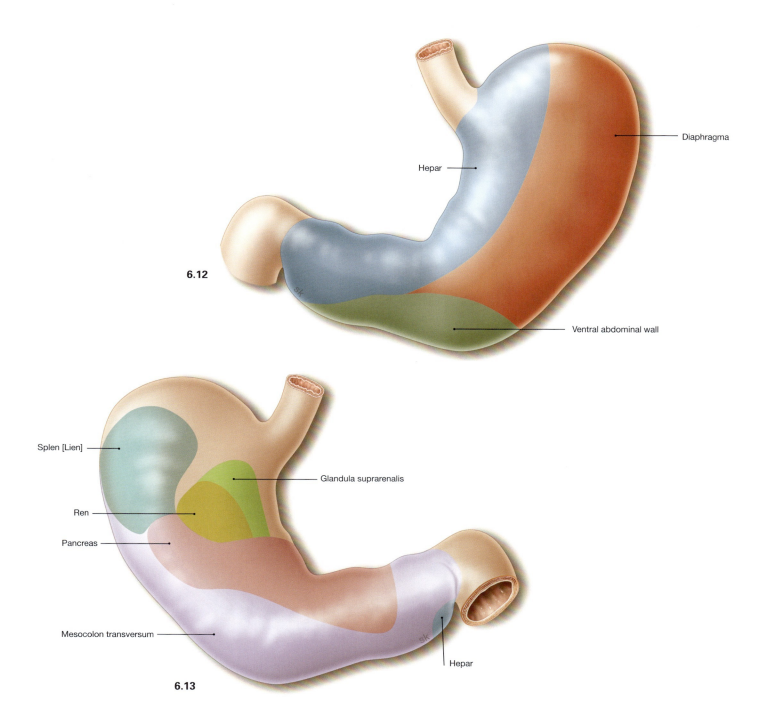

Fig. 6.12 and Fig. 6.13 Contact areas, Facies, of the anterior wall (→ Fig. 6.12) and the posterior wall (→ Fig. 6.13) of the stomach with adjacent organs:
- **ventral:** liver, diaphragm, abdominal wall
- **dorsal:** spleen, kidney, adrenal gland, Pancreas, Mesocolon transversum

The stomach is mobile and, depending on the filling state, has different contact areas with its adjacent organs.

Clinical Remarks

The contact areas have clinical relevance since peptic ulcers may result in **perforation into adjacent organs** resulting in severe damage to these organs and the formation of adhesions which impose difficulties for the surgical removal of tumours.

Viscera of the Abdomen
Development → **Stomach** → Intestines → Liver and gallbladder →

Arteries of the stomach

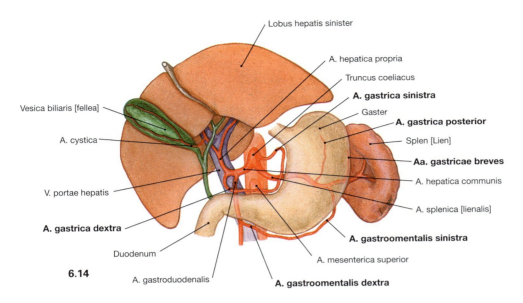

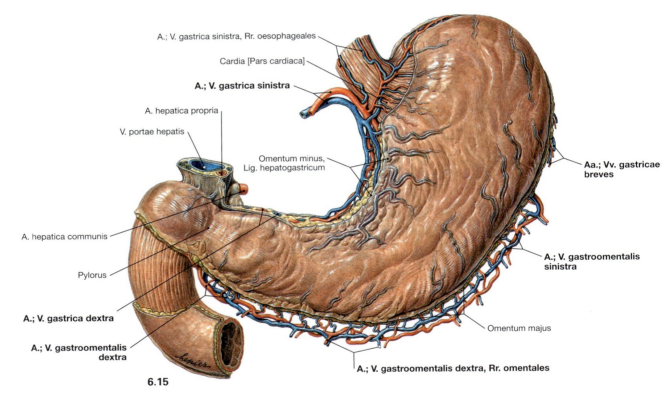

Fig. 6.14 and Fig. 6.15 Arteries of the stomach, Gaster, as schematic illustration (→ Fig. 6.14) and their course along the curvatures of the stomach (→ Fig. 6.15); ventral view.

The three main branches of the Truncus coeliacus (A. gastrica sinistra, A. hepatica communis, A. splenica) collectively give rise to six gastric arteries (→ Table).

Arteries of the Stomach	
Lesser curvature	• A. gastrica sinistra (direct branch of the Truncus coeliacus) • A. gastrica dextra (derived from the A. hepatica propria)
Greater curvature	• A. gastroomentalis sinistra (derived from the A. splenica) • A. gastroomentalis dextra (derived from the A. gastroduodenalis of the A. hepatica communis) These vessels also supply the Omentum majus!
Fundus	• Aa. gastricae breves (derived from the A. splenica in the area of the splenic hilum)
Posterior side	• A. gastrica posterior (present in 30–60%, derives from the A. splenica behind the stomach)

Veins of the stomach

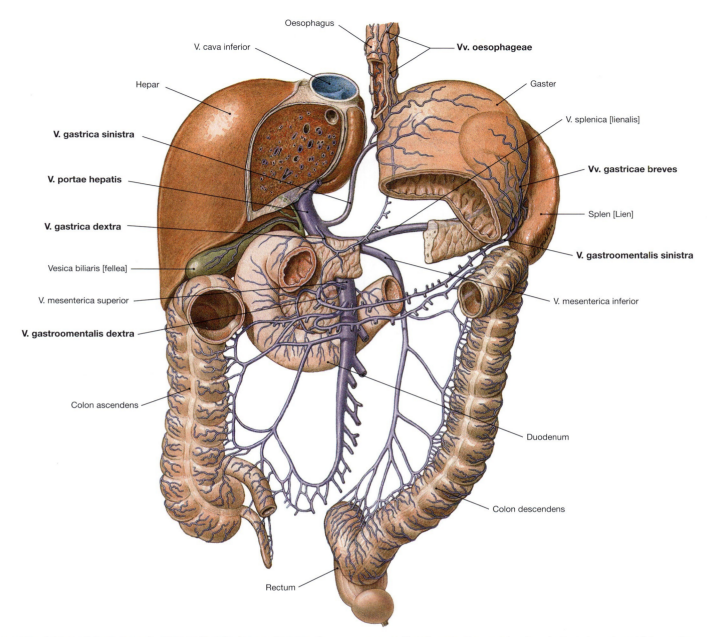

Fig. 6.16 Veins of the stomach, Gaster, in relation to the portal vein, V. portae hepatis; ventral view.
The veins are corresponding to the arteries, but the veins at the lesser curvature directly enter the portal vein, whereas the veins at the greater curvature drain into the larger branches of the portal vein.

Veins of the Stomach	
Lesser curvature	• V. gastrica sinistra • V. gastrica dextra Drainage into the V. portae hepatis: these veins anastomose via the Vv. oesophageae with the azygos system and thus, with the V. cava superior!
Greater curvature	• V. gastroomentalis sinistra (to V. splenica) • V. gastroomentalis dextra (to V. mesenterica superior)
Fundus	• Vv. gastricae breves (to V. splenica)
Posterior side	• V. gastrica posterior (present in 30–60%, to V. splenica)

Clinical Remarks

In cases of increased blood pressure in the portal vein system (portal hypertension), such as in liver cirrhosis, **portocaval anastomoses** may form via the oesophageal veins which may substantially dilate **(oesophageal varices)** and bear the risk for rupture with subsequent potentially life-threatening haemorrhage (→ Fig. 5.81)!

Viscera of the Abdomen Development → **Stomach** → Intestines → Liver and gallbladder →

Lymph vessels of the stomach

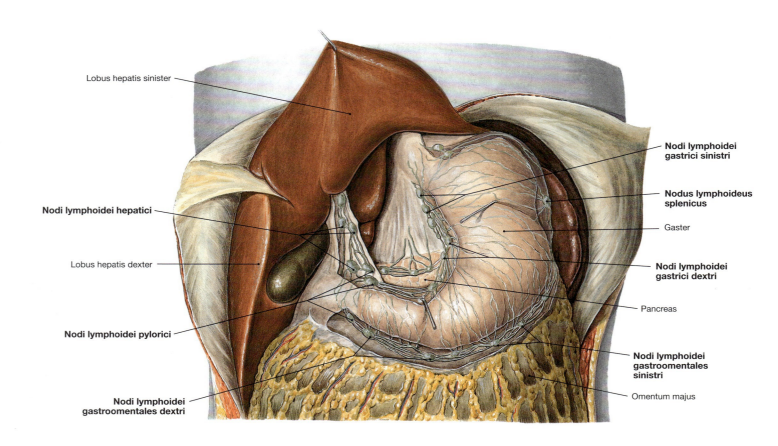

Fig. 6.17 Lymph vessels and lymph nodes of the stomach, Gaster, and the liver, Hepar; ventral view.
The lymph vessels and lymph nodes of the stomach are located alongside both **curvatures** and around the **Pylorus:** the lesser curvature shows the Nodi lymphoidei gastrici, the greater curvature harbours the Nodi lymphoidei splenici and caudal thereof the Nodi lymphoidei gastroomentales. The Nodi lymphoidei pylorici in the region of the Pylorus connect to the Nodi lymphoidei hepatici at the hilum of the liver. Three major lymphatic drainage pathways with three subsequent lymph node stations are distinguished (→ Fig. 6.18).

Clinical Remarks

The lymphatic drainage stations (→ Fig. 6.19) of the stomach are of clinical relevance in the **surgical therapy of gastric cancer.** The lymph nodes of the first and second stations are usually removed together with the stomach. If lymph nodes of the third station are also affected by metastatic cancer cells, curative therapy is not possible. In these cases, total gastrectomy will not be performed.

Lymph vessels of the stomach

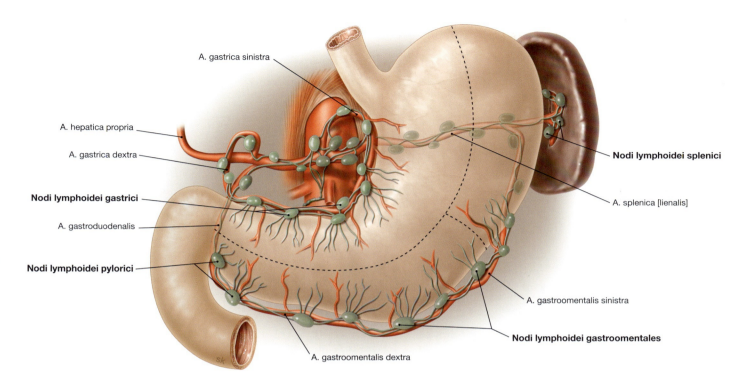

Fig. 6.18 Lymphatic drainage and regional lymph nodes of the stomach, Gaster; ventral view. (according to [1])
The three principle lymphatic drainage pathways which exist for the stomach are marked by dashed lines in this illustration:

- **cardiac area and lesser curvature:** Nodi lymphoidei gastrici
- **upper left quadrant:** Nodi lymphoidei splenici
- **lower two-thirds of the greater curvature and Pylorus:** Nodi lymphoidei gastroomentales and Nodi lymphoidei pylorici

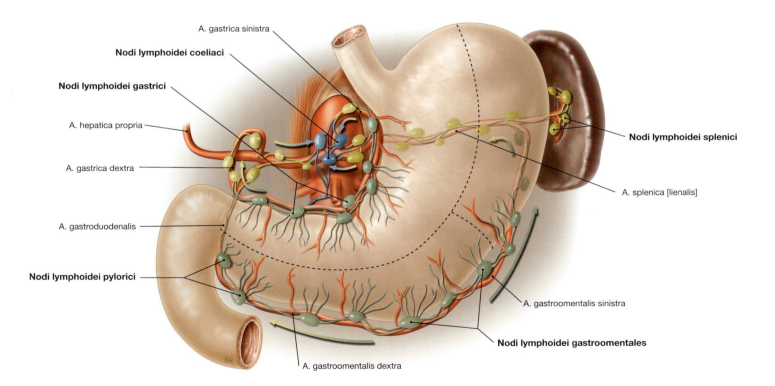

Fig. 6.19 Lymphatic drainage stations of the stomach; ventral view. (according to [1])
Within the three principle lymphatic drainage pathways there are **three subsequent stations**:
- first station (green): lymph nodes along the curvatures (→ Fig. 6.18)
- second station (yellow): lymph nodes along the branches of the Truncus coeliacus
- third station (blue): lymph nodes at the origin of the Truncus coeliacus [Nodi lymphoidei coeliaci]; from here the lymph is drained via the Truncus intestinalis into the Ductus thoracicus.

Viscera of the Abdomen Development → **Stomach** → Intestines → Liver and gallbladder →

Autonomic innervation of the stomach

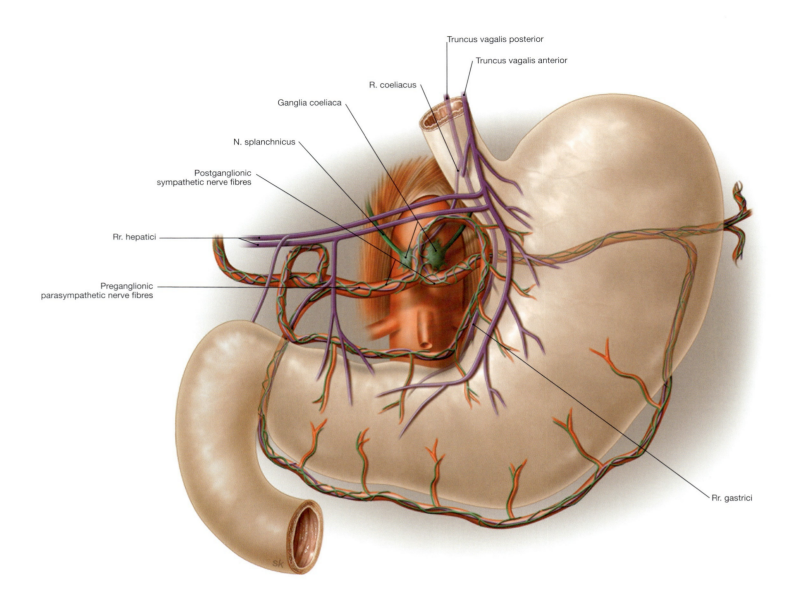

Fig. 6.20 Autonomic innervation of the stomach, Gaster; semischematic illustration. Sympathetic innervation (green), parasympathetic innervation (purple). (according to [1])
Preganglionic **parasympathetic fibres** (Rr. gastrici) reach the stomach as Trunci vagales anterior and posterior descending along the Oesophagus and course along the lesser curvature. As a result of the gastric rotation during development, the anterior Truncus vagalis is predominantly derived from the left, the posterior Truncus vagalis from the right N. vagus [X]. The Pars pylorica is innervated by separate branches (Rr. hepatici) of the Trunci vagales. The postganglionic neurons are located within the muscular layers of the stomach. The **parasympathetic innervation stimulates** the production of gastric acids and promotes the gastric peristalsis.
Preganglionic **sympathetic fibres** traverse the diaphragm on both sides as Nn. splanchnici major and minor and are synapsed to the postganglionic sympathetic neurons in the Ganglia coeliaca located at the origin of the Truncus coeliacus. These postganglionic sympathetic fibres reach the stomach as peri-arterial nerve plexus. The sympathetic innervation counterbalances the parasympathetic influence by reducing gastric acid production, peristalsis, and perfusion.

Clinical Remarks

A former therapy in patients with peptic ulcers was to sever the entire N. vagus [X] inferior to the diaphragm (**total vagotomy**) or its branches to the stomach (**selective vagotomy**) to reduce the production of gastric acid. Nowadays, with the success of oral treatments with antacids and antibiotics to eradicate the causal Helicobacter pylori bacteria, the surgical vagotomy is only rarely performed.

Pancreas → Spleen → Topography → Sections

Stomach, gastroscopy

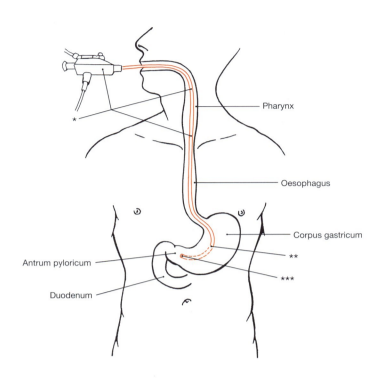

Fig. 6.21 Technique for oesophagoscopy and gastroscopy.

* gastroscope
** gastroscope, tip in the Corpus gastricum (→ Fig. 6.22a)
*** gastroscope, tip in the Antrum pyloricum (→ Fig. 6.22b)

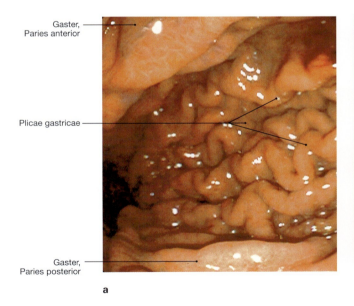

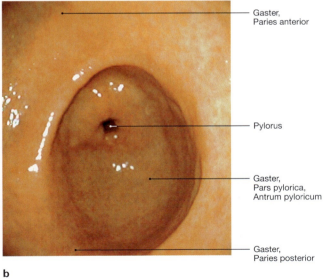

Figs. 6.22a and b Stomach, Gaster; gastroscopy; cranial view.
a view onto the Corpus gastricum showing the longitudinal mucosal folds (Plicae gastricae)
b view onto the Antrum pyloricum showing predominantly smooth mucosa

Clinical Remarks

Gastroscopy enables the **inspection** of the gastric mucosal lining. Pathological findings such as erosive gastric lesions or ulcers (→ Fig. 6.11) require tissue **biopsies** for further pathological diagnostics to distinguish between a benign peptic ulcer and a gastric carcinoma.

6 Viscera of the Abdomen Development → Stomach → Intestines → Liver and gallbladder →

Projection of the small intestine

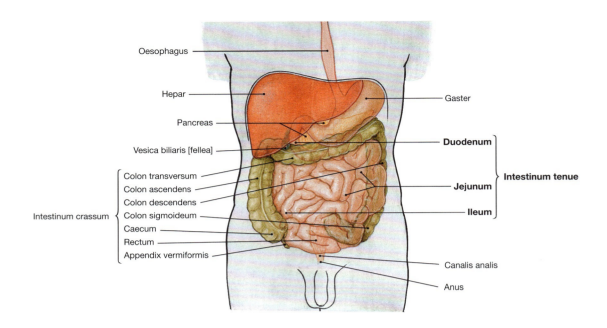

Fig. 6.23 Projection of the abdominal viscera onto the body surface; ventral view.
The small intestine (4–6 m) has three parts:
- Duodenum, 25–30 cm
- Jejunum, two-fifths of the total length
- Ileum, three-fifths of the total length

The Duodenum starts at the Pylorus of the stomach and ends at the Flexura duodenojejunalis. Except for its first part (Pars superior), the Duodenum is fixed in its retroperitoneal position and well separated from the other parts of the small intestine. In contrast, the **intraperitoneal convoluted parts** of the Jejunum and Ileum are not separable macroscopically and reach distally to the Valva iliocaecalis (BAUHIN's valve) at the transition to the large intestine.

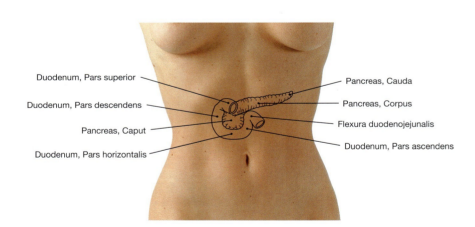

Fig. 6.24 Projection of the duodenum, Duodenum, and pancreas, Pancreas, onto the ventral abdominal wall.
The **intraperitoneal Pars superior** of the Duodenum projects onto the level of the 1st lumbar vertebra. **All other parts** are located **secondary retroperitoneally** and encompass the head of the Pancreas in a C-shaped manner. The head of the Pancreas is adjacent to the Pars descendens of the Duodenum. The Pars horizontalis lies at the level of the 3rd lumbar vertebra and continues as Pars ascendens to the Flexura duodenojejunalis at the level of the 2nd lumbar vertebra. This flexure marks the transition to the intraperitoneal Jejunum.

Structure of the wall of the small intestine

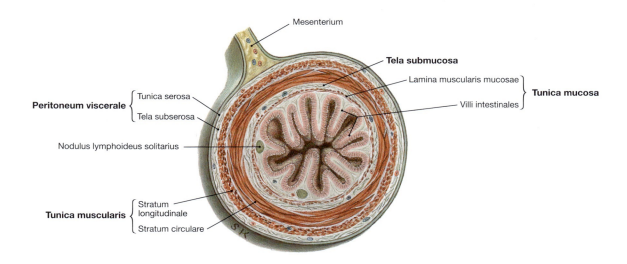

Fig. 6.25 Small intestine, Intestinum tenue; cross-section. The layers are described in → Figure 6.26.

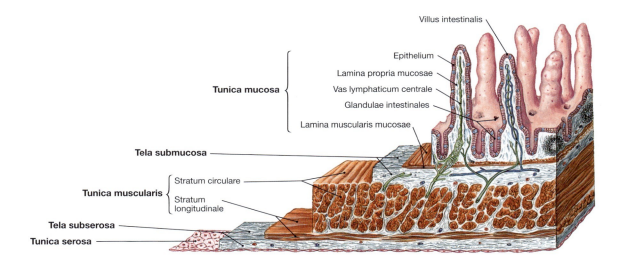

Fig. 6.26 Wall structure of the small intestine, Intestinum tenue; microscopic view.
Similar to other parts of the intestines, the wall of the small intestine consists of the innermost mucosal layer **(Tunica mucosa)** with intestinal villi (Villi intestinales) for surface tenlargement. Separated by a loose connective tissue layer **(Tela submucosa),** the muscular layer **(Tunica muscularis)** consists of the inner circular layer (Stratum circulare) and the outer longitudinal layer (Stratum longitudinale). The intraperitoneal parts (Pars superior of the Duodenum, Jejunum and Ileum) are covered on their outer surface with peritoneum (Peritoneum viscerale) which forms the **Tunica serosa.** Retroperitoneal parts of the Duodenum are anchored by a **Tunica adventitia** within the connective tissue of the retroperitoneal space.

Viscera of the Abdomen Development → Stomach → Intestines → Liver and gallbladder →

Divisions of the duodenum

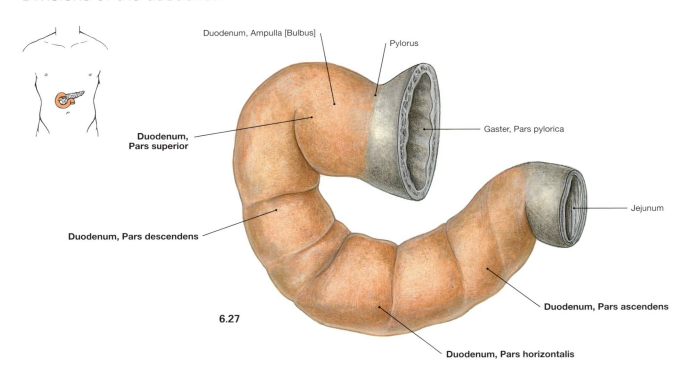

6.27

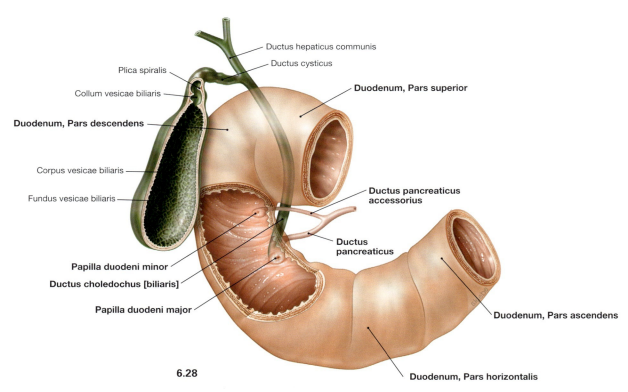

6.28

Fig. 6.27 and Fig. 6.28 Divisions of the duodenum, Duodenum, isolated (→ Fig. 6.27) and together with the extrahepatic bile ducts (→ Fig. 6.28); ventral view.
The Duodenum has **four parts:**
- Pars superior
- Pars descendens
- Pars horizontalis
- Pars ascendens

The **Pars superior** is the only intraperitoneal part and its wider proximal lumen is referred to as Ampulla (Bulbus) duodeni.

The excretory duct of the Pancreas (Ductus pancreaticus, duct of WIRSUNG) enters the **Pars descendens** of the Duodenum frequently together with the common bile duct (Ductus choledochus) on a mucosal papilla (Papilla duodeni major, ampulla of VATER) which is found 8–10 cm distal to the Pylorus. Often, 2 cm proximal to the latter, a smaller Papilla duodeni minor is found into which the Ductus pancreaticus accessorius (SANTORINI's duct) empties its secretion.
The **Pars horizontalis** crosses the vertebral column and continues as **Pars ascendens.**

Pancreas → Spleen → Topography → Sections

Structure of the duodenum

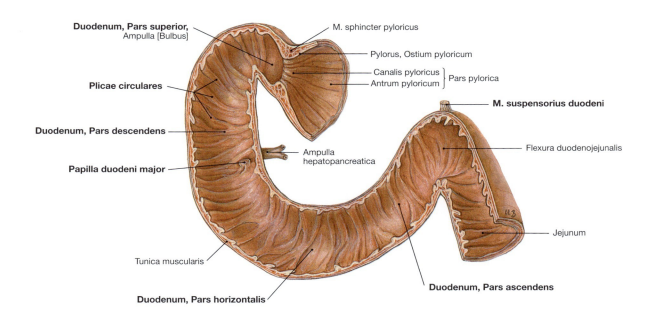

Fig. 6.29 Inner relief of the duodenum, Duodenum; frontal section; ventral view.
The Duodenum has the following four parts: 1. Pars superior, 2. Pars descendens, 3. Pars horizontalis, and 4. Pars ascendens. To increase the absorptive surface, the inner relief of the Duodenum shows circular mucosal folds (Plicae circulares, KERCKRING's folds) similar to other parts of the small intestine. The Pars descendens contains the Papilla duodeni major (ampulla of VATER) at the entrance of the Ductus pancreaticus (duct of WIRSUNG) and the common bile duct (Ductus choledochus), both of which usually merge to form the Ampulla hepatopancreatica. The Pars ascendens is attached to the aorta near the origin of the A. mesenterica superior by smooth muscle fibres (M. suspensorius duodeni, muscle of TREITZ) and dense connective tissue (Lig. suspensorium duodeni), just before the Duodenum transitions into the intraperitoneal Jejunum at the Flexura duodenojejunalis.

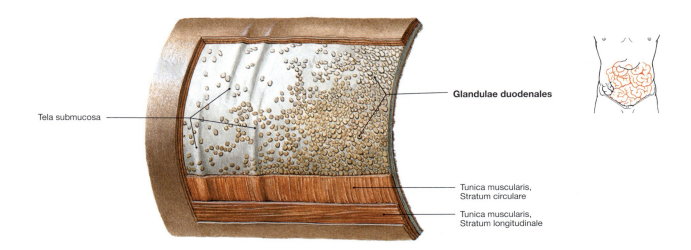

Fig. 6.30 Wall structure of the duodenum, Duodenum, with Glandulae duodenales; view from outside.
The mucous-producing Glandulae duodenales (BRUNNER's glands) are located in the Tela submucosa and allow the identification of the Duodenum in histological sections.

Clinical Remarks

The muscle of TREITZ defines the border between **upper and lower intestinal tract haemorrhages**. This classification is of clinical relevance since both forms of haemorrhage have different common causes and require different diagnostic steps.

6 Viscera of the Abdomen   Development → Stomach → **Intestines** → Liver and gallbladder →

Duodenum, imaging

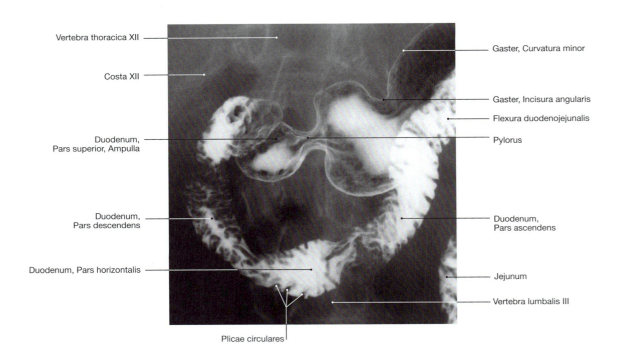

Fig. 6.31 Duodenum, Duodenum; radiograph in anteroposterior (AP) beam projection after oral application of a contrast material; patient in upright position; ventral view.

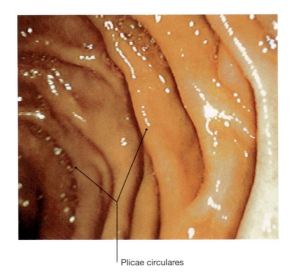

Fig. 6.32 Duodenum, Duodenum; endoscopic image. The circular mucosal folds (Plicae circulares, KERCKRING's folds) are clearly visible.

Clinical Remarks

Similar to the situation in the stomach, **duodenal ulcers** are common and clinically they cannot clearly be distinguished from gastric ulcers (→ p. 78). Malignant tumours, however, are rare in the Duodenum. Several diagnostic approaches can be employed. Conventional **radiology with contrast imaging** is less frequently used because diagnostic **endoscopy** (duodenoscopy) not only enables the direct inspection of the mucosa but also allows the sampling of tissue biopsies.

Structure of the wall of jejunum and ileum

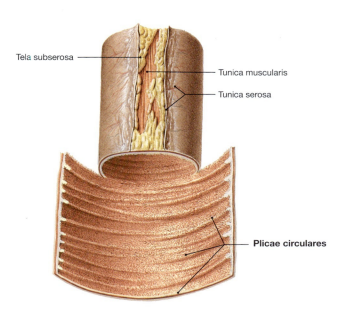

Fig. 6.33 Detail of the jejunum, Jejunum.
The structure of the Jejunum is very similar to the Duodenum but does not contain the Glandulae duodenales (BRUNNER's glands).

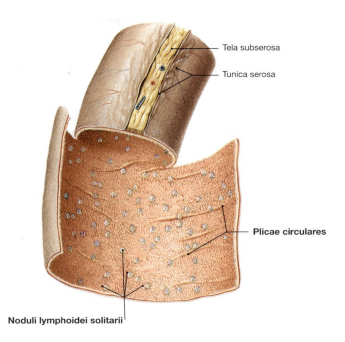

Fig. 6.34 Detail of the proximal ileum, Ileum.
The Plicae circulares (KERCKRING's folds) are much less frequent in the Ileum when compared to the upper small intestine.

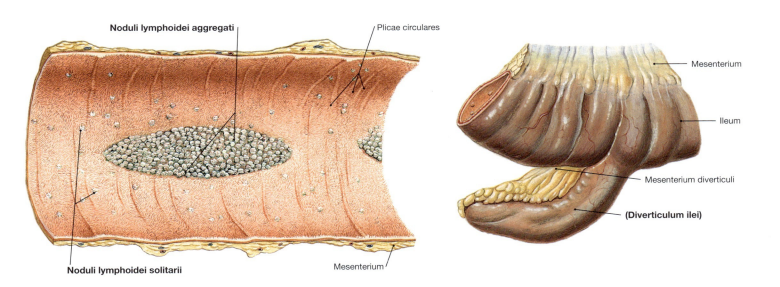

Fig. 6.35 Detail of the distal ileum, Ileum.
The large assemblies of lymph follicles are characteristic for the terminal Ileum. They are a part of the mucosa-associated lymphoid tissue (MALT). The lymph nodes are either located individually (Nodi lymphoidei solitarii; → Fig. 6.34) in the Tela submucosa or are assembled in groups (Noduli lymphoidei aggregati; PEYER's plaques) underneath the elevated mucosa.

Fig. 6.36 MECKEL's diverticulum, Diverticulum ilei.
Up to 3% of people have been diagnosed with a diverticulum, which exists as a remnant of the embryological Ductus vitellinus (→ Fig. 6.2). It is usually located in the Ileum about 100 cm proximal to the ileocaecal valve at the opposite side of the mesentery.
MECKEL's diverticula may contain disseminated gastric mucosa and, when inflamed or bleeding, can mimic the symptoms of an appendicitis.

Viscera of the Abdomen
Development → Stomach → **Intestines** → Liver and gallbladder →

Projection of the large intestine

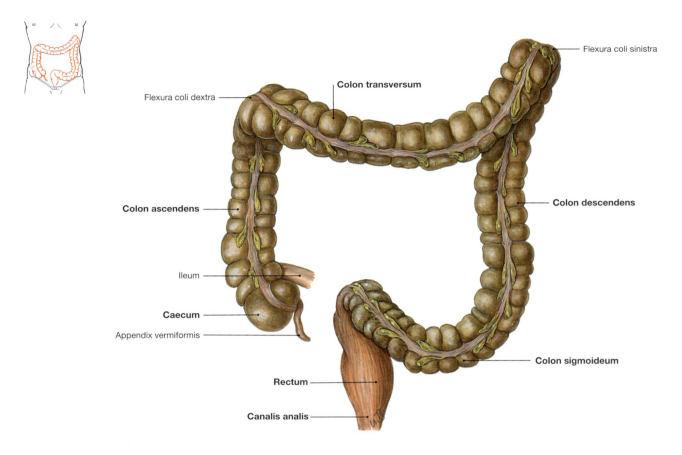

Fig. 6.37 Divisions of the large intestine, Intestinum crassum; ventral view.
The large intestine is about 1.5 m long and consists of **four parts**:
- Caecum (blind gut) with Appendix vermiformis
- Colon with Colon ascendens, Colon transversum, Colon descendens, and Colon sigmoideum
- Rectum
- Canalis analis

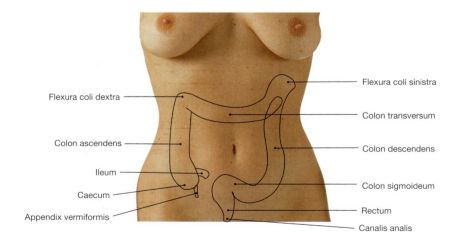

Fig. 6.38 Projection of the large intestine, Intestinum crassum, onto the ventral abdominal wall.
Caecum with Appendix vermiformis, Colon transversum, and Colon sigmoideum are positioned intraperitoneally and have individual mesenteries. Caecum and Appendix vermiformis may also be located retroritoneally (Caecum fixum); in this case they do not have a mesentery. Colon ascendens, Colon descendens, and the major part of the Rectum are usually secondarily retroperitoneal organs, the distal Rectum and the anal canal are subperitoneal. The projections and the length of the individual segments of the large intestine are highly variable and the retroperitoneal segments are usually inconsistently fused with the posterior abdominal wall. Due to the position of the liver on the right side, the left colic flexure (Flexura coli sinistra) is positioned farther cranial than the right colic flexure (Flexura coli dextra; → Fig. 6.53).

Pancreas → Spleen → Topography → Sections

Projection and positional variations of the Appendix vermiformis

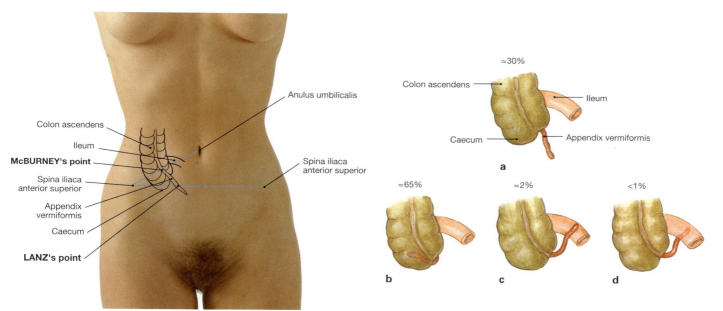

Fig. 6.39 Projection of the caecum, Caecum, and Appendix vermiformis onto the ventral abdominal wall.
The base of the Appendix vermiformis projects onto the **McBURNEY's point** (the transition between the lateral third and the medial two-thirds on a line connecting the umbilicus with the Spina iliaca anterior superior). The location of the tip of the appendix is more variable and projects onto the **LANZ's point** (the transition between the right third and the left two-thirds on a line connecting both Spinae iliacae anteriores superiores; 30%; → Figs. 6.40 and 6.41).

Figs. 6.40a to d Positional variants of the Appendix vermiformis; ventral view.
a descending into the small pelvis
b retrocaecal (most common position)
c pre-ileal
d retro-ileal

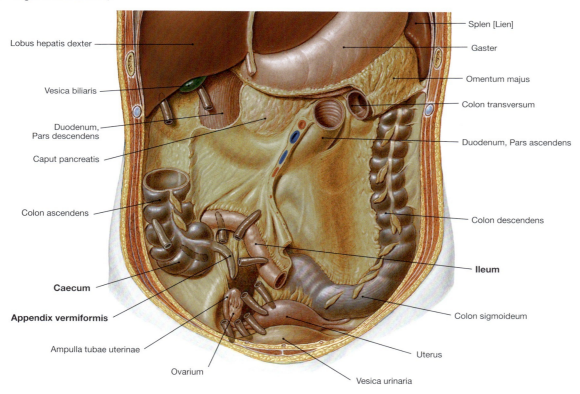

Fig. 6.41 Positional variants of the Appendix vermiformis; ventral view.

Clinical Remarks

The diagnosis of **appendicitis** is often not easy since right lower abdominal pain can also be caused by enteritis or, in women, by inflammatory conditions of the ovary or the fallopian tube. Thus, the pain induced by pressing and releasing (rebound tenderness) the McBURNEY's or the LANZ's point is an important discriminatory sign.

Viscera of the Abdomen Development → Stomach → Intestines → Liver and gallbladder →

Structure of the large intestine

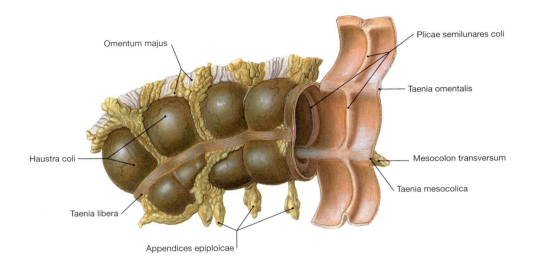

Fig. 6.42 Structural characteristics of the large intestine, Intestinum crassum, the transverse colon taken as an example; ventral caudal view.
The large intestine has four characteristic differences to the small intestine:
- **larger diameter** ("thick" rather than "thin")
- **Taenia:** the longitudinal muscle layer is reduced to three bands. Of these, the Taenia libera is visible, whereas the Taenia mesocolica attaches to the Mesocolon transversum and the Taenia omentalis connects to the greater omentum (Omentum majus).

- **Haustra and Plicae semilunares:** the haustra (Haustra coli) are sacculations of the intestinal wall which correspond to crescent-shaped mucosal folds (Plicae semilunares) at the inner surface.
- **Appendices epiploicae:** fatty projections from the adipose tissue of the Tela subserosa.

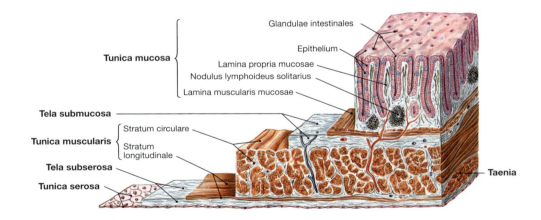

Fig. 6.43 Structure of the wall of the large intestine, Intestinum crassum; microscopic view.
Similar to the other parts of the intestines, the wall of the large intestine consists of an inner mucosal layer **(Tunica mucosa)** which, in contrast to the Duodenum, has no mucosal villi. Separated from the Tunica mucosa by a connective tissue layer **(Tela submucosa)** is the muscular layer **(Tunica muscularis)**. It consists of an inner circular layer **(Stratum circulare)** and an outer longitudinal layer **(Stratum longitudina-** le). However, the longitudinal layer is not continuous but is reduced to three bands **(Taenia)**. At the outside, the intraperitoneal parts (Caecum with Appendix vermiformis, Colon transversum, and Colon sigmoideum) are covered by peritoneum (Peritoneum viscerale) forming the **Tunica serosa.** In contrast, the retroperitoneal parts (Colon ascendens, Colon descendens, and upper rectum) are anchored by the **Tunica adventitia** in the connective tissue of the retroperitoneal space.

Caecum and Appendix vermiformis

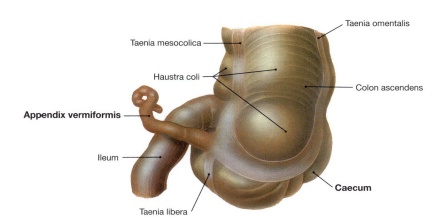

Fig. 6.44 Caecum with Appendix vermiformis, and terminal ileum, Pars terminalis ilei; dorsal view.
The Caecum is approximately 7 cm long. The 8–9 cm long Appendix vermiformis is attached to the Caecum and has its own mesentery (not shown here) with supplying neurovascular structures. The taenia of the Colon converge at the appendix to form a continuous longitudinal muscular layer.

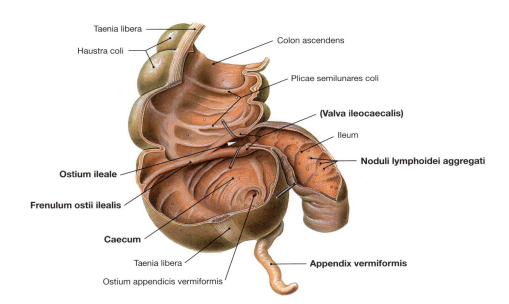

Fig. 6.45 Caecum with Appendix vermiformis, and terminal ileum, Pars terminalis ilei; ventral view; after removal of the anterior parts of the wall.
The Caecum is separated from the terminal ileum by the **ileocaecal valve** (Valva ileocaecalis, BAUHIN's valve). Internally, the two lips of the valve form the Papilla ilealis and border the ileal orifice (Ostium ileale). Laterally, the lips continue in the Frenulum ostii ilealis. The terminal ileum contains aggregations of lymph follicles (Nodi lymphoidei aggregati), referred to as **PEYER's plaques,** which are part of the mucosa-associated lymphoid tissue (MALT). Similarly, the Appendix vermiformis contains large aggregations of lymph follicles and serves the immune defence.

Clinical Remarks

The **appendicitis** is a common disease in the 2nd and 3rd decades of life. The appendicitis is an endogenous inflammation caused usually by the obstruction of the lumen of the appendix by faeces or, in rare cases, by foreign bodies with a resulting transmural inflammation due to intestinal micro-organisms. A perforation may cause a potentially life-threatening peritonitis. Important tasks of the terminal ileum are the absorption of vitamin B$_{12}$ and bile acids as well as its immunological functions. It is frequently affected by CROHN's disease, a chronic inflammatory disease of the intestine with autoimmune component, which, due to a vitamin B$_{12}$ deficiency, may cause anaemia.

Viscera of the Abdomen   Development → Stomach → Intestines → Liver and gallbladder →

Arteries of the small intestine

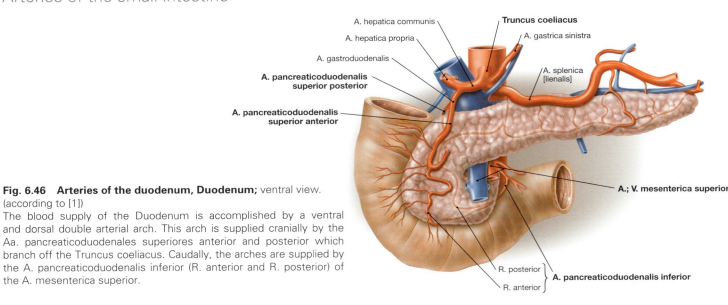

Fig. 6.46 Arteries of the duodenum, Duodenum; ventral view. (according to [1])
The blood supply of the Duodenum is accomplished by a ventral and dorsal double arterial arch. This arch is supplied cranially by the Aa. pancreaticoduodenales superiores anterior and posterior which branch off the Truncus coeliacus. Caudally, the arches are supplied by the A. pancreaticoduodenalis inferior (R. anterior and R. posterior) of the A. mesenterica superior.

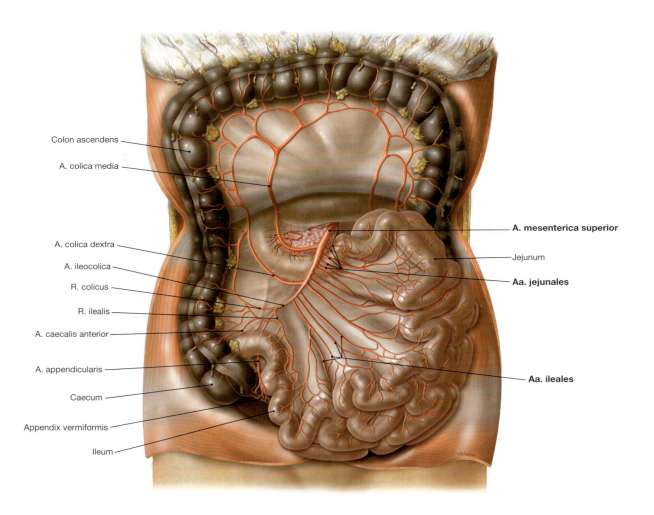

Fig. 6.47 Arteries of the jejunum, Jejunum, and ileum, Ileum; ventral view; Colon transversum reflected superiorly. (according to [1])
The intraperitoneal convolute of the Jejunum and Ileum is supplied by the A. mesenterica superior which distributes its branches (usually four to five Aa. jejunales and twelve Aa. ileales) within the mesentery of the small intestine (→ Fig. 6.115).

Arteries of the large intestine

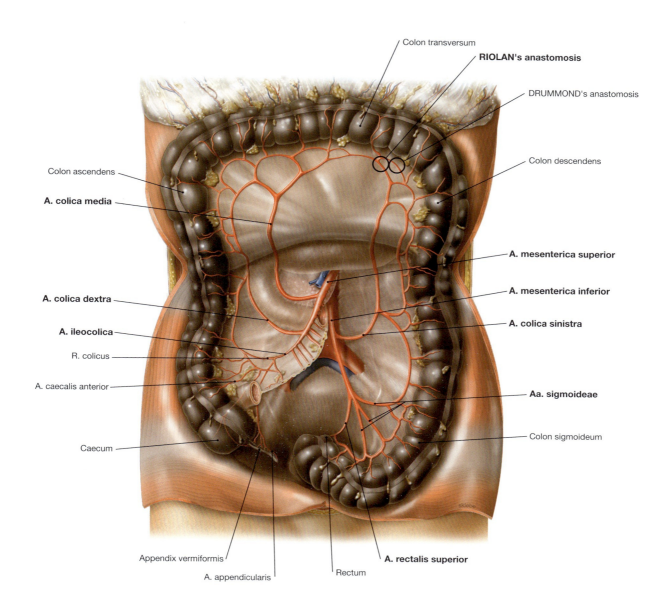

Fig. 6.48 Arteries of the large intestine, Intestinum crassum; ventral view; Colon transversum reflected superiorly. (according to [1])
- **Caecum and Appendix vermiformis: A. ileocolica** with a R. ilealis to the terminal ileum (anastomoses with the last A. ilealis) and with a R. colicus (anastomoses with the A. colica dextra). The artery then divides into the A. caecalis anterior and the A. caecalis posterior on both sides of the Caecum and into the A. appendicularis which courses in the meso-appendix to supply the Appendix vermiformis.
- **Colon ascendens and Colon transversum: A. colica dextra** and **A. colica media** (from the A. mesenterica superior) anastomose with each other. The A. colica media connects to the A. colica sinistra (**RIOLAN's anastomosis**). An occasionally existing anastomosis with one of the arcades at the left colic flexure is referred to as DRUMMOND's anastomosis.
- **Colon descendens and Colon sigmoideum: A. colica sinistra** and **Aa. sigmoideae** from the A. mesenterica inferior. The A. rectalis superior also derives from the A. mesenterica inferior and supplies the upper rectum.

For developmental reasons, the left colic flexure is the watershed for the neurovascular supply. With respect to the arteries: the supply by the A. mesenterica superior for the Colon ascendens and Colon transversum shifts to the supply by the A. mesenterica inferior for the Colon descendens and upper Rectum.

Clinical Remarks

The connections between the A. colica media and the A. colica sinistra, collectively referred to as **RIOLAN's anastomosis,** are clinically important in malperfusions such as in cases of arteriosclerosis or following an arterial occlusion by an embolus. Similar connections exist in the area of the Duodenum and the Rectum (→ Fig. 6.111).

Even the complete occlusion of one of the three unpaired abdominal arteries (Truncus coeliacus, A. mesenterica superior, and A. mesenterica inferior) can largely be compensated for without intestinal infarction. Intestinal malperfusion frequently causes abdominal pain after meals (postprandial pain).

6 Viscera of the Abdomen Development → Stomach → Intestines → Liver and gallbladder →

Veins of the small and large intestine

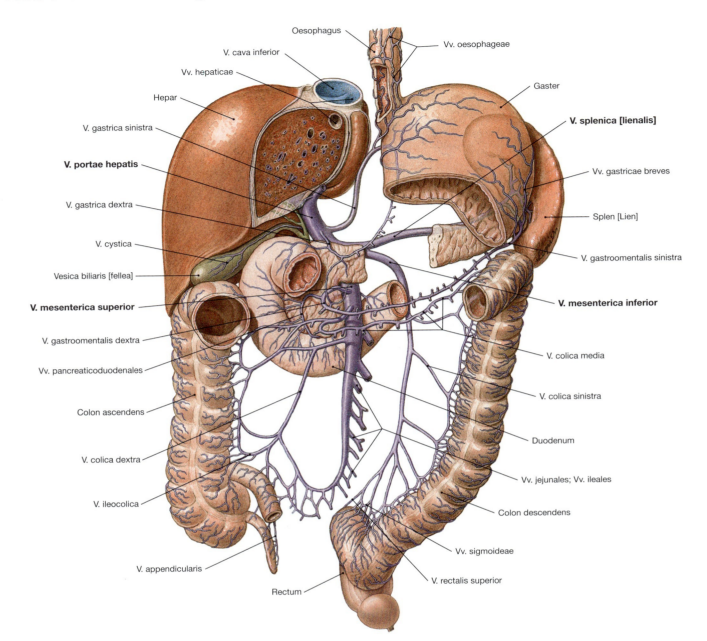

Fig. 6.49 Veins of the small intestine, Intestinum tenue, and the large intestine, Intestinum crassum; ventral view.
Name and course of the intestinal veins are similar to those of the arteries. The veins enter one of the three main tributaries of the portal vein (V. portae hepatis): the V. mesenterica superior merges with the V. splenica behind the pancreatic head to form the V. portae hepatis. The V. mesenterica inferior drains into the V. splenica (70 % of all cases) or into the V. mesenterica superior (30%).

Developmentally, the left colic flexure is the watershed for the neurovascular supply. With respect to the veins: from the Colon ascendens and Colon transversum venous blood drains into the V. mesenterica superior and from the Colon descendens and the upper Rectum the venous blood drains into the V. mesenterica inferior.

Branches of the V. mesenterica superior:
- V. gastroomentalis dextra with Vv. pancreaticoduodenales
- Vv. pancreaticae
- Vv. jejunales and ileales
- V. ileocolica
- V. colica dextra
- V. colica media

Branches of the V. mesenterica inferior:
- V. colica sinistra
- Vv. sigmoideae
- V. rectalis superior: this vein has connections to the V. rectalis media and the V. rectalis inferior, which are tributaries of the V. cava inferior.

Clinical Remarks

In cases of high blood pressure in the portal system (portal hypertension), such as in liver cirrhosis, anastomoses between the venous systems of the V. portae hepatis and the V. cava (**portocaval anastomoses**) may develop (→ Fig. 6.70). These include connections between the V. rectalis superior and the V. rectalis media, and V. rectalis inferior, respectively, which drain into the V. cava inferior. They are clinically less important and are not, as previously assumed, the cause of haemorrhoids. When applying rectal suppositories, it is helpful to know that the drugs are absorbed by the rectal veins to bypass the liver and to enter the general circulation via the V. cava inferior, thus, preventing hepatic metabolism and potential degradation of the drugs in the liver.

Lymph vessels of the intestines

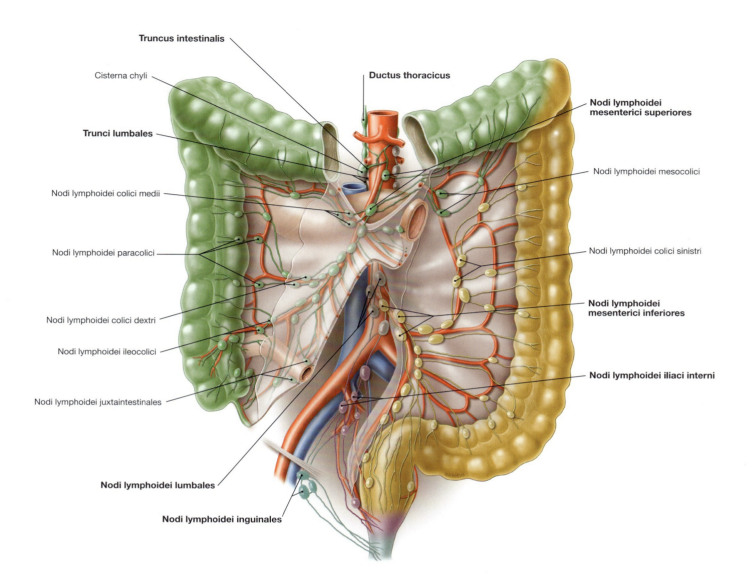

Fig. 6.50 Lymph vessels and regional lymph nodes of the small intestine, Intestinum tenue, and the large intestine, Intestinum crassum.
The respective groups of lymph nodes (a total of 100 to 200 lymph nodes) are coloured differently according to their drainage areas. (according to [1])
Located directly adjacent to the small intestine are the Nodi lymphoidei juxtaintestinales, adjacent to the large intestine the Nodi lymphoidei paracolici. After filtration in several successive lymph stations along the vascular arcades (e.g. Nodi lymphoidei colici dextri, colici medii, colici sinistri, ileocolici, mesocolici), the lymph enters into two major drainage systems:
- From the entire **small intestine** as well as **Caecum, Colon ascendens,** and **Colon transversum,** the lymph drains into the **Nodi lymphoidei mesenterici superiores** at the origin of the A. mesenterica superior and further via the Truncus intestinalis into the Ductus thoracicus (green).

- From the **Colon descendens, Colon sigmoideum,** and **proximal rectum,** the lymph reaches the **Nodi lymphoidei mesenterici inferiores** at the origin of the A. mesenterica inferior (yellow) and further via the retroperitoneal para-aortal lymph nodes (Nodi lymphoidei lumbales, grey) into the Trunci lumbales (grey).

The **distal rectum** and the **anal canal** also drain into the Trunci lumbales. The first lymph node stations, however, are the Nodi lymphoidei iliaci interni, and the Nodi lymphoidei inguinales (pink, turquoise) for the terminal segment of the anal canal, respectively.

Developmentally, the left colic flexure is the watershed for the neurovascular supply. With respect to the lymphatic drainage: the Nodi lymphoidei mesenterici superiores are the regional lymph nodes for the Colon ascendens and Colon transversum, whereas the Nodi lymphoidei mesenterici inferiores drain the Colon descendens.

Clinical Remarks

The **lymphatic drainage** plays a clinically important role in the diagnosis of colon carcinomas since the therapeutic approach depends on the stage of the disease (staging). Lymph node metastases of tumours in the area of the Colon ascendens or Colon transversum are expected to appear in the Nodi lymphoidei mesenterici superiores.

Carcinomas in the Colon descendens, however, metastasise into the Nodi lymphoidei mesenterici inferiores along the retroperitoneal A. mesenterica inferior and often connect to other retroperitoneal lymph nodes.

6 Viscera of the Abdomen   Development → Stomach → Intestines → Liver and gallbladder →

Innervation of the intestines

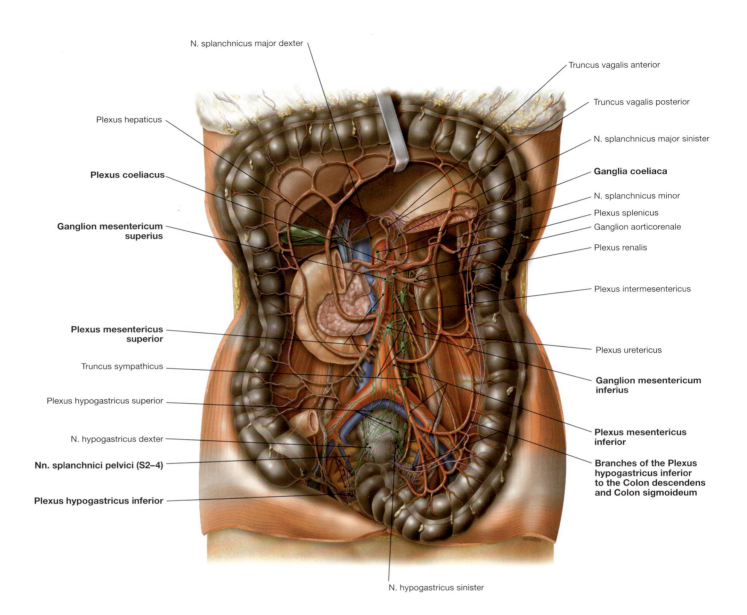

Fig. 6.51 Autonomic innervation of the small intestine, Intestinum tenue, and large intestine, Intestinum crassum; ventral view. (according to [1])

The autonomic nerves of the sympathetic (green) and parasympathetic (purple) nervous system generate a plexus at the anterior side of the Aorta **(Plexus aorticus abdominalis).** These nerve fibres continue along the major branches of the Aorta to reach the target organs. Small and large intestines are innervated by fibres derived from the plexus around the three major visceral branches of the Aorta (**Plexus coeliacus, Plexus mesentericus superior** and **Plexus mesentericus inferior**).

The perikarya of the **preganglionic sympathetic neurons** are located in the intermediolateral cell column of the spinal cord. Their axons reach the sympathetic trunk (Truncus sympathicus) and course without synapsing in the Nn. splanchnici major and minor to the plexus around the Aorta, where they finally synapse in the respective ganglia (**Ganglion coeliacum, Ganglia mesenterica superius** and **inferius**) to postganglionic neurons. Axons of the postganglionic neurons travel along the arteries to reach the intestines.

Preganglionic parasympathetic neurons of the **Nn. vagi [X]** course along the Oesophagus as Trunci vagales anterior and posterior, pass through the diaphragm and reach the visceral nerve plexus of the Aorta abdominalis. They pass through the ganglia without synapsing to reach the postganglionic neurons within the wall or in the vicinity of the target organs. The innervation area of the Nn. vagi [X] ends in the Plexus mesentericus superior and, thus, in the area of the left colic flexure.

The Colon descendens is innervated by the **sacral division of the parasympathetic nervous system.** The preganglionic parasympathetic neurons are localised at the S2–S4 spinal cord level and the nerve fibres leave the spinal nerves as Nn. splanchnici pelvici. They are synapsed in the ganglia of the Plexus hypogastricus inferior in the vicinity of the Rectum. The postganglionic nerve fibres either ascend to the Plexus mesentericus inferior (not shown) or directly reach the Colon descendens.

The **parasympathetic** innervation **stimulates,** and the **sympathetic** innervation **inhibits** peristalsis and perfusion of the intestines.

For developmental reasons, the left colic flexure is the watershed for the neurovascular supply. With respect to the autonomic innervation: Colon ascendens and Colon transversum are innervated from the Plexus mesentericus superior, whereas the Colon descendens is innervated by the Plexus mesentericus inferior (cranial/sacral division of the parasympathetic system).

Pancreas → Spleen → Topography → Sections

Large intestine, imaging

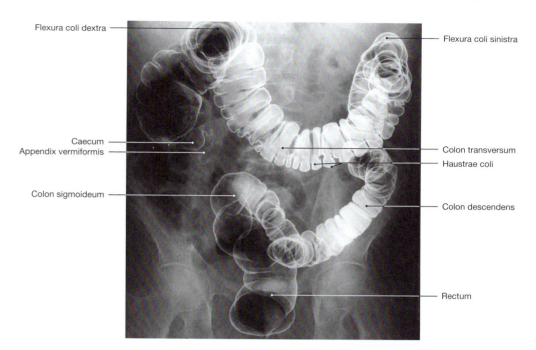

Fig. 6.52 Large intestine, Intestinum crassum; radiograph in anteroposterior (AP) beam projection after application of contrast medium and air (double contrast barium enema). Positional variations of the Colon transversum can be detected (→ Fig. 6.53).

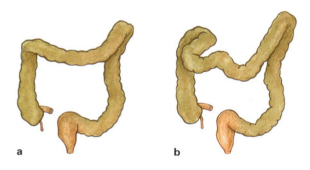
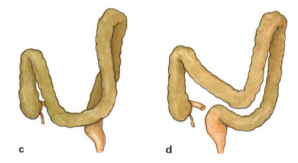

Figs. 6.53a to d Positional variations of the transverse colon, Colon transversum; ventral view.

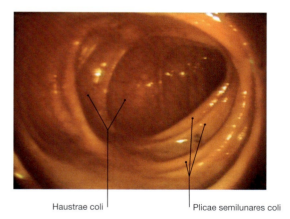

Fig. 6.54 Ascending colon, Colon ascendens; endoscopy of the colon (coloscopy).
In contrast to the circular mucosal folds of the small intestine, the mucosal folds of the large intestine are crescent-shaped (Plicae semilunares).

Clinical Remarks

Malignant tumours of the colon (**colon carcinomas**) are among the most common malignancies in both, men and women, and therefore contribute substantially to the causes of death in the Western world. With preventive medical check-ups the number of deaths could be reduced. Coloscopy is recommended as diagnostic method of choice for the detection of colon carcinoma and the costs are covered by the public health system. Not only does coloscopy enable the inspection of the mucosa but it also allows taking biopsies for definite diagnostics by a pathologist. The importance of the radiological contrast imaging has declined. However, this conventional radiological method allows to obtain a reliable diagnosis based on characteristic alterations of the shape and position of the lumen in cases where endoscopy is not possible (e.g. obstructing tumours or diseases located beneath the mucosal lining).

6 Viscera of the Abdomen Development → Stomach → **Intestines** → Liver and gallbladder →

Projection of liver and gallbladder

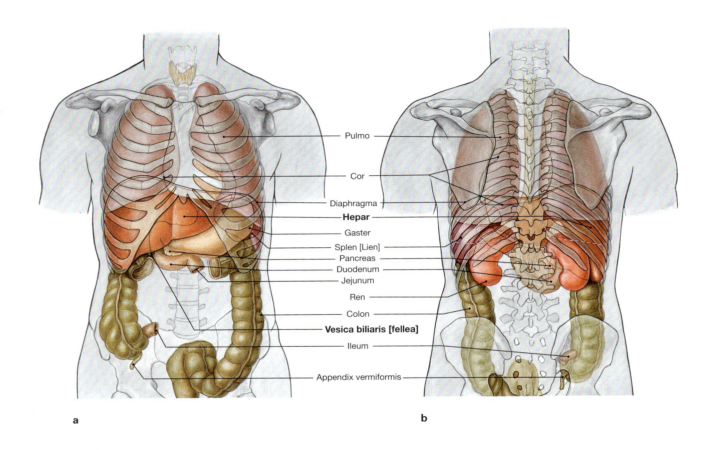

Figs. 6.55a and b Projection of the viscera onto the body surface; ventral (**a**) and dorsal (**b**) views.

The liver and gallbladder are located **intraperitoneally** in the right epigastrium. The fundus of the gallbladder projects onto the right midclavicular line at the level of rib IX. The left lobe of the liver is located in the left Epigastrium (up to the left midclavicular line) anterior to the stomach. The position of the liver varies with respiration (lower with inspiration, higher with expiration) because its Area nuda is attached to the diaphragm. Therefore, its position is also dependent on the size of the lung. Because of the dome-shaped diaphragm, the anterior and posterior side of the liver is covered in part by the pleural cavity (→ Fig. 6.124). Up to the midclavicular line, the inferior margin of the liver usually co-locates with the right inferior costal margin and, thus, the liver is not palpable. With an enlarged lung, such as with pulmonary emphysema in a smoker, the liver may be palpable without being enlarged. The topography of the liver is also important for diagnostic procedures such as liver biopsies (→ Fig. 6.75).

Clinical Remarks

A complete physical examination includes the palpation of the liver to determine its size. Changes in consistency and size may already suggest certain conditions such as a **fatty liver** (diabetes mellitus, alcohol abuse), **inflammation** (hepatitis) due to viral infections or alcoholism, or **liver cirrhosis** as the terminal stage of almost all liver pathologies. Palpation of the liver margin alone is not sufficient to determine the size of the liver, since the anatomy of the lung and the position of the diaphragm influence the position of the liver margins. Therefore the palpation of the inferior liver margin during inhalation is complemented by the percussion of the liver to determine the upper margin of the liver underneath the rib cage. The craniocaudal diameter of a normal liver should not exceed 12 cm in the midclavicular line.

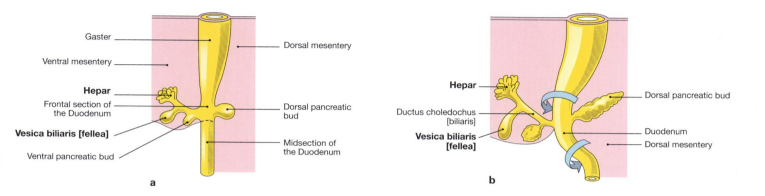

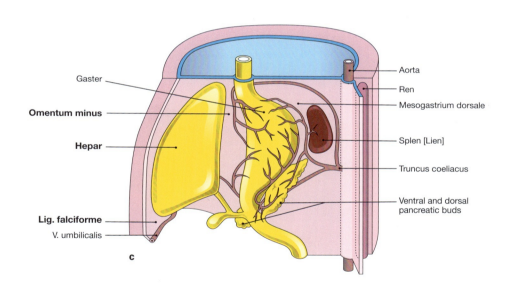

Figs. 6.56a to c Developmental stages of the liver, Hepar, and the gallbladder, Vesica biliaris, in weeks 4 to 5. [20]
The epithelial tissues of liver and gallbladder derive from the endoderm of the primordial gut at the level of the future Duodenum. In week 4 (from day 22 on) the endoderm forms a thickening (**hepatic diverticulum**) which divides into a superior liver primordium and an inferior primordium for the bile system (**a** and **b**). The epithelium of the liver primordium grows into the connective tissue of the Septum transversum in which islets of haematopoiesis develop. This way, the connective tissue components and the intrahepatic blood vessels (sinusoids) intermingle with the liver primordium. The liver then grows into the Mesogastrium ventrale (**c**) and, thus, splits it into a Mesohepaticum ventrale and a Mesohepaticum dorsale (→ Fig. 6.1). The Mesohepaticum ventrale develops into the **Lig. falciforme hepatis** and connects to the ventral body wall. The Mesohepaticum dorsale becomes the **Omentum minus** connecting the liver with the stomach and the Duodenum.

Viscera of the Abdomen Development → Stomach → Intestines → Liver and gallbladder →

Liver, overview

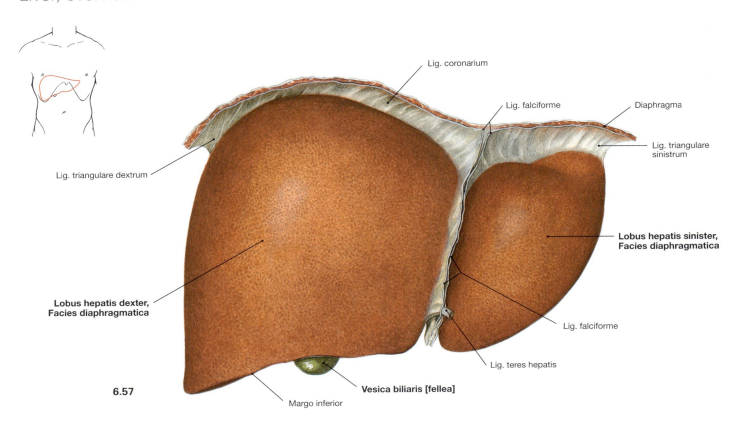

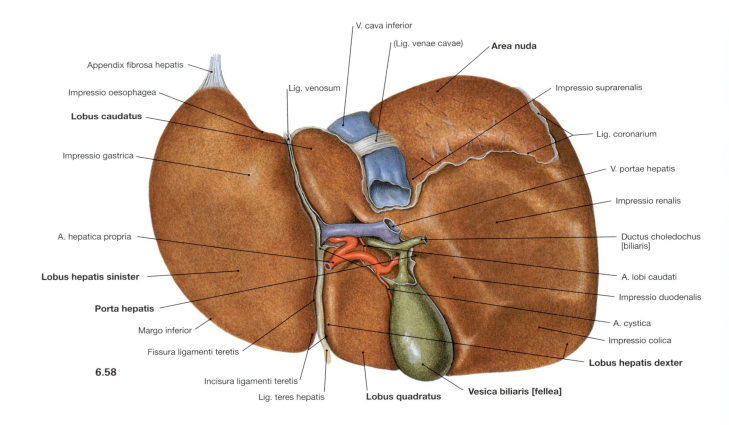

Fig. 6.57 and Fig. 6.58 Liver, Hepar; ventral (→ Fig. 6.57) and dorsal caudal (→ Fig. 6.58) views. For explanations → Figure 6.59.

Liver, overview

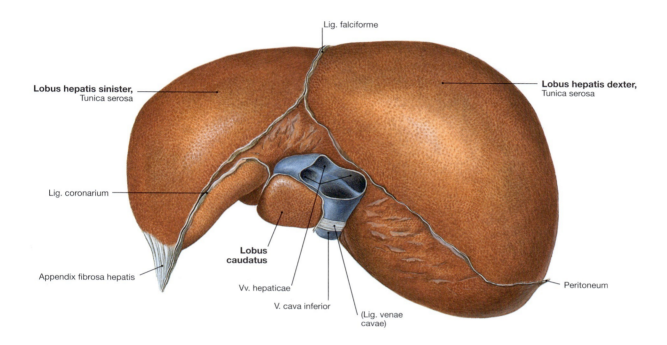

Fig. 6.59 Liver, Hepar; cranial view.
The liver is the largest gland (1200–1800 g) and the main metabolic organ of the body. The Facies diaphragmatica is adjacent to the diaphragm and the Facies visceralis with the anterior lower margin (Margo inferior) points towards the abdominal viscera (→ Figs. 6.57 and 6.58).
The **Facies diaphragmatica** is partly adherent to the diaphragm and lacks the peritoneal lining in this area **(Area nuda).** The liver is divided in a larger right and a smaller left lobe **(Lobus dexter** and **Lobus sinister)** which are separated ventrally by the Lig. falciforme. The latter continues as Lig. coronarium which then becomes the right and left Lig. triangulare connecting to the diaphragm. The Lig. triangulare sinistrum continues into the fibrous Appendix fibrosa hepatis. The free margin of the Lig. falciforme contains the Lig. teres hepatis (remnant of the prenatal V. umbilicalis). Both ligaments connect to the ventral abdominal wall.
At the **Facies visceralis** the Fissura ligamenti teretis hepatis continues to the Porta hepatis which harbours the vascular structures to and from the liver (V. portae hepatis, A. hepatica propria, Ductus hepaticus communis). Cranially, the Lig. venosum (remnant of the prenatal Ductus venosus) is shown. On the right side of the Porta hepatis (hilum of the liver), the V. cava inferior is located in a superior groove and the gallbladder **(Vesica biliaris)** is embedded in the inferior Fossa vesicae biliaris. The Lig. teres hepatis, Lig. venosum, V. cava inferior, and gallbladder delineate two rectangular areas on both sides of the Porta hepatis at the inferior side of the right hepatic lobe, the ventral **Lobus quadratus** and the dorsal **Lobus caudatus.** The liver is not covered by peritoneum in four larger areas: Area nuda, Porta hepatis, bed of the gallbladder, and groove of the V. cava inferior.
In vivo, the liver is deformable and adjusts to the shape of the surrounding organs. In fixed condition, adjacent organs cause impressions which are fixation artifacts without further relevance, although they provide positional information about the liver.

6 Viscera of the Abdomen Development → Stomach → Intestines → Liver and gallbladder →

Structure of the liver

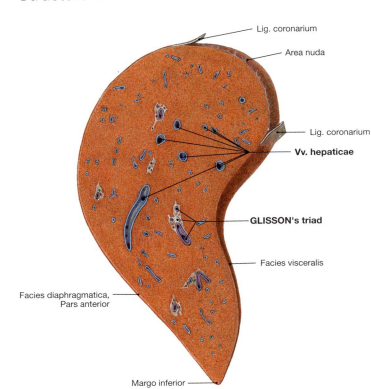

Fig. 6.60 Liver, Hepar; sagittal section through the right lobe of the liver.
The vascular and bile duct structures entering the liver at the hilum (V. portae hepatis, A. hepatica propria, Ductus hepaticus communis) are surrounded by connective tissue. They branch within the parenchyma of the liver, and create the GLISSON's triad (portal triad) in the portal tracts (portal canals) (→ Fig. 6.61).
The liver veins (Vv. hepaticae) and their tributaries which drain the blood from the liver into the V. cava inferior course separately from the vessels of the GLISSON's triad.

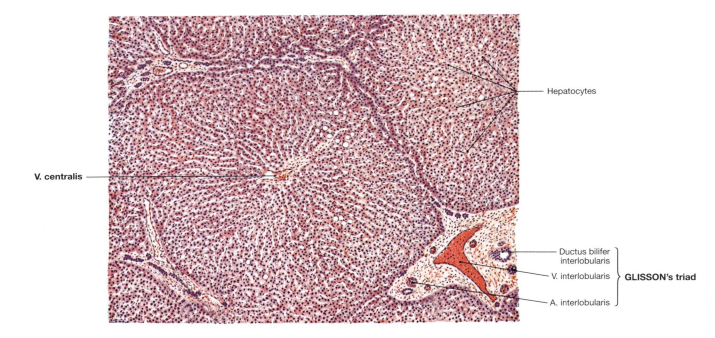

Fig. 6.61 Structure of the liver, Hepar; microscopic view. [24]
The structural unit of the liver parenchyma is the hepatic lobule which consists of radially oriented trabeculae of **hepatocytes**. The classical almost hexagonal **hepatic lobule** is surrounded by **portal tracts** at three to six corners. Three structures referred to collectively as **GLISSON's triad (portal triad)** are always found in the portal tract, embedded in connective tissue (A. and V. interlobularis, Ductus bilifer interlobularis). The centrilobular venule **(V. centralis)** is located in the centre of the hepatic lobule and collects the blood from the liver sinusoids which originally derives the arteries and veins at the periphery of the lobule. The centrilobular venule then drains into the Vv. sublobulares, which are branches of the Vv. hepaticae. The slow radial blood flow in the sinusoids enables hepatocytes to absorb nutrients and metabolites and to secrete synthesised proteins as for example plasma proteins.

Clinical Remarks

The blood flow in the hepatic lobules is extremely important for the liver function. In **liver cirrhosis,** the structure of the hepatic lobules is altered by nodular connective tissue remodelling of the parenchyma which compromises the blood flow. The high parenchymal resistance in the liver results in an increased blood pressure in the portal vein **(portal hypertension).** This condition may re-canalise or open **portocaval anastomoses** (→ Fig. 6.70).

Pancreas → Spleen → Topography → Sections

Segments of the liver

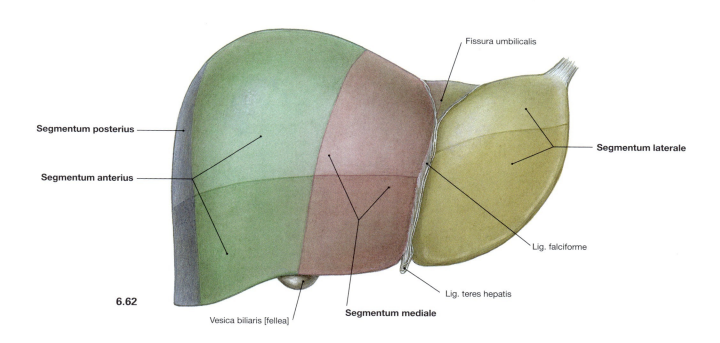

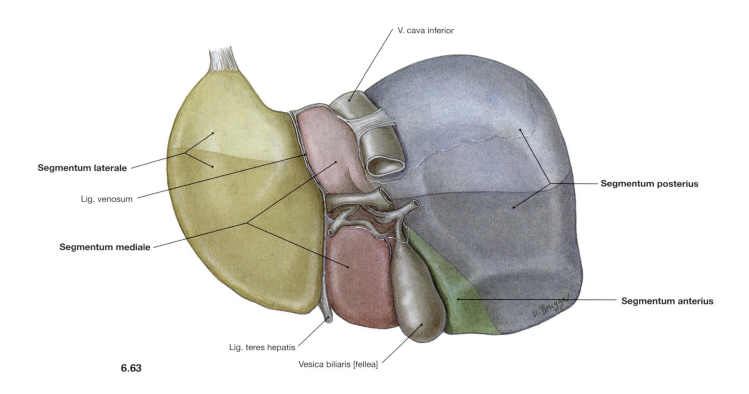

Fig. 6.62 and Fig. 6.63 Segments of the liver, Hepar; ventral (→ Fig. 6.62) and dorsal (→ Fig. 6.63) views. Individual liver segments are coloured differently.
The **three** almost vertically oriented **liver veins** (Vv. hepaticae, → Fig. 6.64) divide the liver into four adjacent segments. The **Segmentum laterale** corresponds to the anatomical left lobe of the liver and is bordered by the Lig. falciforme hepatis, which is adjacent to the left liver vein. The **Segmentum mediale** is located between the Lig. falciforme and the gallbladder at the level of the middle liver vein. To the right side, the **Segmentum anterius** and the **Segmentum posterius** follow and are separated by the right liver vein, which is not visible on the liver surface. The structures of the **portal triad** organise these liver segments into **eight functional** and clinically important **liver segments** (→ Fig. 6.64) which are indicated here by different colourations.

Viscera of the Abdomen Development → Stomach → Intestines → Liver and gallbladder →

Segments of the liver

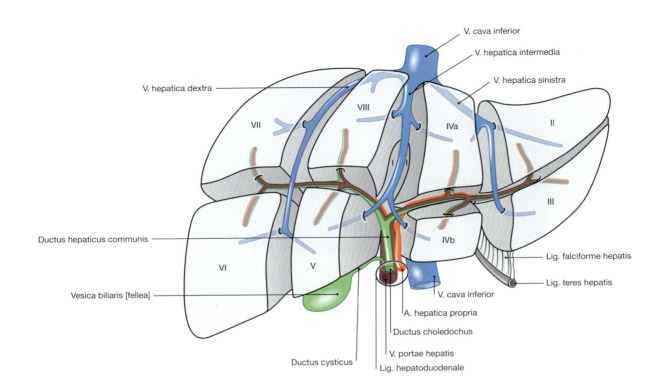

I	Lobus caudatus
II	Segmentum laterale superius
III	Segmentum laterale inferius
IVa	Segmentum mediale superius
IVb	Segmentum mediale inferius
V	Segmentum anterius inferius
VI	Segmentum posterius inferius
VII	Segmentum posterius superius
VIII	Segmentum anterius superius

Fig. 6.64 Schematic illustration of the liver segments and their relations to the intrahepatic blood vessels and the bile ducts; ventral view. (according to [1])
The liver is divided into **eight functional segments** which are supplied by one branch of the portal triad (V. portae hepatis, A. hepatica propria, Ductus hepaticus communis) each and therefore are functionally independent. Two segments each are combined by the vertically oriented three liver veins to four adjacent liver segments (→ Figs. 6.62 and 6.63).

It is of functional importance that **segments I to IV** are supplied by branches of the left portal triad and can be combined to a functional **left liver lobe. The segments V to VIII** are supplied by branches of the right portal triad and represent the **functional right liver lobe.** As a result, the border between the functional right and left liver lobes is located in the sagittal plane between the V. cava inferior and gallbladder and not at the level of the Lig. falciforme hepatis.

Clinical Remarks

In **visceral surgery,** the liver segments are clinically of great relevance. The existence of liver segments allows the resection of individual segments and their supplying vessels without extensive blood loss. Localised liver pathologies, such as solitary liver metastases, can be treated by the surgical resection of individual segments in different parts of the liver without compromising the liver function as a whole. The ligation of the individual branches of the supplying vessels and the subsequent discolouration of the respective segment due to lack of perfusion enables the surgeon to identify each segment.

Pancreas → Spleen → Topography → Sections

Segments of the liver

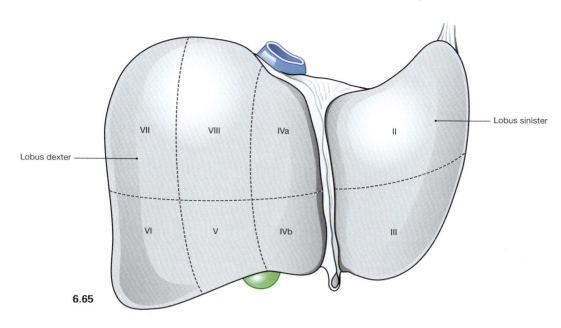

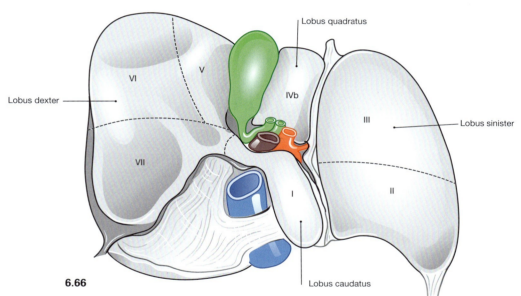

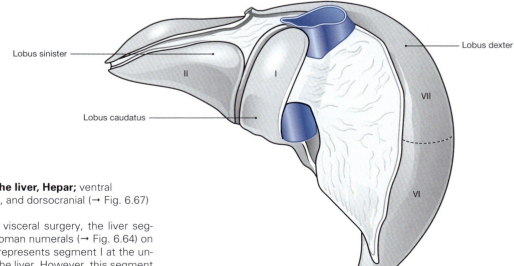

Fig. 6.65 to Fig. 6.67 Segments of the liver, Hepar; ventral (→ Fig. 6.65), dorsocaudal (→ Fig. 6.66), and dorsocranial (→ Fig. 6.67) view. (according to [1])
Because of their clinical relevance for visceral surgery, the liver segments are marked in this figure with Roman numerals (→ Fig. 6.64) on the liver surface. The Lobus caudatus represents segment I at the underside of the anatomical right lobe of the liver. However, this segment functionally belongs to the left lobe of the liver.

6 Viscera of the Abdomen Development → Stomach → Intestines → Liver and gallbladder →

Arteries of the liver and gallbladder

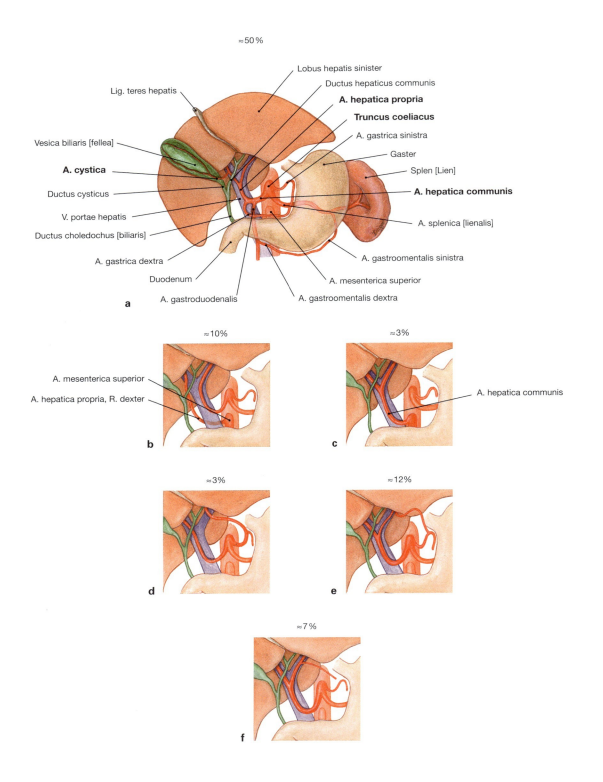

Figs. 6.68a to f Arteries of the liver, Hepar, and the gallbladder, Vesica biliaris.
The liver is supplied by the **A. hepatica propria** derived from the A. hepatica communis, a direct arterial branch of the Truncus coeliacus. After giving off the A. gastrica dextra, the A. hepatica propria courses within the Lig. hepatoduodenale together with the V. portae hepatis and the common bile duct (Ductus choledochus) to the hilum of the liver. Here, this artery divides into the R. dexter and the R. sinister to the liver lobes. The R. dexter gives rise to the **A. cystica** to the gallbladder. In 10–20% of all cases, the A. mesenterica superior contributes to the blood supply of the right liver lobe, and the A. gastrica sinistra contributes to the supply of the left liver lobe.

Variations of the blood supply of the liver:
a textbook case
b contribution of the A. mesenterica superior to the blood supply of the right liver lobe
c origin of the A. hepatica communis by the A. mesenterica superior
d blood supply of the left liver lobe by the A. gastrica sinistra
e contribution of a branch of the A. gastrica sinistra to the blood supply of the left liver lobe in addition to the R. sinister of the A. hepatica propria
f blood supply of the lesser curvature of the stomach by an accessory branch of the A. hepatica propria

Veins of the liver and gallbladder

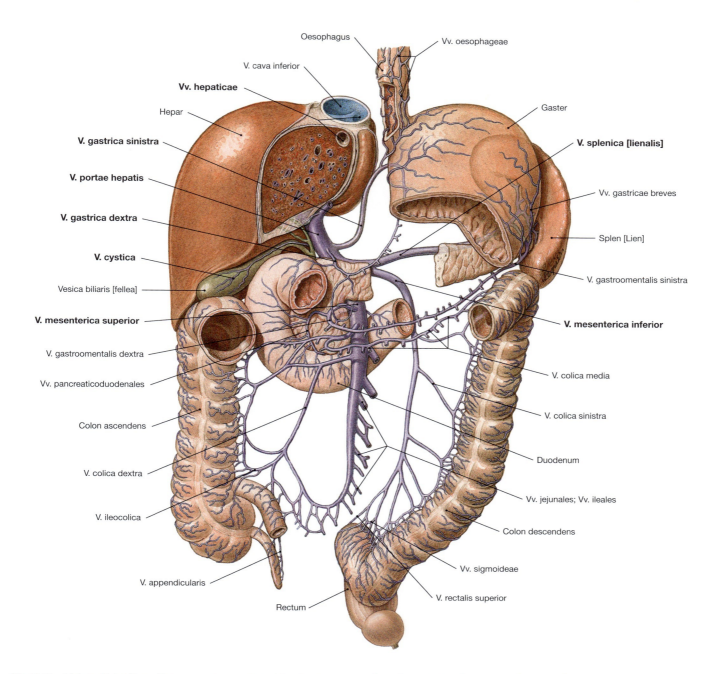

Fig. 6.69 Veins of the liver, Hepar, and the gallbladder, Vesica biliaris; ventral view.
The liver has an incoming and an outgoing venous system. The **portal vein** (V. portae hepatis) collects the nutrient-rich blood from the unpaired abdominal organs (stomach, intestines, Pancreas, spleen) and feeds this blood, together with the arterial blood from the A. hepatica communis, into the sinusoids of the liver lobules. Three **liver veins** (Vv. hepaticae, → Fig. 6.60) transport the blood from the liver to the V. cava inferior.
The portal vein has three main tributaries: Behind the head of the Pancreas, the V. mesenterica superior merges with the V. splenica to form the V. portae hepatis. In most cases (70 %), the V. mesenterica inferior drains into the V. splenica; in the remaining cases (30%) it drains into the V. mesenterica superior.

Branches of the V. splenica (collecting blood from the spleen and from parts of the stomach and Pancreas):
- Vv. gastricae breves
- V. gastroomentalis sinistra
- Vv. pancreaticae (from the pancreatic tail and body)

Branches of the V. mesenterica superior (collecting blood from parts of the stomach and Pancreas, from the entire small intestine, the Colon ascendens, and Colon transversum):
- V. gastroomentalis dextra with Vv. pancreaticoduodenales
- Vv. pancreaticae (from the pancreatic head and body)
- Vv. jejunales and ileales
- V. ileocolica
- V. colica dextra
- V. colica media

Branches of the V. mesenterica inferior (collecting blood from the Colon descendens, and the upper Rectum):
- V. colica sinistra
- Vv. sigmoideae
- V. rectalis superior: the vein anastomoses with the V. rectalis media and the V. rectalis inferior, which drain into the V. cava inferior.

In addition, there are veins which drain **directly into the portal vein** once the main venous branches have merged:
- V. cystica (from the gallbladder)
- Vv. paraumbilicales (via veins in the Lig. teres hepatis from the abdominal wall around the Umbilicus)
- Vv. gastricae dextra and sinistra (from the lesser curvature of the stomach)

Viscera of the Abdomen
Development → Stomach → Intestines → Liver and gallbladder →

Portocaval anastomoses

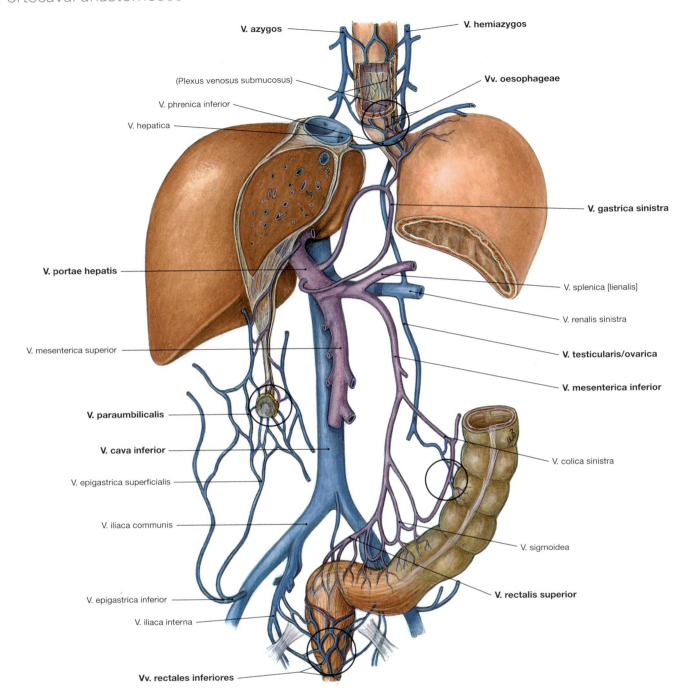

Fig. 6.70 Portocaval anastomoses (connections between the portal vein and the V. cava superior/inferior). Tributaries to the V. cava superior/inferior (blue), tributaries to the V. portae hepatis (purple).
There are four possible collateral circulations via portocaval anastomoses (marked by black circles):
- Vv. gastricae dextrae and sinistrae via oesophageal veins and veins of the azygos system to the V. cava superior. This may result in the dilation of submucosal veins of the Oesophagus (**oesophageal varices**).
- Vv. paraumbilicales via veins of the ventral abdominal wall (deep: Vv. epigastricae superior and inferior; superficial: V. thoracoepigastrica and V. epigastrica superficialis) to the V. cava superior and inferior. Dilation of the superficial veins may appear as **Caput medusae**.
- V. rectalis superior via veins of the distal rectum and anal canal and via the V. iliaca interna to the V. cava inferior
- retroperitoneal anastomoses via the V. mesenterica inferior to the V. testicularis/ovarica with connection to the V. cava inferior

Clinical Remarks

Increased blood pressure in the portal system (**portal hypertension;** e.g. in liver cirrhosis) may cause the dilation or the opening of the above mentioned venous connections to the systemic venous system (**portocaval anastomoses**). Clinically important are the connections to the **oesophageal veins** because rupture of oesophageal varices may result in **life-threatening haemorrhage,** the most common cause of death in patients with liver cirrhosis. The connections to superficial veins of the ventral abdominal wall are only of diagnostic value. Although the **Caput medusae** is rare, the appearance is so characteristic that a liver cirrhosis cannot be overlooked. The anastomoses to the retroperitoneal veins and to the veins of the inferior rectum and anal canal are clinically not important.

Lymph vessels of the liver and gallbladder

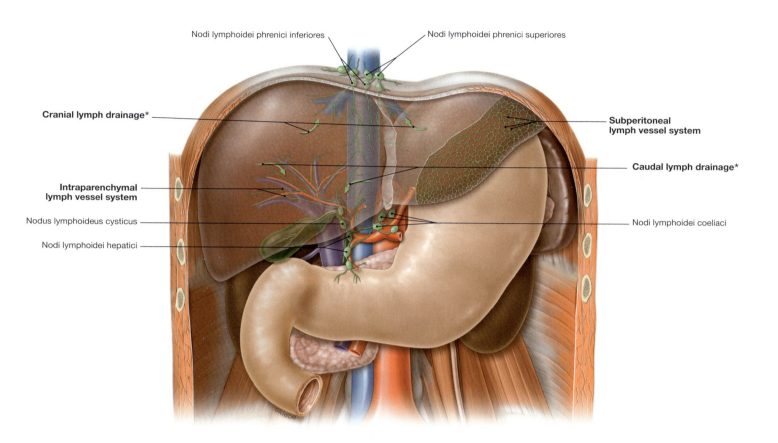

Fig. 6.71 Lymph vessels and lymph nodes of the liver and bile duct system.
The **liver** has **two lymph vessel systems**:
- the subperitoneal system at the surface of the liver
- the intraparenchymal system alongside the structures in the portal triad to the hilum of the liver

With respect to the regional lymph nodes, there are **two major lymph drainage routes**:
- in **caudal direction to the hilum of the liver** (most important) via the Nodi lymphoidei hepatici at the hilum of the liver (→ Fig. 6.17) and from there via the Nodi lymphoidei coeliaci to the Truncus intestinalis
- in **cranial direction passing the diaphragm** via the Nodi lymphoidei phrenici inferiores and superiores into the Nodi lymphoidei mediastinales anteriores and posteriores which drain into the Trunci bronchomediastinales; using this drainage pathway, carcinomas of the liver may also metastasise into thoracic lymph nodes.

There are **two minor lymph drainage route**:
- to the anterior abdominal wall via the lymph vessels in the Lig. teres hepatis to the inguinal and axillary lymph nodes
- to the stomach and Pancreas from the left lobe of the liver

The **gallbladder** usually has its own Nodus lymphoideus cysticus in the area of the neck, which drains into the lymph nodes at the hilum of the liver (in the caudal direction).

* The arrows depict the direction of lymph drainage from the parenchyma via the cranial or caudal route.

6 Viscera of the Abdomen Development → Stomach → Intestines → Liver and gallbladder →

Liver, imaging

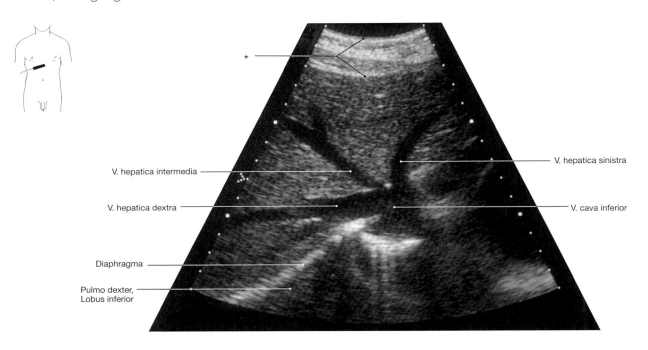

Fig. 6.72 Confluence of the liver veins, Vv. hepaticae, with the V. cava inferior; ultrasound image; caudal view.

* abdominal wall

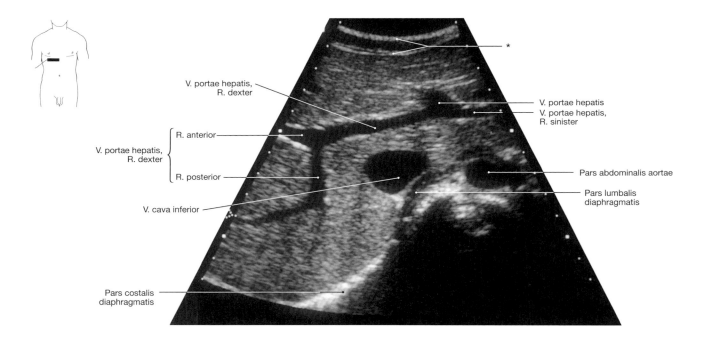

Fig. 6.73 Liver, Hepar, V. portae hepatis; demonstration of the branching of the portal vein; ultrasound image; caudal view.

* abdominal wall

Clinical Remarks

Ultrasonic examination (sonography) of the liver is a standard diagnostic tool used by specialists in internal medicine and by radiologists. Sonography enables a noninvasive investigation of the liver parenchyma and allows the detection of structural changes, for example by the local or general increased echogenicity in cases of a fatty liver degeneration in hepatitis or liver cirrhosis. Focal tumours or cysts are also detectable. Subsequently, liver biopsies (→ Fig. 6.75) or a laparoscopic investigation of the liver (→ Fig. 6.76) may be performed to reach a diagnosis.

Pancreas → Spleen → Topography → Sections

Liver biopsy

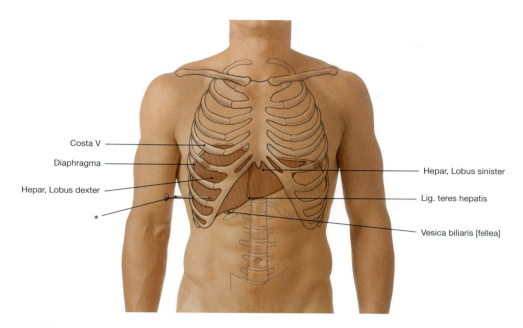

Fig. 6.74 Projection of the liver, Hepar, and the gallbladder, Vesica biliaris, onto the ventral abdominal wall in mid-respiration position.

* position of the needle during liver puncture

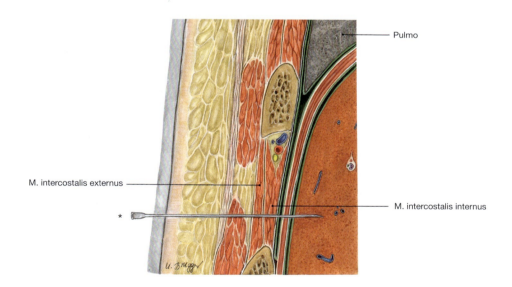

Fig. 6.75 Layers of the chest wall and the liver, Hepar; frontal section; liver puncture biopsy.
The ultrasound-guided puncture is performed in expiration through one of the lower intercostal spaces. Since the liver is partly covered by the pleural cavity this access reduces the risk of a pneumothorax. To spare the intercostal neurovascular structures, the puncture is always performed at the superior costal margin. The peritoneal lining covering the liver capsule receives sensory innervation by the N. phrenicus (C3–C5) from the Plexus cervicalis. This explains why patients often experience **referred pain** in the area of the right shoulder.

* position of the needle during liver puncture

Clinical Remarks

A liver puncture biopsy is performed to determine the nature of suspicious **tumours,** or the stage of a **hepatitis** or **liver cirrhosis,** respectively. Only the biopsy enables the definitive diagnosis by a pathologist.

6 Viscera of the Abdomen Development → Stomach → Intestines → Liver and gallbladder →

Liver and gallbladder, imaging

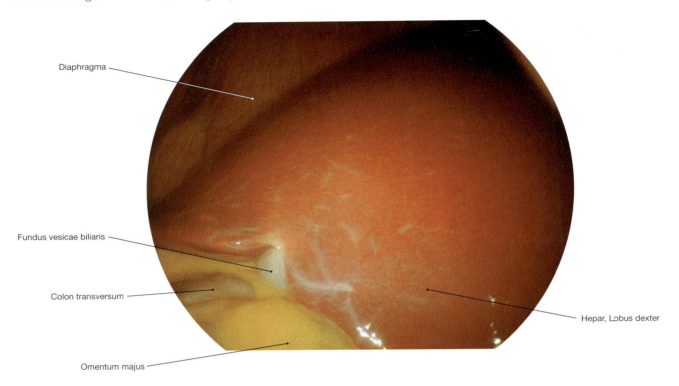

Fig. 6.76 Liver, Hepar, and gallbladder, Vesica biliaris; laparoscopic image; oblique caudal view from the left side.

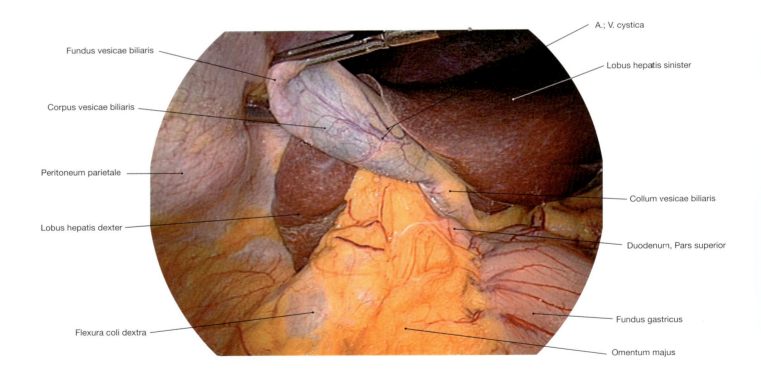

Fig. 6.77 Liver, Hepar, and gallbladder, Vesica biliaris; laparoscopic image; ventral view.

Clinical Remarks

Laparoscopy is the final opportunity to inspect the liver or to take biopsy material prior to the surgical opening of the abdominal wall. Using a laparoscope and one or two additional entrance ports for light sources, camera, or biopsy instruments, the entire abdominal cavity can be inspected and biopsies can be taken under visual control.

Pancreas → Spleen → Topography → Sections

Structure of the gallbladder and extrahepatic bile ducts

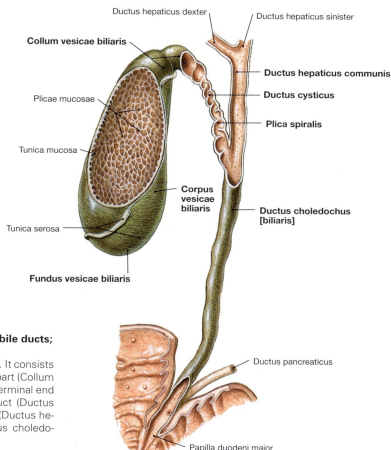

Fig. 6.78 Gallbladder, Vesica biliaris, and extrahepatic bile ducts; ventral view.
The gallbladder usually holds approximately 40–70 ml of bile. It consists of a body (Corpus vesicae biliaris) with a fundus and a neck part (Collum vesicae biliaris). A spiral fold (Plica spiralis HEISTER) at the terminal end of the neck closes the opening of the excretory cystic duct (Ductus cysticus), which then fuses with the common hepatic duct (Ductus hepaticus communis) to form the common bile duct (Ductus choledochus).

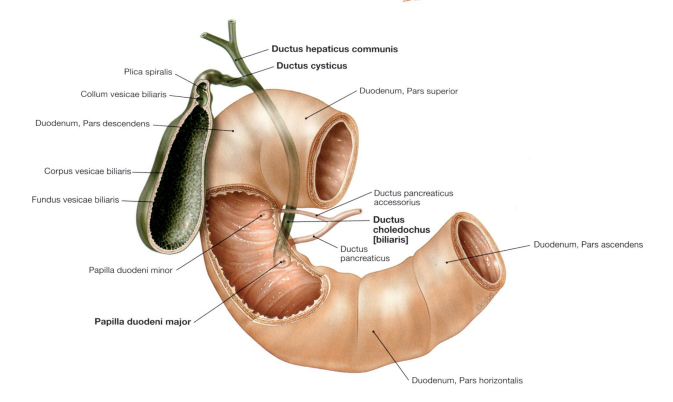

Fig. 6.79 Gallbladder, Vesica biliaris, extrahepatic bile ducts and duodenum, Duodenum; ventral view.
The common bile duct (Ductus choledochus) is usually 6 cm long and 0.4–0.9 cm in diameter. It courses within the Lig. hepatoduodenale ventral to the portal vein, then runs behind the Pars superior of the Duodenum to traverse the head of the Pancreas and reach the descending part of the Duodenum. In 60% of all cases, the common bile duct fuses with the Ductus pancreaticus to form the Ampulla hepatopancreatica, which enters the Duodenum at the Papilla duodeni major (Papilla VATERI). At its distal end, smooth muscles of the common bile duct (Ductus choledochus) create the M. sphincter ductus choledochi. The inferior part thereof, also referred to as M. sphincter ampullae (ODDI), encompasses the ampulla and the entrance of the Duodenum.

Viscera of the Abdomen
Development → Stomach → Intestines → Liver and gallbladder →

CALOT's triangle

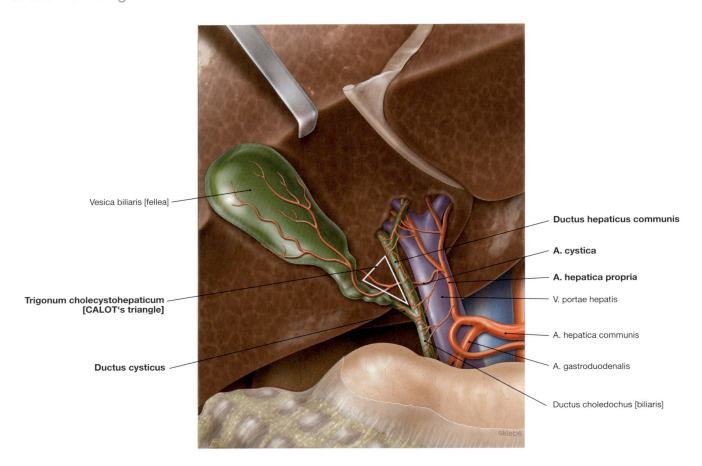

Fig. 6.80 CALOT's triangle, Trigonum cholecystohepaticum; caudal view. (according to [1])
The Ductus cysticus, the Ductus hepaticus communis and the inferior area of the liver together form the Trigonum cholecystohepaticum, also referred to as CALOT's triangle. In 75% of all cases, the A. cystica originates in this triangle from the R. dexter of the A. hepatica propria and courses posteriorly through this triangle to reach the Ductus cysticus and the neck of the gallbladder.

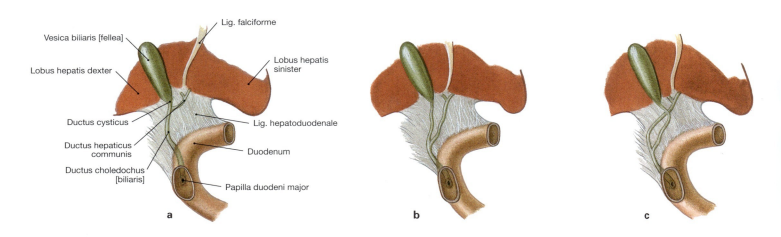

Figs. 6.81a to c Variations of the bile ducts regarding the confluence of the Ductus hepaticus communis and Ductus cysticus.
- **a** high junction
- **b** low junction
- **c** low junction with crossing

Clinical Remarks

The CALOT's triangle is an important landmark during the **surgical removal of the gallbladder.** Prior to removal of the gallbladder, all structures are identified before the A. cystica and the Ductus cysticus are ligated. This way, the risk of an accidental ligation of an the Ductus choledochus with subsequent stasis of the bile (cholestasis) is reduced.

Pancreas → Spleen → Topography → Sections

Gallbladder and extrahepatic bile ducts, imaging

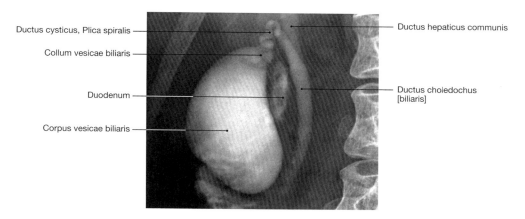

Fig. 6.82 **Gallbladder, Vesica biliaris, extrahepatic bile ducts;** radiograph in anteroposterior (AP) beam projection after application of contrast medium; patient in upright position; ventral view.

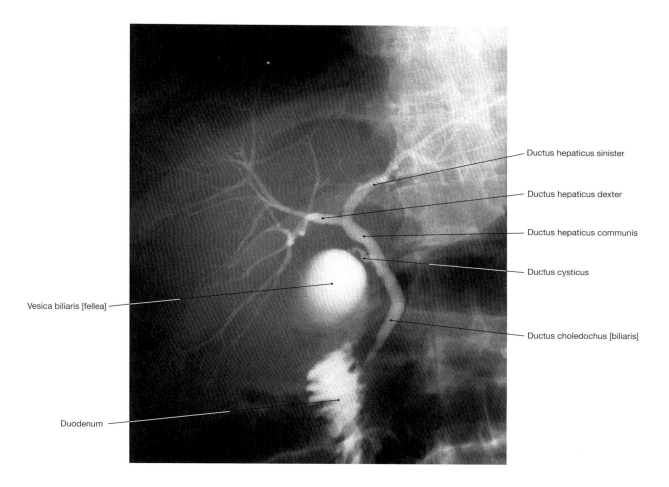

Fig. 6.83 **Gallbladder, Vesica biliaris, as well as intra- and extrahepatic bile ducts;** radiograph in anteroposterior (AP) beam projection after application of contrast medium; patient in upright position; ventral view.

Clinical Remarks

Radiography after intravenous application of contrast medium allows the visualisation of the gallbladder and bile ducts, including the detection of noncalcified bile concrements. Malignant tumours of the bile ducts (cholangiocarcinomas) or of the Pancreas (pancreatic carcinomas) may cause cholestasis which appears as dilation of the bile ducts.

6 Viscera of the Abdomen Development → Stomach → Intestines → Liver and gallbladder →

Projection of the pancreas

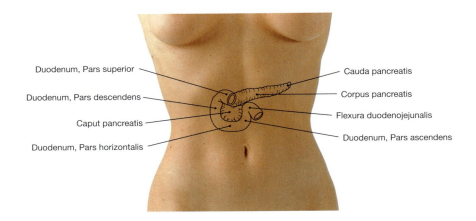

Fig. 6.84 Projection of the pancreas, Pancreas, and the duodenum, Duodenum, on the ventral abdominal wall.
The Pancreas is in a **secondary retroperitoneal** position and projects roughly onto the 1st or 2nd lumbar vertebra. The head (Caput pancreatis) is adjacent to the Pars descendens of the Duodenum and continues as pancreatic body (Corpus pancreatis) which crosses the vertebral column to continue as pancreatic tail (Cauda panceatis) to the hilum of the spleen.

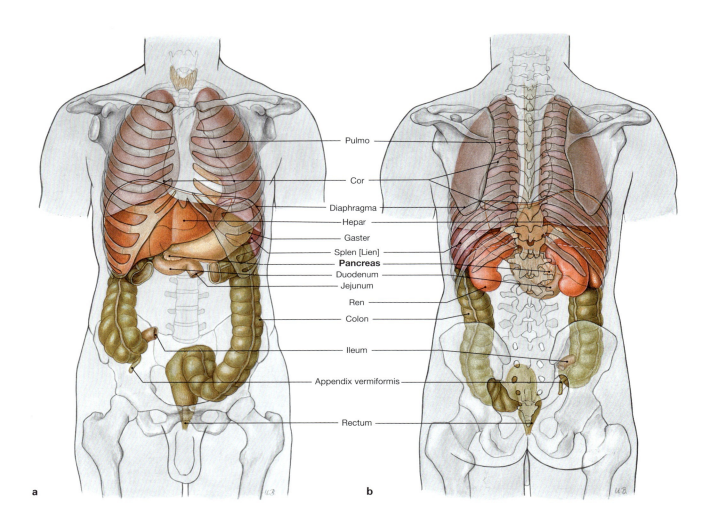

Figs. 6.85a and b Projection of the viscera onto the body surface; ventral (**a**) and dorsal (**b**) views.

Clinical Remarks

The **inflammation of the Pancreas** (pancreatitis) is most commonly caused by an obstruction of the duodenal papilla by a gallstone with resulting stasis of bile or by chronic alcohol abuse. It frequently causes a belt-like radiating abdominal pain.

Development of the pancreas

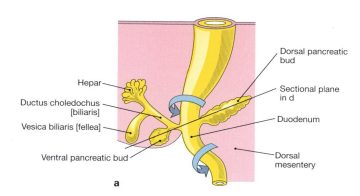

Figs. 6.86a to f Development of the pancreas, Pancreas, in weeks 5 to 8. [20]

a to **c** ventral view
d to **f** schematic cross-sections through to Duodenum and Pancreas primordium; rotations marked by arrows

On day 28, a ventral and a dorsal pancreatic bud emerge from the endoderm of the primordial gut (**a, d**) inferior to the primordium of liver and gallbladder at the level of the future Duodenum. The ventral pancreatic bud moves dorsally (**b,e**) and, in weeks 6 to 7, fuses with the dorsal pancreatic bud, including their respective excretory ducts (**d, f**). The excretory pancreatic duct is formed by the union of the distal dorsal pancreatic duct and the ventral pancreatic duct and enters the Papilla duodeni major. The proximal portion of the dorsal pancreatic duct develops (65% of all cases) into the accessory pancreatic duct which joins the Duodenum at the Papilla duodeni minor.

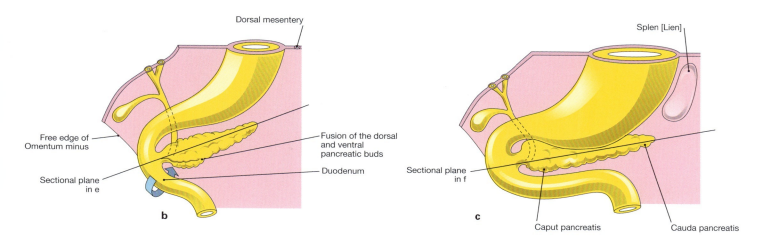

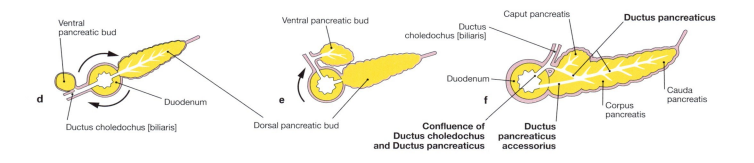

Clinical Remarks

If the fusion of both pancreatic buds is incomplete (**Pancreas divisum**) the dorsal pancreatic duct may constitute the main excretory duct (10% of all cases) which may cause repetitive pancreatitis due to a stasis of secretions. If the pancreatic parenchyma grows as a circular gland around the Duodenum (**annular pancreas**), ileus with vomiting may occur which is particularly evident in newborns. In these cases, the Duodenum is mobilised, cut, and positioned next to the Pancreas or surgically bypassed.

6 Viscera of the Abdomen Development → Stomach → Intestines → Liver and Gallbladder →

Structure and topographical relationships of the pancreas

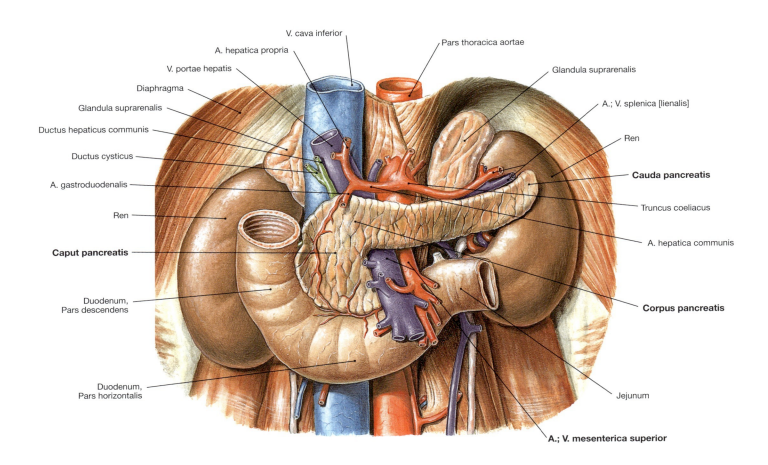

Fig. 6.87 Retroperitoneal organs of the epigastrium: pancreas, Pancreas, duodenum, Duodenum, and on both sides kidney, Ren, and adrenal gland, Glandula suprarenalis; ventral view.
The Pancreas is in a **secondary retroperitoneal** position. The head (Caput pancreatis) is adjacent to the Pars descendens of the Duodenum and has a dorsal uncinate process (Proc. uncinatus) which embraces the A. and V. mesenterica superior. Caudally, the Pars horizontalis of the Duodenum is adjacent.
To the left side, the pancreatic head continues as the pancreatic body (Corpus pancreatis) which traverses the vertebral column. The subsequent pancreatic tail (Cauda pancreatis) passes over the left kidney to reach the hilum of the spleen.

The Pancreas has an anterior and a posterior surface (Facies anterior and Facies posterior) which are separated by the dull upper and lower border (Margo superior and Margo inferior). The anterior aspect of the Pancreas is covered by parietal peritoneum and forms the posterior wall of the Bursa omentalis. The posterior aspect of the Pancreas is fused to the original parietal peritoneum of the posterior abdominal wall because the Pancreas was repositioned into the retroperitoneal space during its development. The fused area appears as a fascia during dissection.

Clinical Remarks

The close topographical relationship of the pancreatic head with the A. and V. mesenterica superior and the portal vein imposes the risk of injury to these vessels during **endoscopic manipulation of the Papilla duodeni major.** Damage to these structures may occur during endoscopic procedures when removing a bile concrement or during application of contrast medium for an endoscopic retrograde cholangiopancreatography (ERCP) to visualise the bile and pancreatic ducts. In case of injury emergency surgical treatment is required.

Pancreas → Spleen → Topography → Sections

Structure of the pancreas

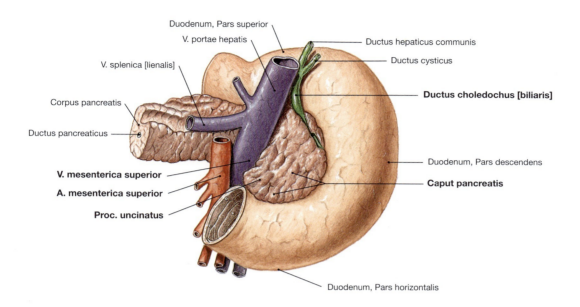

Fig. 6.88 Pancreas, Pancreas, and duodenum, Duodenum; dorsal view.
The figure illustrates the pancreatic head (Caput pancreatis) located in the C-shaped Pars descendens of the duodenum where it is obliquely pierced by the common bile duct (Ductus choledochus) in its course to the Papilla duodeni major. Dorsally, the uncinate process (Proc. uncinatus) of the pancreatic head embraces the A. and V. mesenterica superior.

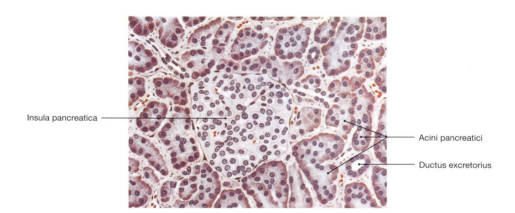

Fig. 6.89 Structure of the pancreas, Pancreas; microscopic view. [26]
The pancreas is a mixed exocrine and endocrine gland. In the acini, the **exocrine** part produces digestive enzymes which are delivered as inactive precursors via the duct system to reach the lumen of the intestine.

The **endocrine** part consists of the islets of LANGERHANS (Insulae pancreaticae) and is embedded within the parenchyma of the exocrine gland, particularly in the pancreatic tail. Besides other hormones, the islets produce insulin and glucagon which are secreted into the blood and serve the regulation of the blood glucose level.

Clinical Remarks

The function of the Pancreas explains why tissue damage (necrosis) in the pancreatic parenchyma has exocrine and endocrine consequences; inflammatory diseases **(pancreatitis)** for example, will result in **digestive problems** and fatty stools and may in cases of severe tissue loss (80–90%) also cause **diabetes mellitus** due to the insufficient insulin production.

Viscera of the Abdomen   Development → Stomach → Intestines → Liver and gallbladder →

Excretory ducts of the pancreas

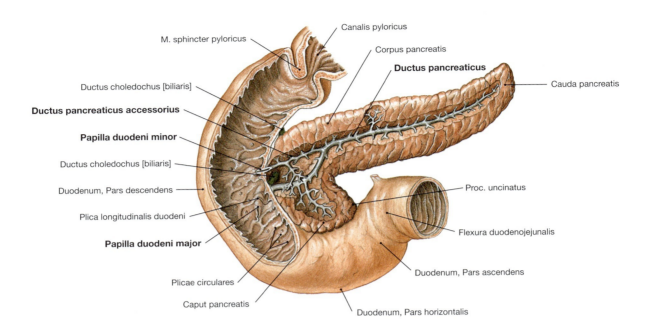

Fig. 6.90 Excretory duct system of the pancreas, Pancreas; ventral view; Ductus pancreaticus after partial resection of the Duodenum and the ventral Pancreas.

The main excretory duct (Ductus pancreaticus [duct of WIRSUNG]) fuses with the terminal segment of the common bile duct (Ductus choledochus) in 60% of all cases to form the Ampulla hepatopancreatica.

The latter enters the Pars descendens of the Duodenum at the Papilla duodeni major (papilla of VATER). Developmentally (→ Fig. 6.86), an accessory duct (Ductus pancreaticus accessorius [SANTORINI's duct]) exists in 65% of all cases which opens into the Duodenum 2 cm proximal to the Papilla duodeni minor.

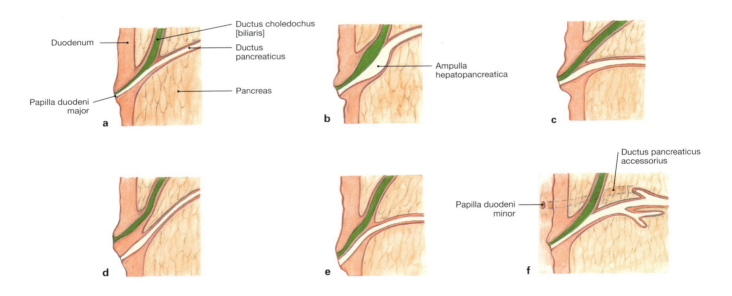

Figs. 6.91a to f Variations of the junction of the Ductus pancreaticus and Ductus choledochus.
a long common portion
b ampullary dilation of the terminal part (60% of all cases)
c short common portion
d separate entrance
e common entrance with septated common duct
f accessory duct (Ductus pancreaticus accessorius, 65% of all cases)

Clinical Remarks

The variations in the confluence of the excretory pancreatic ducts and the bile ducts influence the **course of pancreatic diseases.** Besides alcohol abuse, an obstructive bile concrement in the Papilla duodeni major is the most common cause for inflammatory conditions of the Pancreas (pancreatitis). The main risk here is the autodigestion of the gland by prematurely activated enzymes of the exocrine Pancreas. In the cases of obstruction of the papilla of VATER, a separate Ductus pancreaticus accessorius may allow sufficient secretion and, thus, prevent a pancreatitis.

Arteries of the pancreas

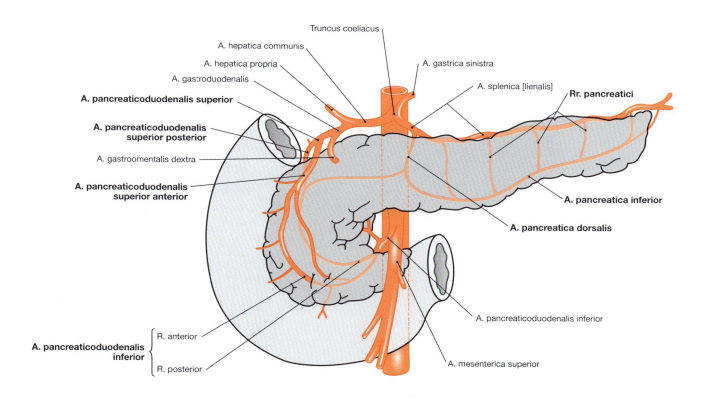

Fig. 6.92 Arteries of the pancreas, Pancreas; schematic illustration. (according to [1])
The Pancreas is supplied by **two separate arterial systems** for the pancreatic head, and the pancreatic body and tail, respectively.
- **head:** double arterial arches from the Aa. pancreaticoduodenales superiores anterior and posterior (from the A. gastroduodenalis) and from the A. pancreaticoduodenalis inferior with a R. anterior and a R. posterior (from the A. mesenterica superior).
- **body and tail:** Rr. pancreatici from the A. splenica which give rise to an A. pancreatica dorsalis behind the Pancreas and an A. pancreatica inferior at the inferior border of the gland.

This extensive perfusion of the gland may explain why infarction of the Pancreas is rare.
The **veins** of the Pancreas correspond to the arteries and drain via the V. mesenterica superior and the V. splenica into the portal vein (→ Fig. 6.69).

Lymph vessels of the pancreas

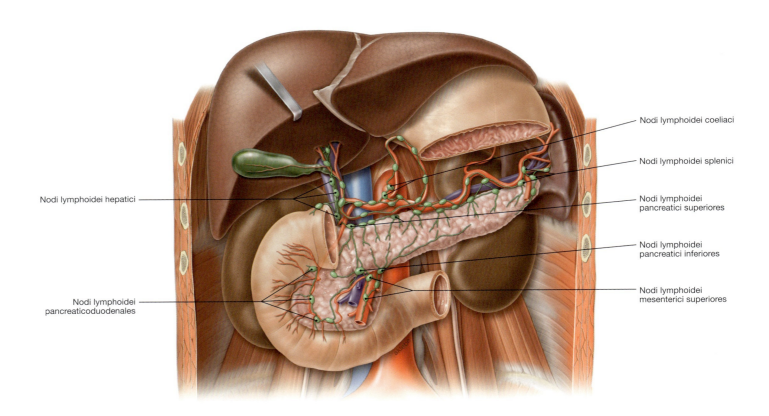

Fig. 6.93 Lymphatic drainage pathways of the pancreas, Pancreas; ventral view.
The distinct parts of the pancreas have separate regional lymph nodes.
- **head:** Nodi lymphoidei pancreaticoduodenales anteriores and posteriores along the identically named arteries (Aa. pancreaticoduodenales superiores anterior and posterior), then via Nodi lymphoidei hepatici to the Nodi lymphoidei coeliaci or directly to the Nodi lymphoidei mesenterici superiores and finally to the Truncus intestinalis
- **body:** Nodi lymphoidei pancreatici superiores and inferiores along the A. and V. splenica; from there to the Nodi lymphoidei coeliaci and to the Nodi lymphoidei mesenterici superiores. There are also connections to the retroperitoneal Nodi lymphoidei lumbales.
- **tail segment:** Nodi lymphoidei splenici

Clinical Remarks

The diverse lymphatic drainage pathways explain why in cases of **pancreatic carcinoma** usually extensive **lymph node metastases** exist at the time of diagnosis. Since these metastases cannot be completely removed, curative surgery is not possible.

Pancreas → Spleen → Topography → Sections

Pancreas, imaging

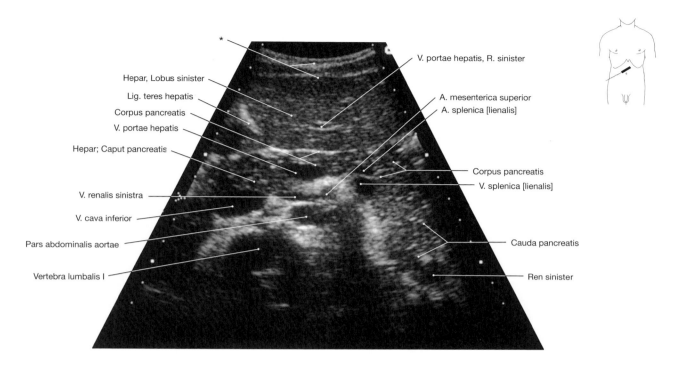

Fig. 6.94 Pancreas, Pancreas; ultrasound image; oblique caudal view in deep inspiration.

The ultrasonic examination of the Pancreas frequently is unsatisfactory as the retroperitoneal Pancreas is usually obscured by air-filled bowels

* abdominal wall

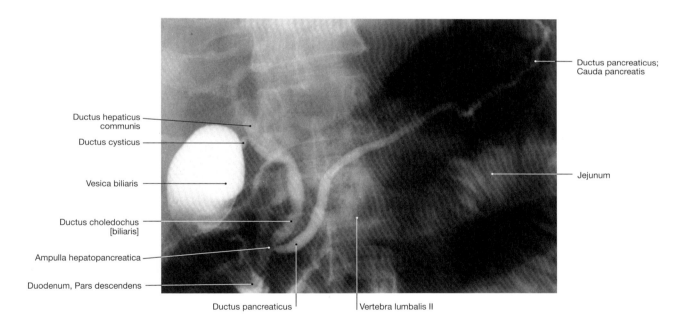

Fig. 6.95 Pancreas, Pancreas, and bile ducts; endoscopic retrograde cholangiopancreatography (ERCP); ventral view. To visualise the duct systems in the radiograph, the excretory duct of the Pancreas and the Ductus choledochus were filled with contrast medium from the Papilla duodeni major via an endoscope.

Clinical Remarks

For the **imaging of the Pancreas** ultrasound is performed initially to detect a potential swelling of the organ as an indication for pancreatitis. In cases of a non-conclusive ultrasound image, computer tomography is performed. With ERCP the diagnosis of a Pancreas divisum as potential reason for recurrent pancreatitis is possible. Contrast filling defects of the pancreatic duct may indicate a pancreatic carcinoma.

6 Viscera of the Abdomen   Development → Stomach → Intestines → Liver and gallbladder →

Projection of the spleen

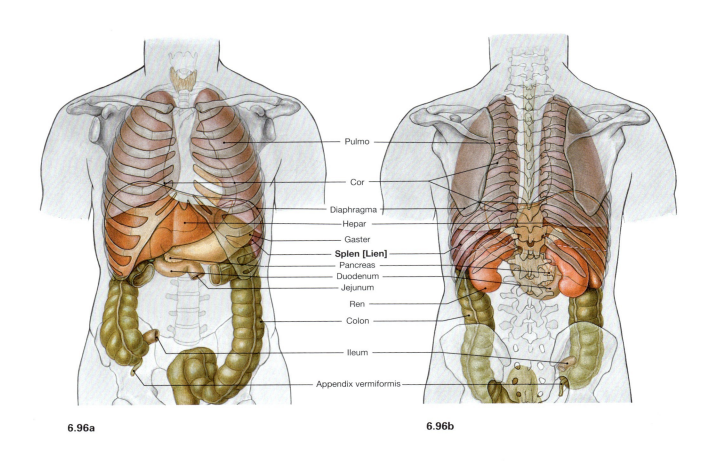

6.96a   6.96b

Fig. 6.96 and Fig. 6.97 Projection of the viscera onto the body surface; ventral (→ Fig. 6.96a) and dorsal (→ Fig. 6.96b) views, and view from the left side (→ Fig. 6.97).

The spleen is located **intraperitoneally** in the left epigastrium. Its longitudinal axis projects onto rib X. A normal-sized spleen is not palpable beyond the costal margin. Due to its large contact area with the diaphragm, the position of the spleen is dependent on respiration. The spleen lies in the so-called splenic niche which is confined inferiorly by the Lig. phrenicocolicum between the left colic flexure and diaphragm (→ Fig. 6.102).

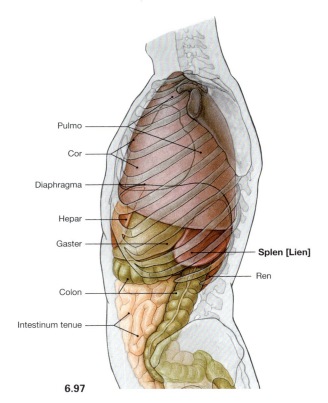

6.97

Pancreas → **Spleen** → Topography → Sections

Structure of the spleen

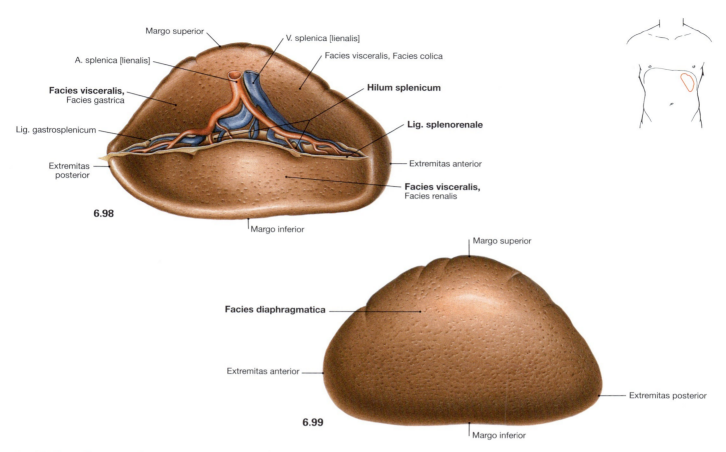

Fig. 6.98 and Fig. 6.99 Spleen, Splen [Lien]; medial ventral (→ Fig. 6.98) and lateral cranial (→ Fig. 6 99) views.
The spleen is a **secondary lymphatic organ** and plays a role in the immune system as well as in filtering of the blood. The spleen weighs 150 g, is 11 cm long, 7 cm wide and 4 cm high. Its convex side, Facies diaphragmatica, is adjacent to the diaphragm, its concave side, Facies visceralis, is facing the abdominal viscera, especially the left kidney, the left colic flexure, and the stomach. The superior border (Margo superior) shows indentations, whereas the inferior border (Margo inferior) is rather smooth. The blood vessels enter and exit at the splenic hilum (Hilum splenicum). The branching pattern of the blood vessels reflects the segmentation of the spleen, although the segments can not be identified at the surface. The spleen is anchored to the surroundings by two **peritoneal duplicatures**, both of which insert at the splenic hilum. The Lig. gastrosplenicum connects the spleen to the stomach and continues as Lig. splenorenale to the posterior wall of the trunk.

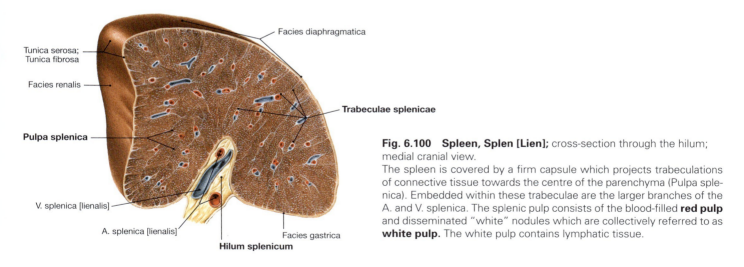

Fig. 6.100 Spleen, Splen [Lien]; cross-section through the hilum; medial cranial view.
The spleen is covered by a firm capsule which projects trabeculations of connective tissue towards the centre of the parenchyma (Pulpa splenica). Embedded within these trabeculae are the larger branches of the A. and V. splenica. The splenic pulp consists of the blood-filled **red pulp** and disseminated "white" nodules which are collectively referred to as **white pulp.** The white pulp contains lymphatic tissue.

Clinical Remarks

Following a traumatic injury to the abdomen, a **rupture of the spleen** may occur. A rupture may result in life-threatening haemorrhage. Because of the segmental structure of the spleen, longitudinal lacerations will affect several splenic segments and cause intense bleeding; transverse lacerations bleed weakly since splenic arteries are terminal arteries. This also explains the wedge-shaped area of **infarction** between the segmental borders.

Viscera of the Abdomen Development → Stomach → Intestines → Liver and gallbladder →

Greater omentum

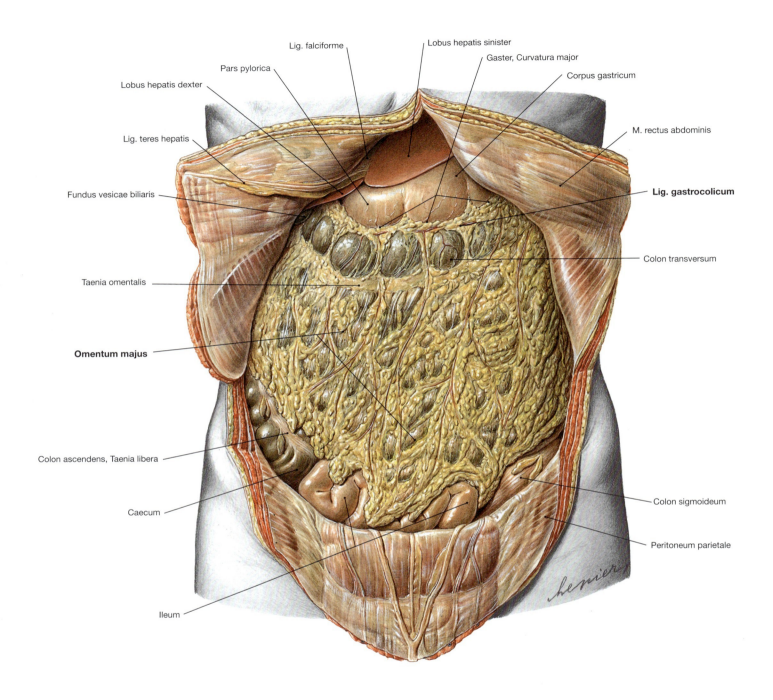

Fig. 6.101 Position of the viscera, Situs viscerum, in the Epigastrium and the greater omentum, Omentum majus; ventral view.
The abdominal cavity is opened and the Umbilicus was cut from the left side to preserve the Lig. teres hepatis between the liver and the ventral abdominal wall. The horizontal Colon transversum divides the abdomen in epigastrium and hypogastrium. The viscera of the lower abdomen are almost completely covered by the greater omentum which is attached to the greater curvature of the stomach. The Omentum is associated with the Epigastrium because its blood supply is derived from the vessels of the greater curvature of the stomach (Rr. omentales of the Aa. gastroomentales; → Fig. 6.116). The Omentum majus is a peritoneal duplicature composed of the Lig. gas-trocolicum, the Lig. gastrosplenicum and a free apron-like portion. The greater omentum plays a role not only in the mechanical protection and thermal insulation but also in the secretion and absorption of peritoneal fluids. It also contains lymphatic tissue and has immunological functions.

Pancreas → Spleen → **Topography** → Sections

Epigastrium

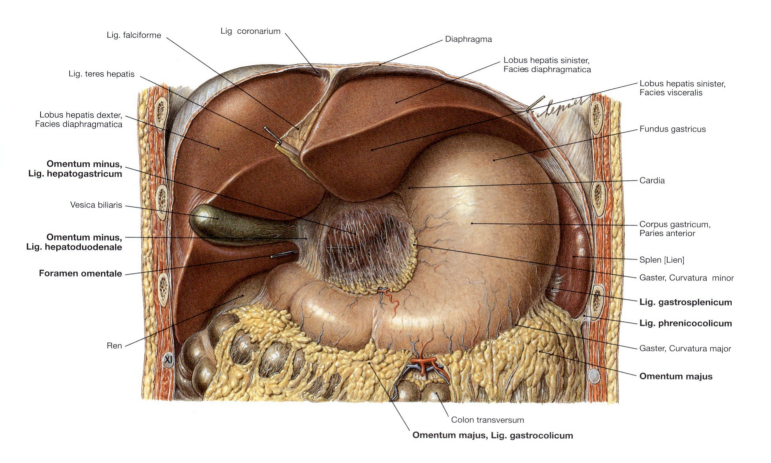

Fig. 6.102 Position of the viscera, Situs viscerum, in the Epigastrium; ventral view.
The liver was reflected cranially to visualise the lesser omentum **(Omentum minus)**. It spans between the liver and the lesser curvature of the stomach and the Pars superior of the Duodenum. The Omentum minus consists of the Lig. hepatogastricum and the Lig. hepatoduodenale. The latter guides the common bile duct (Ductus choledochus), the portal vein (V. portae hepatis), and the A. hepatica propria to the Porta hepatis (the hilum of the liver). Behind the Lig. hepatoduodenale is the entrance to the Bursa omentalis (Foramen omentale, marked here by a probe), a sliding space between stomach and pancreas anteriorly confined by the Omentum minus.

The **Omentum majus** is attached to the greater curvature of the stomach and to the Taenia omentalis of the transverse colon. It is subdivided into the Lig. gastrocolicum (to the Colon transversum) and the Lig. gastrosplenicum (to the spleen). The spleen resides in the splenic niche and rests on the Lig. phrenicocolicum between the left colic flexure and diaphragm.

6 Viscera of the Abdomen → Development → Stomach → Intestines → Liver and gallbladder →

Epigastrium with Bursa omentalis

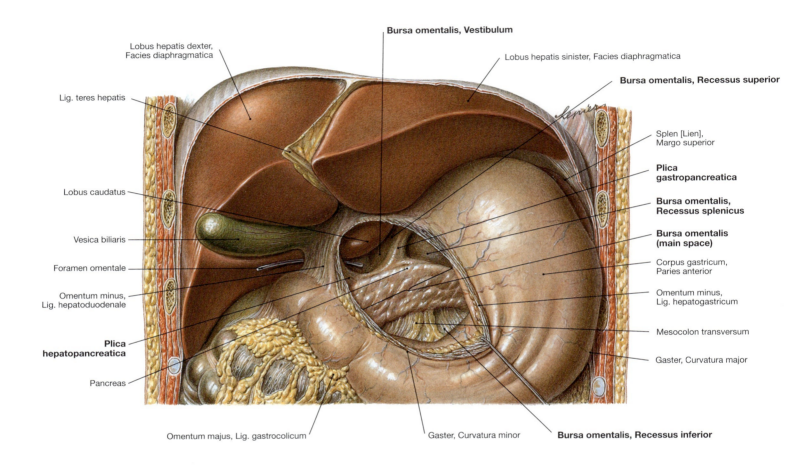

Fig. 6.103 Position of the viscera, Situs viscerum, in the Epigastrium; ventral view.
The lesser omentum (Omentum minus) between the liver and the lesser curvature of the stomach was separated to show the Bursa omentalis.
The Bursa omentalis is a sliding space between stomach and Pancreas and exclusively communicates with the abdominal cavity through the Foramen omentale behind the Lig. hepatoduodenale. Due to its confined position, the Bursa omentalis is also referred to as the "lesser sac of the peritoneal cavity".
The Bursa omentalis is subdivided into four parts:
- **Foramen omentale:** The entrance to the Bursa omentalis is confined anteriorly by the Lig. hepatoduodenale, cranially by the Lobus caudatus, caudally by the Bulbus duodeni, and posteriorly by the V. cava inferior.

- **Vestibulum:** The vestibule is confined by the Omentum minus ventrally and its Recessus superior extends behind the liver.
- **Isthmus:** The narrowing between vestibule and main space is confined by two peritoneal folds: on the right side by the Plica hepatopancreatica which is created by the A. hepatica communis, and on the left side by the Plica gastropancreatica which marks the course of the A. gastrica sinistra.
- **Main space:** This space is located between the stomach (anterior) and the Pancreas and the Mesocolon transversum (posterior), respectively. On the left side, the Recessus splenicus extends to the hilum of the spleen; the Recessus inferior lies behind the Lig. gastrocolicum and extends to the origin of the Mesocolon at the Colon transversum.

→ dissection link

Pancreas → Spleen → **Topography** → Sections

Epigastrium with Bursa omentalis

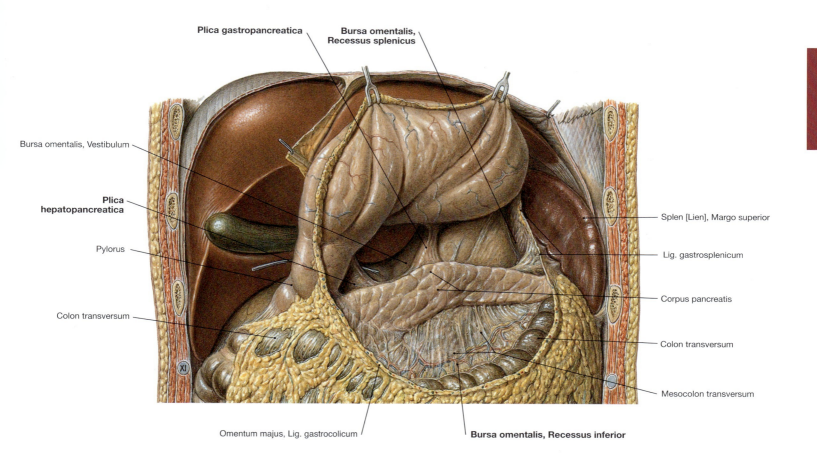

Fig. 6.104 Position of the viscera, Situs viscerum, in the Epigastrium; ventral view.
The Lig. gastrocolicum was sectioned and the stomach reflected cranially to show the main space of the Bursa omentalis. The posterior wall of the bursa is created by the Pancreas and the Mesocolon transversum. On the left side, it extends to the hilum of the spleen (Recessus splenicus), inferiorly to the origin of the Mesocolon at the Colon transversum (Recessus inferior).

Clinical Remarks

Similar to the other recesses of the peritoneal cavity, the Bursa omentalis is of clinical relevance. Herniation of small intestinal loops **(internal hernias),** dissemination of malignant tumours **(peritoneal carcinosis),** or bacteria **(peritonitis)** can involve the omental bursa. Therefore, during abdominal surgery, the surgeon usually inspects the Bursa omentalis.

During **surgical treatment** in the epigastrium (e.g. interventions at the Pancreas), the surgeon can access the Bursa omentalis **in three different ways:**
- via the Omentum minus (→ Fig. 6.103)
- via the Lig. gastrocolicum
- via the Mesocolon transversum

6 Viscera of the Abdomen Development → Stomach → Intestines → Liver and gallbladder →

Hypogastricum

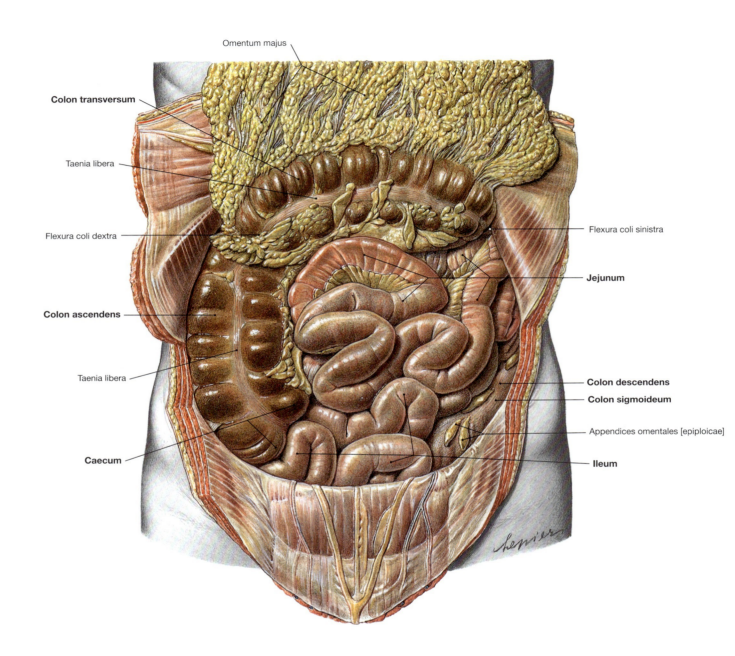

Fig. 6.105 Position of the viscera, Situs viscerum, in the Hypogastrium; ventral view.
The Omentum majus was reflected cranially to visualise the small and large intestines in the Hypogastrium. Thus, the intraperitoneal segments are visible: Jejunum and Ileum of the small intestine, Caecum, Colon transversum, and Colon sigmoideum of the large intestine. This figure also shows that the retroperitoneal segments of the colon are relocated to the posterior wall of the abdomen to a variable extent. In this case, the Colon ascendens is clearly visible, but the Colon descendens is shifted further dorsally and is partially covered by the small intestine. The large intestine frames the convolute of Jejunum and Ileum.

134 → *dissection link*

Pancreas → Spleen → **Topography** → Sections

Hypogastricum

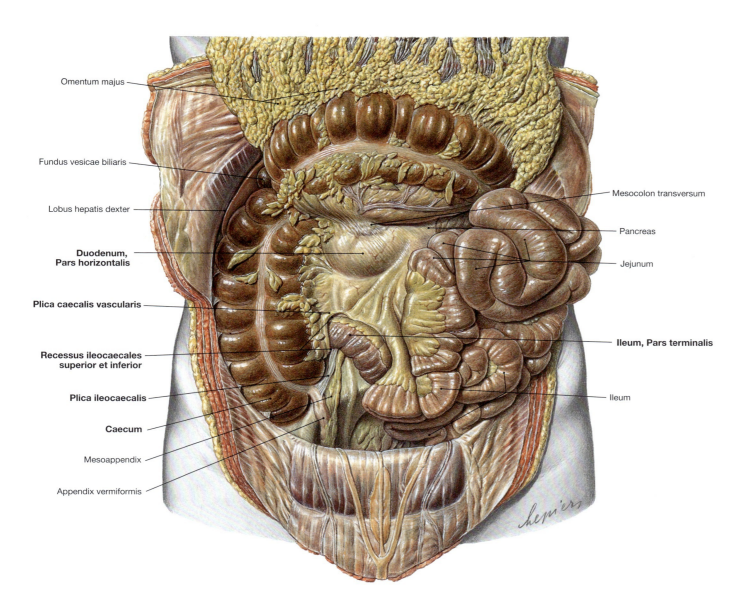

Fig. 6.106 Position of the viscera, Situs viscerum, in the Hypogastrium; ventral view.
The Omentum majus was reflected cranially and the loops of the small intestine were reflected to the left side to visualise the secondary retroperitoneal Pars horizontalis of the Duodenum. At the transition between the Ileum and the Caecum there are two spaces: the **Recessus ileocaecalis superior** is covered by the Plica caecalis vascularis (contains a branch of the A. ileocolica), the **Recessus ileocaecalis inferior** is covered by the Plica ileocaecalis between the Ileum and the Appendix vermiformis. Similar to the Bursa omentalis and other abdominal recessus, small intestinal loops may be trapped here (internal hernias).

→ *dissection link*

6 Viscera of the Abdomen Development → Stomach → Intestines → Liver and gallbladder →

Hypogastricum

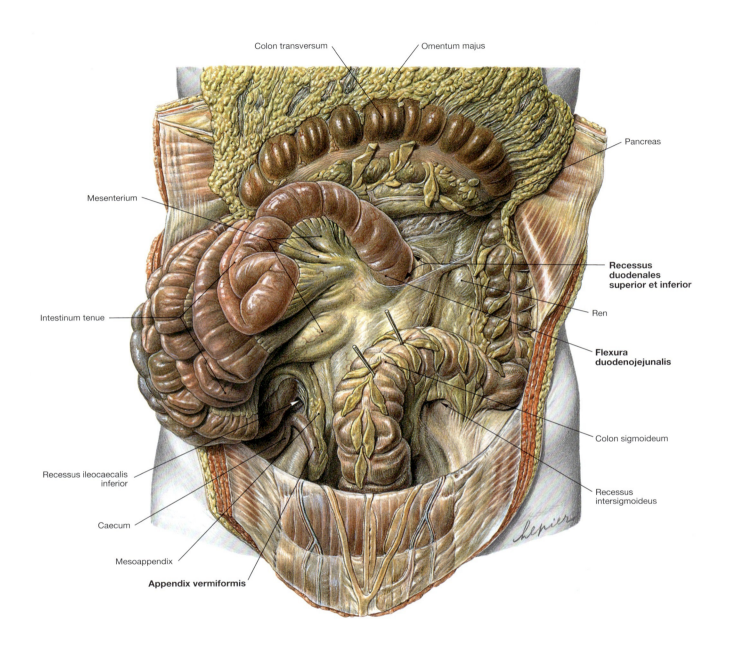

Fig. 6.107 Position of the viscera, Situs viscerum, in the Hypogastrium; ventral view.
The Omentum majus was reflected cranially and the loops of the small intestine were reflected to the right side to demonstrate the Flexura duodenojejunalis which marks the transition of the retroperitoneal Duodenum into the intraperitoneal Jejunum. This area also contains two recesses: **Recessus duodenales superior** and **inferior.** In the right Hypogastrium, the Appendix vermiformis is visible, the tip of which descends into the small pelvis (descending type).

Clinical Remarks

The Recessus duodenales superior and inferior are the most common sites for the herniation of small intestinal loops (**TREITZ's hernias**). This herniation may result in an intestinal obstruction (ileus) or intestinal infarction.

136 → dissection link

Pancreas → Spleen → **Topography** → Sections

Mesenteries

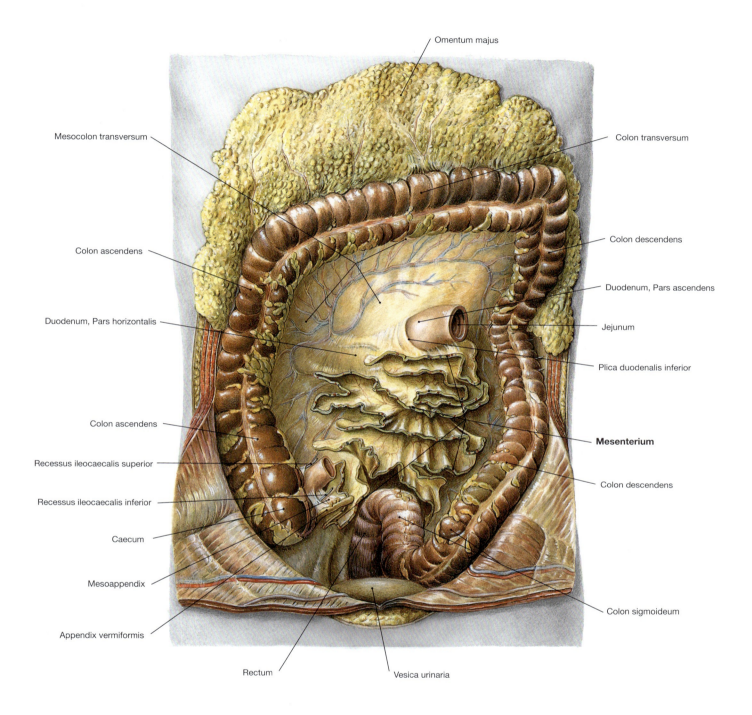

Fig. 6.108 Mesenteries of the small intestine, Mesenterium, and large intestine, Intestinum crassum; ventral view.
The Omentum majus and the Colon transversum were reflected cranially. The intraperitoneal small intestinal convolute of Jejunum and Ileum was resected at the mesentery. The mesentery consists of a duplicature of the peritoneal membranes, contains the neurovascular structures to supply the small intestine, and serves as mobile attachment of the small intestine to the posterior abdominal wall.

→ *dissection link* 137

6 Viscera of the Abdomen Development → Stomach → Intestines → Liver and gallbladder →

Secondary retroperitoneal organs

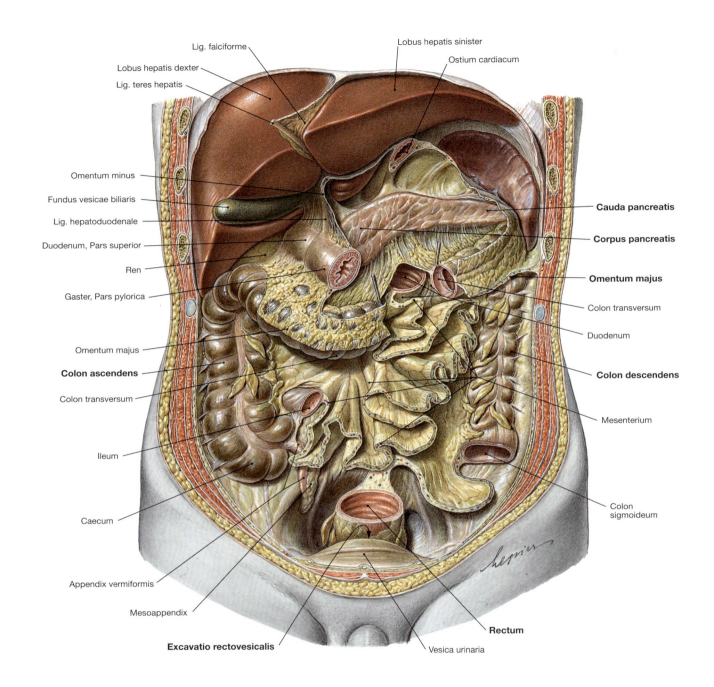

Fig. 6.109 Position of the secondary retroperitoneal organs; ventral view.
The stomach was removed, Jejunum and Ileum were resected at the mesentery, and Colon transversum and Colon sigmoideum were sectioned. Most of the secondary retroperitoneal organs are now visible. These include the Duodenum (except for the Pars superior), the Pancreas, the Colon ascendens, and the Colon descendens, and the Rectum to the Flexura sacralis. Anterior to the Rectum, the opening of the Excavatio rectovesicalis can be seen. This peritoneal pouch is the most inferior part of the peritoneal cavity in men.

Clinical Remarks

In an upright position (seldom in bedridden patients), in the most inferior extension of the peritoneal cavity, the **Excavatio rectovesicalis** in men, and the **Excavatio rectouterina** (pouch of DOUGLAS) in women (→ Fig. 6.110), may accumulate inflammatory exudate or pus in cases of inflammatory events in the Hypogastrium. By ultrasound (abdominal, transvaginal) examination, this can be detected as free fluid in the abdomen.

→ dissection link

Pancreas → Spleen → **Topography** → Sections

Posterior wall of the peritoneal cavity

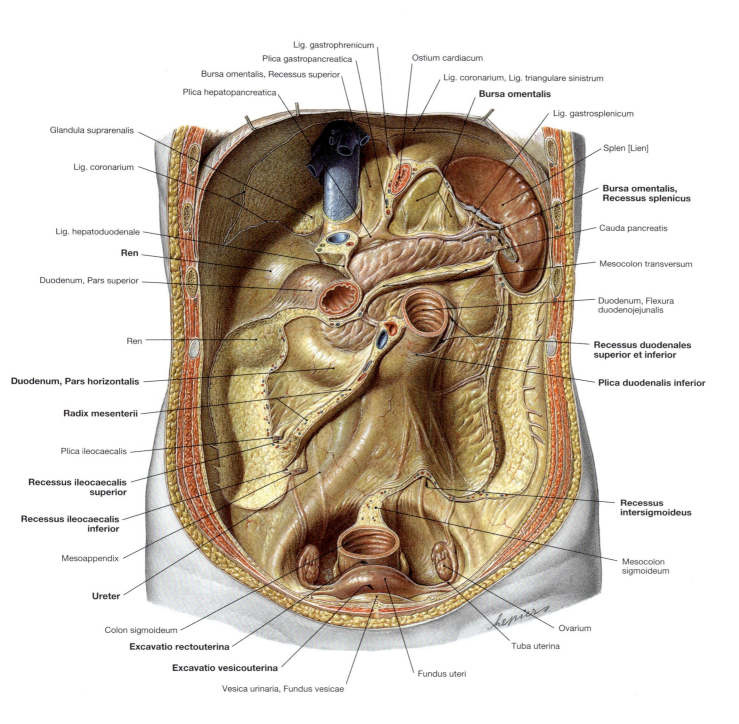

Fig. 6.110 Dorsal wall of the peritoneal cavity, Cavitas peritonealis, with recesses, Recessus, and spleen, Splen [Lien]; ventral view.

Liver, small and large intestines were removed except for the Duodenum to expose the dorsal wall of the peritoneal cavity. The peritoneal lining over the right kidney and the Pars descendens of the Duodenum is clearly visible due to its shiny surface. The attachment areas of the secondary retroperitoneal Colon ascendens and Colon descendens are lacking this peritoneal lining.

The peritoneal duplicatures form the relief of the dorsal wall of the peritoneal cavity as folds (Plicae) and ligaments and create diverse recesses (Recessus). The largest of them is the **Bursa omentalis** (→ Fig. 6.103), the portions and extensions thereof are visible here. At the area of the Flexura duodenojejunalis, the Plicae duodenales superior and inferior form two recesses (**Recessus duodenales superior** and **inferior**). Further recesses (peritoneal gutters) are located at the entrance of the terminal ileum into the Caecum (**Recessus iliocaecales superior** and **inferior**) and occasionally another recess is located inferior to the Mesocolon sigmoideum (**Recessus intersigmoideus**).

Anterior to the rectum, a deep peritoneal space exists which is confined by the uterus and the broad ligament at the ventral side. This **Excavatio rectouterina** (pouch of DOUGLAS) is the most caudal recess of the peritoneal cavity in women. The ventrally positioned **Excavatio vesicouterina** between urinary bladder and Uterus does not extend downwards as deeply as the Excavatio rectouterina. Between the Flexura duodenojejunalis and the right Fossa iliaca, the 12–16 cm long root of the mesentery (Radix mesenterii) is attached. It contains the blood vessels supplying the small intestine (A./V. mesenterica superior). The root of the mesentery traverses the Pars horizontalis of the Duodenum and the right Ureter.

6 Viscera of the Abdomen Development → Stomach → Intestines → Liver and gallbladder →

Arteries of the abdomen

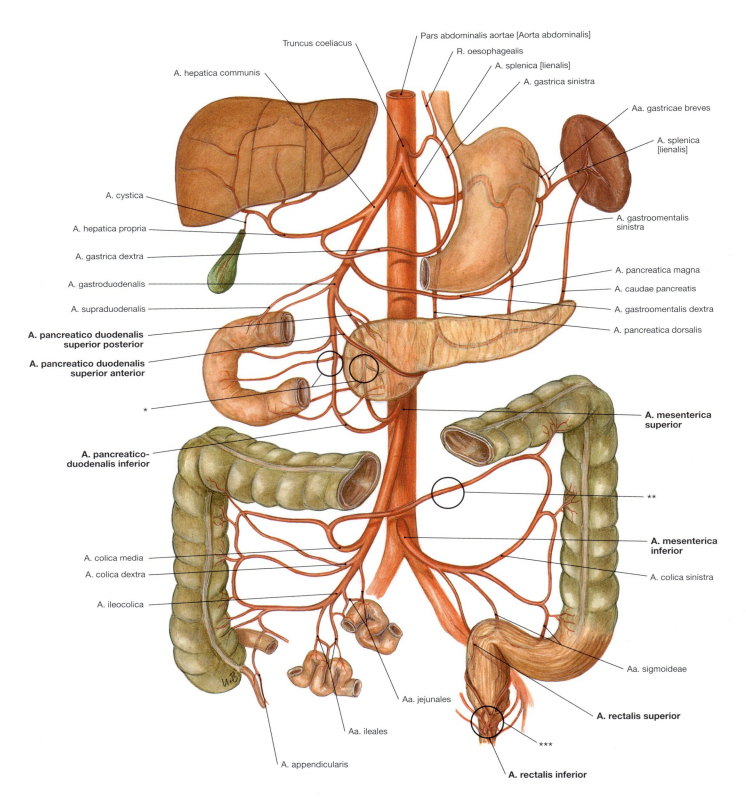

Fig. 6.111 Arteries of the abdominal viscera; semischematic illustration; ventral view.
The most important anastomoses are marked by black circles. The three unpaired arteries to the abdominal viscera derived from the Aorta abdominalis are the Truncus coeliacus, the A. mesenterica superior, and the A. mesenterica inferior. The A. mesenterica superior has its origin directly below the Truncus coeliacus (here not shown due to semischematic presentation). Its respective branches are described on the following pages. All three arteries anastomose with each other and with branches of the A. iliaca interna. This may prevent ischemic infarction in cases of an occlusion of one of these vessels.

The **anastomoses** are:
- connections between the Truncus coeliacus and the A. mesenterica superior via Aa. pancreaticoduodenales (*).
- connections between the Aa. mesentericae superior and inferior: RIOLAN's anastomosis between the A. colica media and A. colica sinistra (**).
- Plexus of rectal arteries: here the A. rectalis superior from the A. mesenterica inferior connects to the Aa. rectales media and inferior from the A. iliaca interna (***).

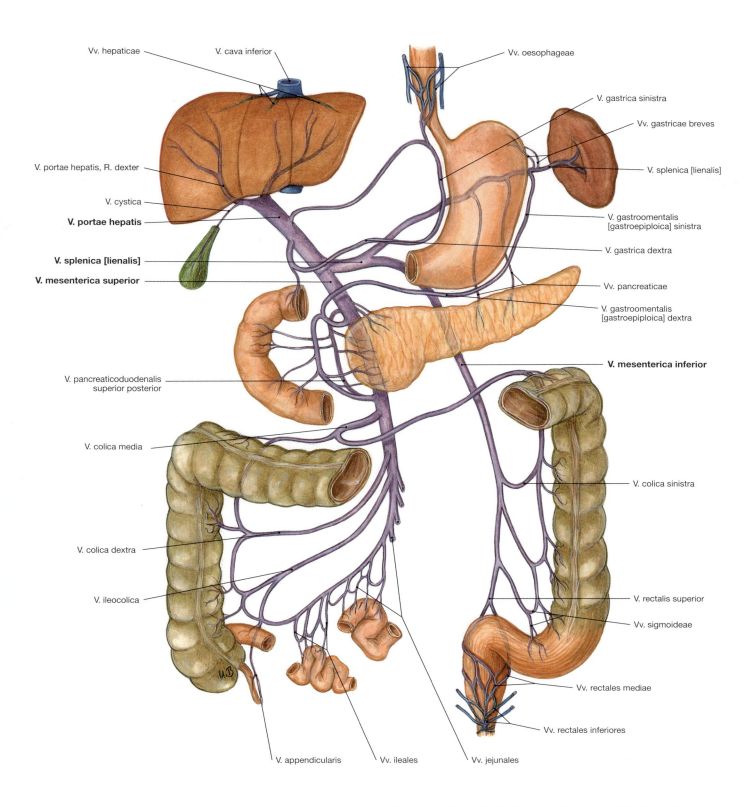

Fig. 6.112 Portal vein, V. portae hepatis, with tributaries; semischematic illustration; ventral view.
The tributaries of the portal vein are described in detail in → Figure 6.69.

6 Viscera of the Abdomen Development → Stomach → Intestines → Liver and gallbladder →

Truncus coeliacus

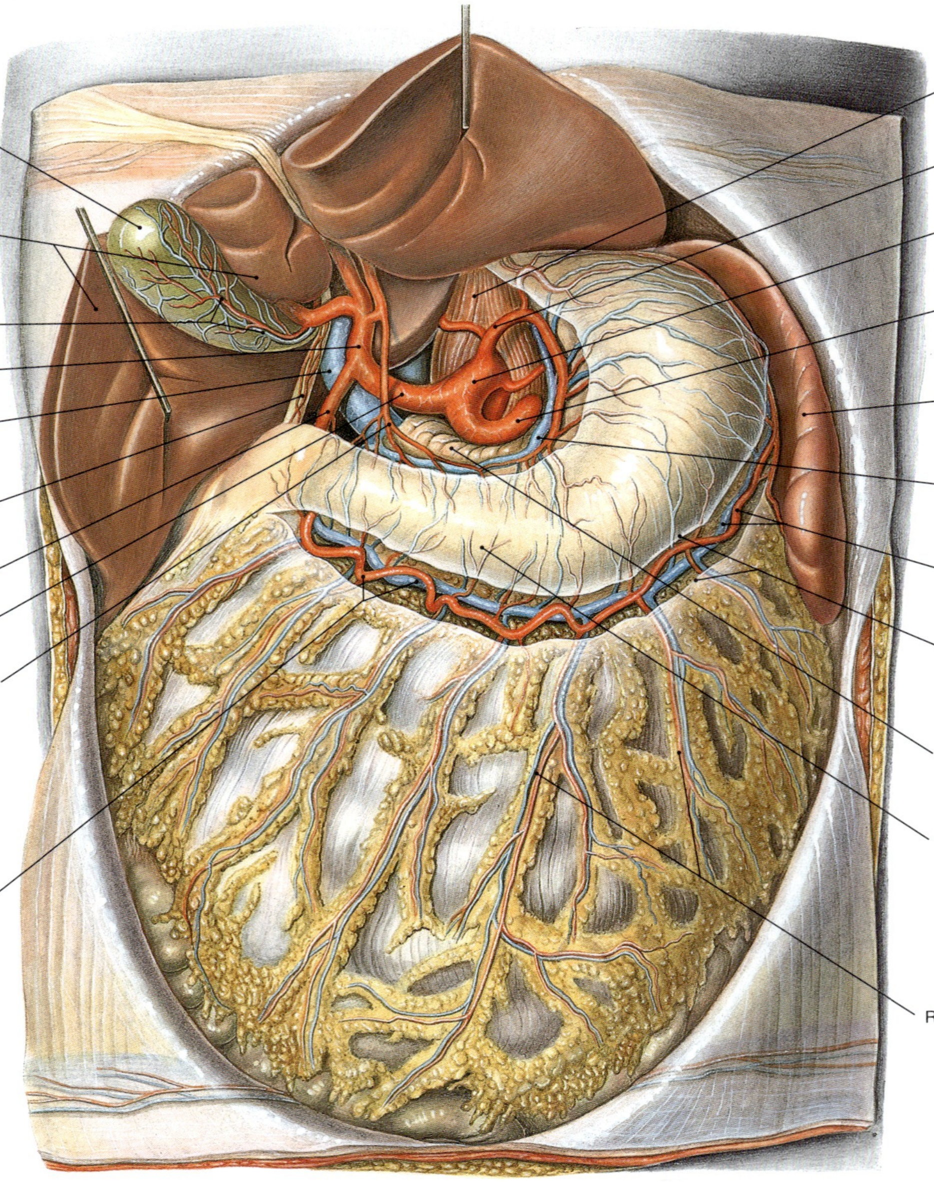

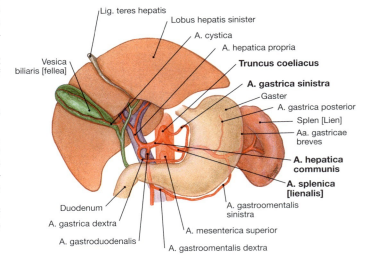

Fig. 6.113 Truncus coeliacus; ventral view; after removal of the Omentum minus.

The Truncus coeliacus derives as first unpaired branch from the Aorta abdominalis. In the retroperitoneal space behind the Bursa omentalis its short (mostly 2–3 cm) trunk divides into the three major arteries which supply the viscera of the Epigastrium (Gaster, Duodenum, Hepar, Vesica biliaris, Pancreas and Splen):

- **A. gastrica sinistra:** branches off to the left and superior side. It anastomoses with the A. gastrica dextra at the lesser curvature of the stomach and is usually the stronger vessel.
- **A. hepatica communis:** turns to the right side and divides into:
  – A. hepatica propria: releases the A. gastrica dextra and supplies liver and gallbladder (A. cystica)
  – A. gastroduodenalis: descends behind the Pylorus or Duodenum, divides into the A. gastroomentalis dextra to the greater curvature of the stomach and the Aa. pancreaticoduodenales superiores anterior and posterior which anastomose with the A. pancreaticoduodenalis inferior from the A. mesenterica superior to supply the head of the Pancreas and the Duodenum.
- **A. splenica:** courses to the inferior left side at the superior border of the Pancreas and releases the following branches during its course to the spleen:
  – Rr. pancreatici for the Pancreas
  – A. gastrica posterior to the stomach (30–60% of all cases)
  – A. gastroomentalis sinistra: courses from the left side to the greater curvature of the stomach and anastomoses with the A. gastroomentalis dextra
  – Aa. gastrici breves: short branches to the fundus of the stomach
  – Rr. splenici: terminal branches to the spleen

Fig. 6.114 Branches of the Truncus coeliacus.

142 → dissection link

Pancreas → Spleen → **Topography** → Sections

A. mesenterica superior

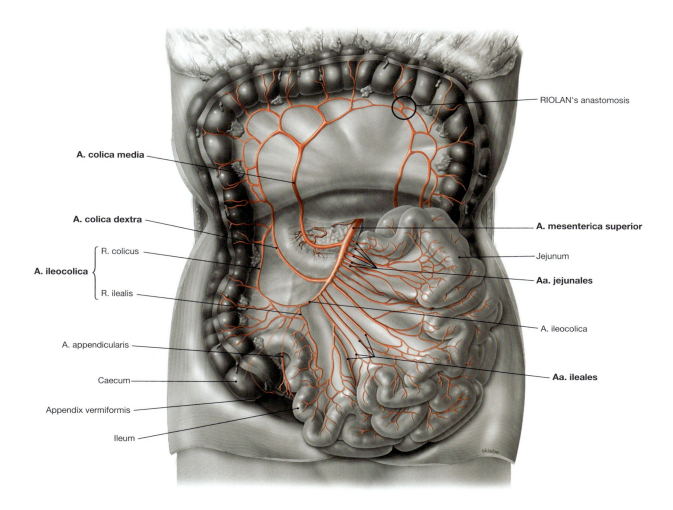

Fig. 6.115 A. mesenterica superior; ventral view; Colon transversum reflected cranially. (according to [1])
The unpaired A. mesenterica superior branches off the Aorta abdominalis directly below the Truncus coeliacus, courses retroperitoneally behind the Pancreas and then enters the mesentery. Its branches can be displayed if the mesentery is opened and the adipose tissue between the vascular arcades is removed. It supplies parts of the Pancreas and Duodenum, the entire small intestine, and the large intestine up to the left colic flexure.

Branches of the A. mesenterica superior:
- **A. pancreaticoduodenalis inferior:** branches off to the superior right side; R. anterior and R. posterior anastomose with the Aa. pancreaticoduodenales superiores anterior and posterior (→ Fig. 6.116).
- **Aa. jejunales** (4–5) and **Aa. ileales** (12): directed to the left side
- **A. colica media:** originates on the right side and anastomoses with the A. colica dextra and with the A. colica sinistra (RIOLAN's anastomosis)
- **A. colica dextra:** courses to the Colon ascendens
- **A. ileocolica:** supplies the distal Ileum, Caecum and Appendix vermiformis (A. appendicularis)

6 Viscera of the Abdomen Development → Stomach → Intestines → Liver and gallbladder →

A. mesenterica superior

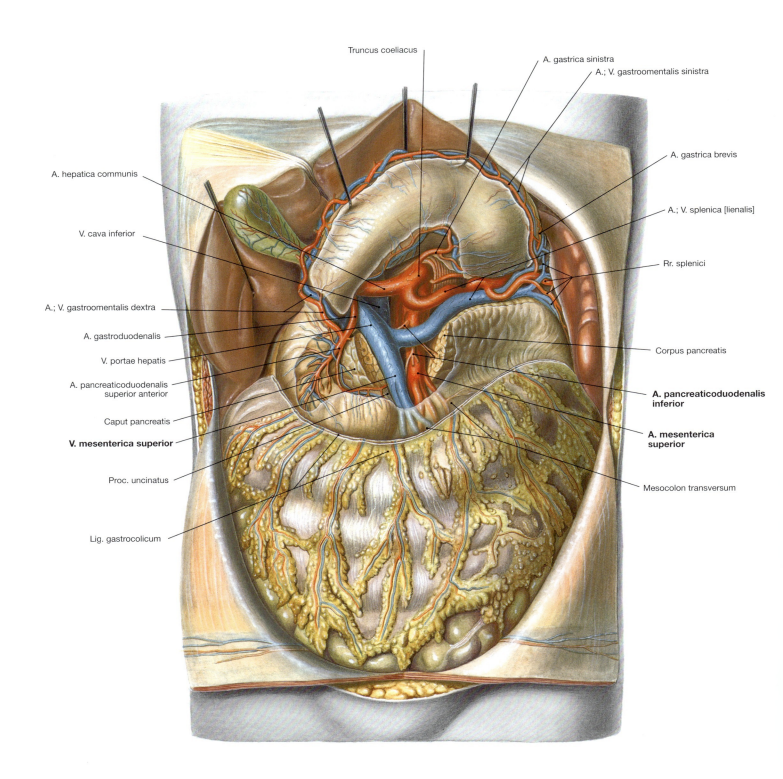

Fig. 6.116 Origins of the A. mesenterica superior and Truncus coeliacus; ventral view; after reflecting the stomach cranially and dissecting the Pancreas.
Following its origin from the Aorta abdominalis inferior to the Truncus coeliacus, the A. mesenterica superior descends behind the Pancreas and enters the mesentery anterior to the Duodenum. The Pancreas was sectioned to show the A. and V. mesenterica superior ventral to the Proc. uncinatus of the Pancreas. The A. mesenterica superior supplies the A. pancreaticoduodenalis inferior as its first branch to the right side.

A. mesenterica superior

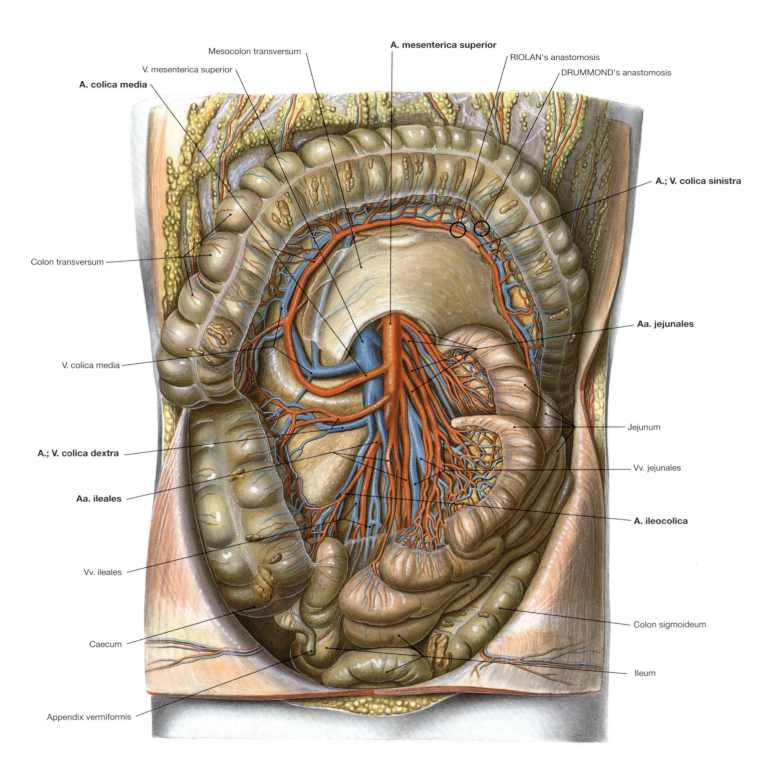

Fig. 6.117 Course of the A. and V. mesenterica superior; ventral view; after opening of the mesentery with the Colon transversum reflected cranially.
Within the mesentery, the A. mesenterica superior gives rise to the following branches: Aa. jejunales and Aa. ileales to the left side, A. colica media, A. colica dextra, and A. ileocolica to the right side. All arteries form arcades at different levels of their divisions. This allows the mobility of the intestinal loops. At the left colic flexure, the A. colica media forms a **functionally important anastomosis (RIOLAN's anastomosis)** with the A. colica sinistra from the A. mesenterica inferior. This facilitates the formation of collateral circulations in the case of occlusion of one of the arteries. The anastomosis between the two arteries in one of the arcades close to the intestines is occasionally referred to as DRUMMOND's anastomosis. In the clinical jargon, all anastomoses in the area of the left colic flexure are summarised as RIOLAN's anastomosis.
The venous branches correspond to the arteries.

6 Viscera of the Abdomen Development → Stomach → Intestines → Liver and gallbladder →

A. mesenterica inferior

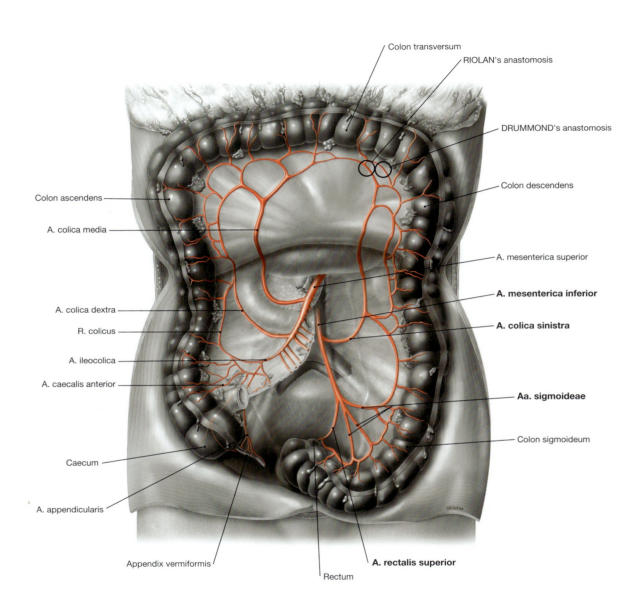

Fig. 6.118 A. mesenterica inferior; ventral view; Colon transversum reflected cranially. (according to [1])
The unpaired A. mesenterica inferior branches off the abdominal aorta approximately 5 cm above its bifurcation and turns to the left side. With the exception of a short terminal section, the A. mesenterica inferior descends into the retroperitoneal space to supply the Colon descendens and the upper Rectum.

Branches of the A. mesenterica inferior:
- **A. colica sinistra:** ascends along the Colon descendens and anastomoses via the A. colica sinistra with the A. colica media from the A. mesenterica superior (RIOLAN's anastomosis)
- **Aa. sigmoideae:** several branches to the Colon sigmoideum
- **A. rectalis superior:** supplies Rectum and the rectal cavernous bodies in the submucosa (Corpus cavernosum recti) which are a part of the continence mechanism.

A. mesenterica inferior

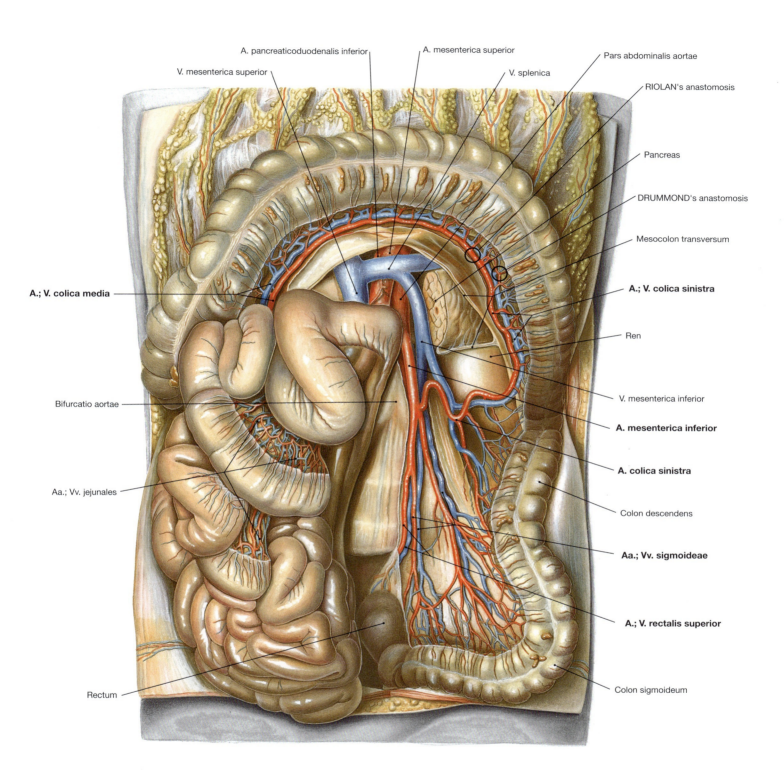

Fig. 6.119 Course of the A. and V. mesenterica inferior in the retroperitoneal space; ventral view; Colon transversum reflected cranially and small intestinal loops to the right side.
Following its origin above the aortic bifurcation, the A. mesenterica inferior descends in the retroperitoneal space and releases first the A. colica sinistra to the left side, then several Aa. sigmoideae and finally the unpaired A. rectalis superior.

The A. colica sinistra ascends along the Colon descendens, forms arcades and anastomoses with the A. colica media derived from the A. mesenterica superior **(RIOLAN's anastomosis).** The anastomosis between the two arteries in one of the arcades close to the intestines is occasionally referred to as DRUMMOND's anastomosis.

6 Viscera of the Abdomen Development → Stomach → Intestines → Liver and gallbladder →

Abdomen and pelvis, median section

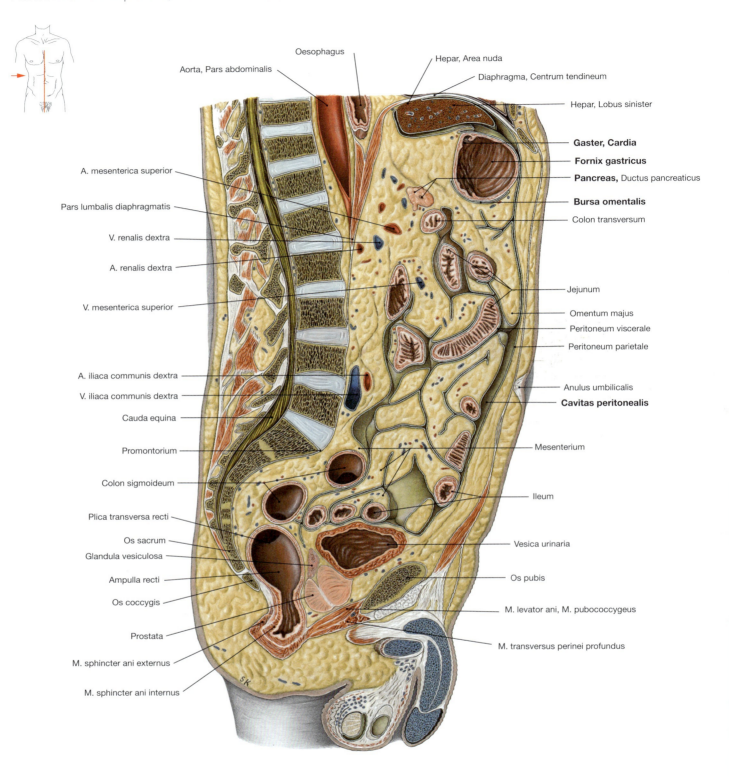

Fig. 6.120 Abdomen, Abdomen, and pelvis, Pelvis, of a man; median section; view from the right side.
This illustration shows clearly that the peritoneal cavity (Cavitas peritonealis) is not a wide empty space, but rather consists of small recesses between the intraperitoneal viscera. Also the Bursa omentalis between the stomach and the Pancreas is only a narrow space with peritoneal lining. A large portion of the abdominal cavity is occupied by the mesentery which may accumulate plenty of adipose tissue.

Pancreas → Spleen → Topography → Sections

Abdomen and pelvis, sagittal section

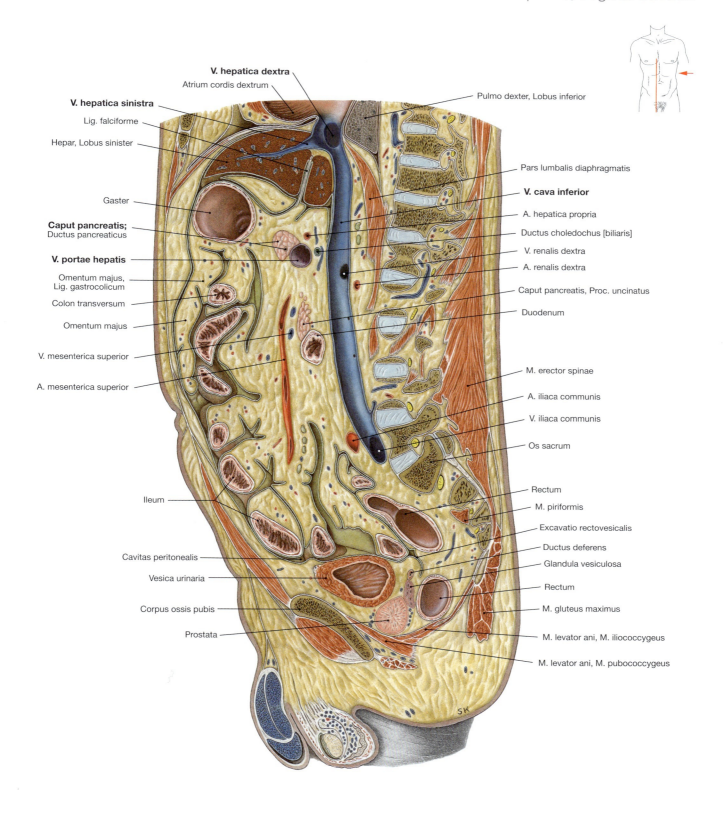

Fig. 6.121 Abdomen, Abdomen, and pelvis, Pelvis, of a man; sagittal section; view from the left side.
This is a right paramedian section at the level of the V. cava inferior. Thus, the confluence of the liver veins (Vv. hepaticae), which drain the venous blood from the liver, is clearly visible. The portal vein (V. portae hepatis), which brings the nutrient-rich blood from the unpaired viscera to the liver, arises from the confluence of the two main tributaries behind the pancreatic head.

6 Viscera of the Abdomen Development → Stomach → Intestines → Liver and gallbladder →

Abdomen and pelvis, frontal section

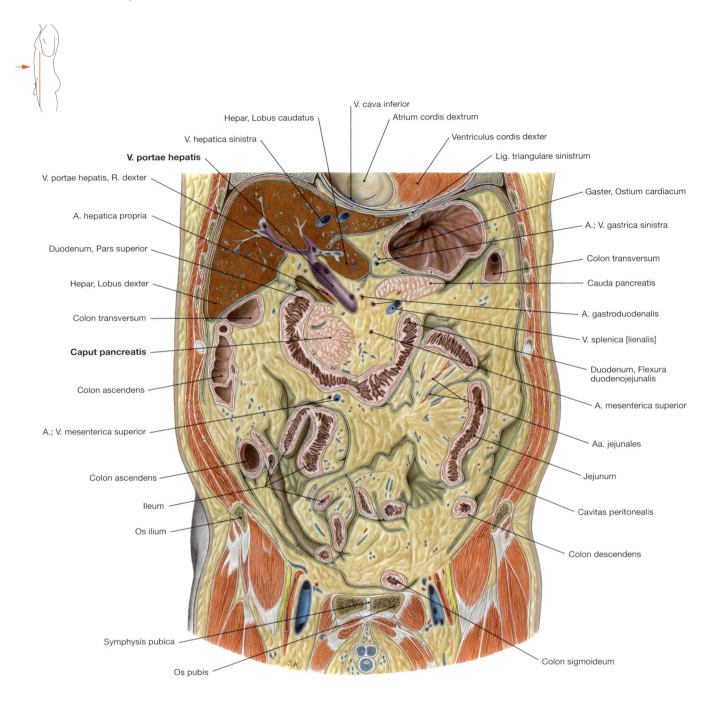

Fig. 6.122 Abdomen, Abdomen, and pelvis, Pelvis, of a man; frontal section through the anterior part; ventral view.

This is a frontal section through the portal vein (V. portae hepatis) which courses above the pancreatic head (Caput pancreatis) to the hilum of the liver and divides into a right and a left branch.

Pancreas → Spleen → Topography → **Sections**

Epigastrium, frontal section

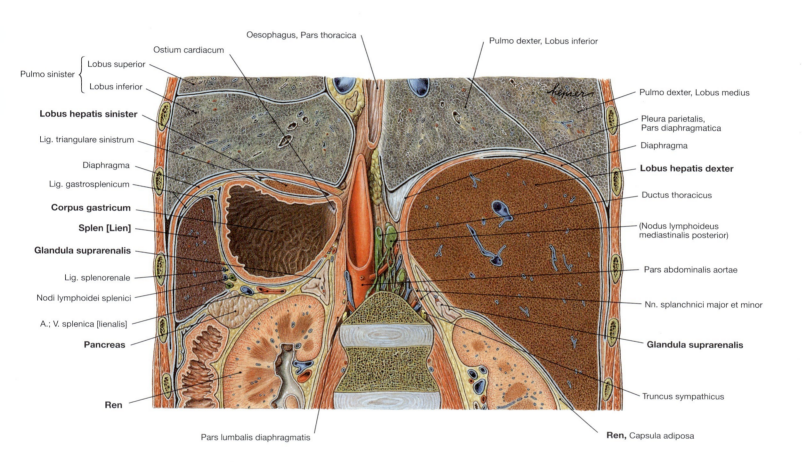

Fig. 6.123 Abdominal cavity, Cavitas abdominalis, and inferior thorax, Cavitas thoracis; frontal section at the level of the kidneys; dorsal view.
The section shows the topographical relationships of the epigastric viscera. The right Epigastrium is entirely occupied by the right lobe of the liver (Lobus hepatis dexter) which contacts the right kidney (Ren) and the right adrenal gland (Glandula suprarenalis) at its caudal aspect. On the left side, the cranial part of the left hepatic lobe covers the stomach (Gaster) which, in turn, contacts the spleen and caudally the left kidney, the left adrenal gland and the Pancreas. The pancreatic tail extends towards the spleen.

6 Viscera of the Abdomen Development → Stomach → Intestines → Liver and gallbladder →

Epigastrium, sagittal section

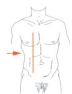

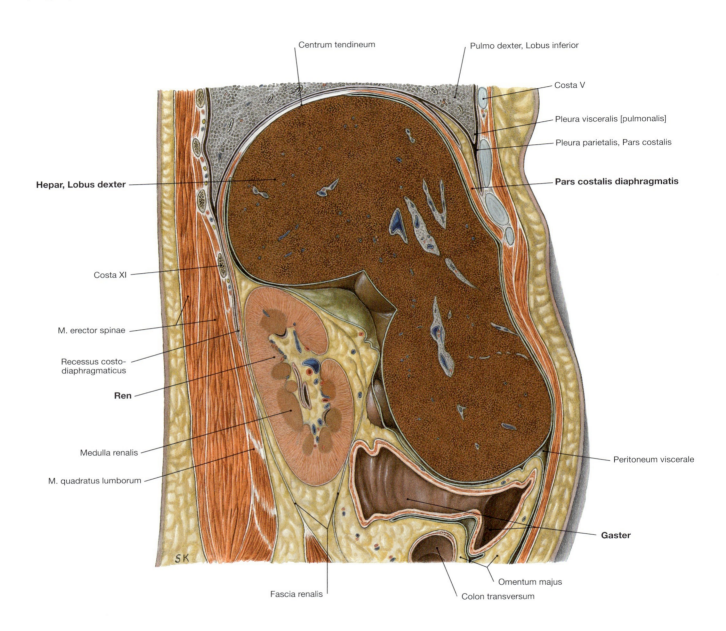

Fig. 6.124 Abdomen, Abdomen; sagittal section through the right epigastrium at the level of the kidney; view from the right side.
The right epigastrium contains the right lobe of the liver (Hepar, Lobus dexter) which has extensive contacts with the inferior aspect of the diaphragm. Dorsal and inferior to the liver, the kidney (Ren) is located in the retroperitoneal space; ventral thereof the Pass pylorica of the stomach (Gaster) is located in the intraperitoneal cavity.

Pancreas → Spleen → Topography → **Sections**

Epigastrium, sagittal section

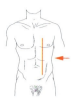

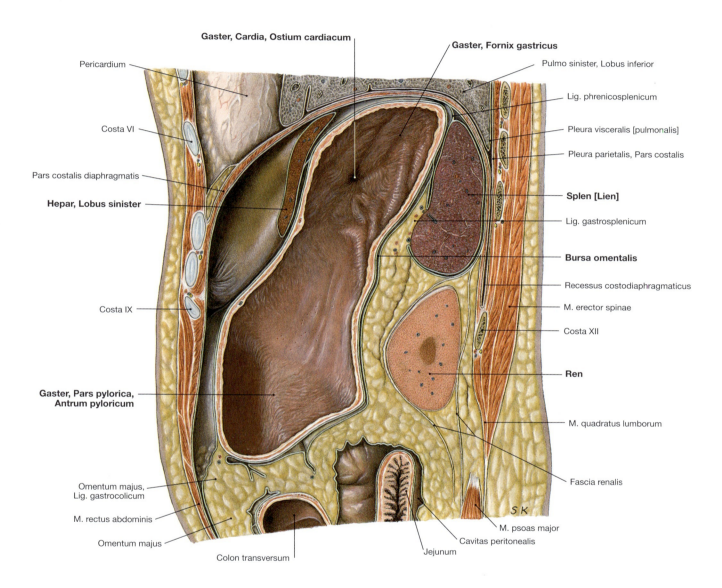

Fig. 6.125 Abdomen, Abdomen; sagittal section through the left epigastrium at the level of the spleen; view from the left side. The stomach (Gaster) occupies the major part of the left Epigastrium. It is covered ventrally by the left lobe of the liver (Hepar, Lobus sinister) and contacts the spleen and the left kidney (Ren) at its dorsal side; the left kidney is located in the retroperitoneal space. Lined by peritoneum, the Bursa omentalis forms a small recess behind the stomach.

Viscera of the Abdomen
Development → Stomach → Intestines → Liver and gallbladder →

Epigastrium, transverse sections

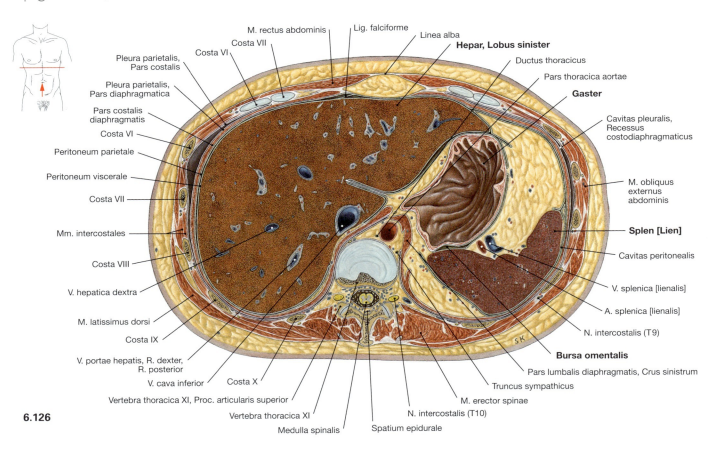

6.126

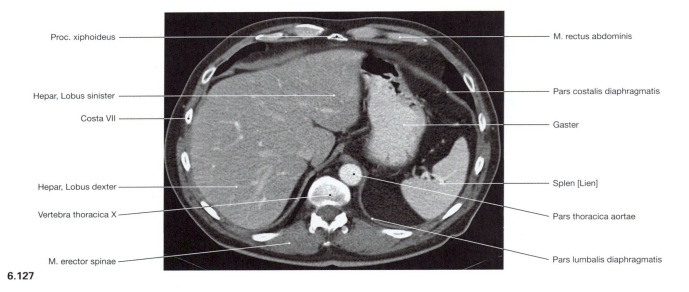

6.127

Fig. 6.126 and Fig. 6.127 Abdominal cavity, Cavitas abdominalis; transverse section at the level of the 11th thoracic vertebra (→ Fig. 6.126) and corresponding computed tomographic section (CT; → Fig. 6.127); caudal view.

The liver occupies the entire right epigastrium and with its left lobe extends to the left anterior side of the stomach (Gaster). Posterior to the stomach and lined by peritoneum is the Bursa omentalis. The spleen is cut in the left Epigastrium.

Clinical Remarks

Sectional imaging as shown here for **computed tomography** (CT) is established routinely in diagnostic procedures. It allows the imaging of soft tissues without contrast medium and is less prone to disturbances than ultrasound imaging which may suffer from decreased resolution by certain conditions such as air-filled intestinal loops. Therefore, CT imaging is used as additional diagnostic tool and in preoperative planning. According to convention, CT images are **always shown in caudal view.** For didactic and practical purposes, it is advisable to study anatomical sections also in caudal view.

Pancreas → Spleen → Topography → Sections

Epigastrium, transverse sections

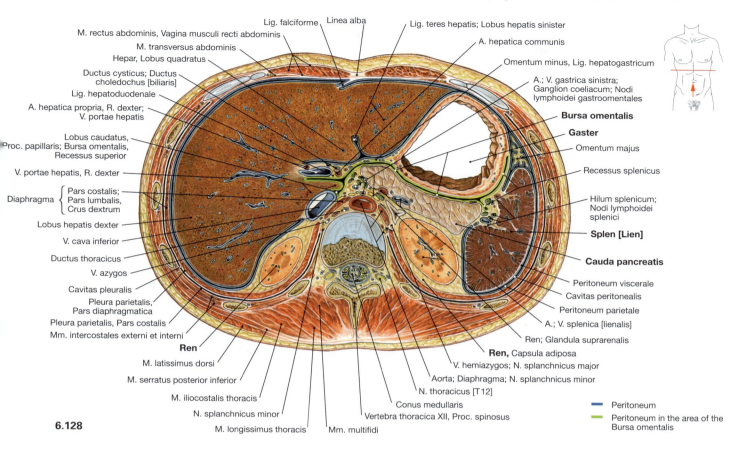

6.128

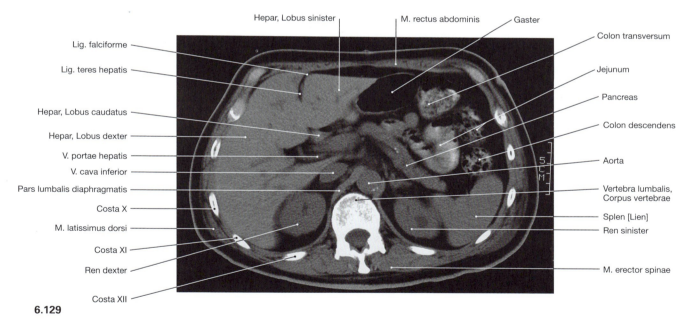

6.129

Fig. 6.128 and Fig. 6.129 Abdominal cavity, Cavitas abdominalis; transverse section at the level of the 1st lumbar vertebra (→ Fig. 6.128) and corresponding computed tomographic section (CT; → Fig. 6.129); caudal view.

At the level of the 1st lumbar vertebra, additional viscera are visible, such as the superior poles of the kidneys (Ren) and the Pancreas. The Pancreas is located posterior to the stomach, separated by the Bursa omentalis, and extends to the left side until it reaches the hilum of the spleen.

Clinical Remarks

For the examination of the Pancreas, ultrasound imaging is often not very informative due to the air-filled intestinal loops. The CT is performed to find or confirm the diagnosis of pancreatic conditions such as inflammatory disease (pancreatitis), when oedematous or cystic swelling of the organ is detected. CT imaging is also used to monitor the progress of pancreatic diseases.

Viscera of the Abdomen

Epigastrium, transverse sections

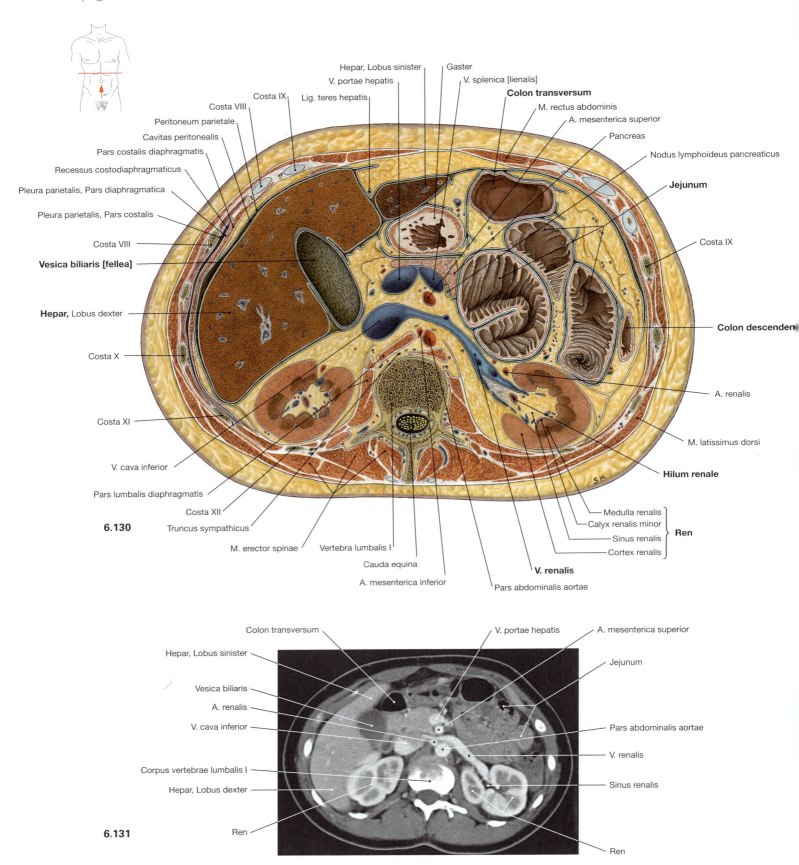

Fig. 6.130 and Fig. 6.131 Abdominal cavity, Cavitas abdominalis; transverse section at the level of the 1st lumbar vertebra (→ Fig. 6.130) and corresponding computed tomographic section (CT; → Fig. 6.131); caudal view.

Typically, the hilum of the kidney (Ren) is located at the level of the first two lumbar vertebrae (recognizable by the confluence of the left V. renalis). The gallbladder (Vesica biliaris) is sectioned at the inferior border of the liver (Hepar). In the left Epigastrium, portions of the small intestinal Loops (Jejunum) and portions of the large intestine (Colon transversum and Colon descendens) are visible.

Pelvis and Retroperitoneal Space

Kidney and Adrenal Gland 160

Efferent Urinary System 174

Genitalia. 182

Rectum and Anal Canal 220

Topography 228

Sections 236

7

Pelvis and Retroperitoneal Situs

The **pelvis** (Pelvis) is designed to fulfil two purposes: On the one hand, it has to bear the weight of the viscera in humans exhibiting an erected posture. Hence, a solid, weight bearing, possibly bony floor would be reasonable at the caudal aspect of the abdominal cavity (Cavitas abdominalis). On the other hand, with regards to the elimination of products by the intestines and the kidneys, the act of procreation, and in particular childbirth, a rigid closure is not practical. The "constructive" compromise is the Diaphragma pelvis: a funnel-shaped group of muscles at the bottom of the pelvis, which is perforated in the midsagittal plane by the Urethra, the Rectum, and the Vagina in females.

To review the **retroperitoneal situs of the abdomen** – including the organs, which are not situated in the abdominal cavity, but at the dorsal wall – along with the pelvis, has a good (ontogenetic) reason. The kidneys, the major organs of the retroperitoneal space, initially originate from the pelvis and ascend to a level just inferior to the ribs. Conversely, the gonads, i.e. testicles (Testes) and ovaries (Ovaria), descend from the abdomen into the pelvis and in men even further down into the Scrotum. Thus, the subperitoneal (see below) connective tissue spaces of the pelvis and the retroperitoneal space form a continuum.

In order to gain insight into the regions addressed in the following, radical dissection steps are necessary to some extent: The small and large intestines have to be removed or at least mobilised so that they can be cleared from the posterior abdominal wall. Some dissectors even remove all organs of the epigastric region at once.

The View into the Pelvis

The so-called **greater pelvis** (Pelvis major, between the wings of the ilium) seems to be almost empty after the removal of the intestines. The psoas major muscle (M. psoas major) is accompanied by the Vasa iliaca externa and spans from the lumbar spine down to the inguinal region flanking the entrance to the lesser pelvis (Pelvis minor).

In contrast, the caudally narrowing funnel-shaped **lesser pelvis** is not vacant, especially in women. Ventrally, immediately behind the Symphysis pubica, lies the fundus of the urinary bladder (Vesica urinaria). In women, the Fundus of the Uterus is located immediately posterior to the urinary bladder. Bilaterally, two uterine (FALLOPIAN) tubes (Tubae uterinae) ascend from the Uterus towards the ovaries (Ovaria), which they embrace with their fimbriated projections. The ovaries are located bilaterally at the pelvic wall, just inferior to the boundary between the greater and the lesser pelvis. The rectum (Rectum) is positioned between the urinary bladder, the Uterus, and the dorsal pelvic wall (i.e. the sacrum), respectively.

The body of the Uterus as well as the uterine tubes and the ovaries are located in separate peritoneal duplicatures/mesenteries ("Mesos") in the abdominopelvic cavity **(Cavitas peritonealis pelvis)** which project at various depths towards the actual pelvic floor. In women, there is a particularly deep recess between the rear wall of the Uterus and the frontal wall of the Rectum, the Excavatio rectouterina. The fundus of the bladder and the upper portion of the Rectum are covered by peritoneum. Incising the peritoneum and dissecting the above-mentioned pelvic organs reveals the subperitoneal space of the pelvis **(Spatium extraperitoneale pelvis)**. The lower parts of urinary bladder, Uterus, and Rectum are located within this connective tissue, as well as the female Vagina and the male accessory sex glands (in particular the prostate gland [Prostata] and the seminal vesicles [Glandulae vesiculosae]), respectively. Branches of the A. iliaca interna and numerous nerves that supply the pelvic organs, but also the lower extremities, extend into this subperitoneal connective tissue.

Mobilisation of the blood vessels and organs exposes a muscular pelvic floor, the **Diaphragma pelvis,** which is perforated by the Urethra and Vagina (if present). It is like a deep, laterally compacted funnel. At the deepest point of the cone, the Rectum perforates the funnel. The M. levator ani is the muscle that forms a large part of the pelvic floor, and is able to (voluntarily!) raise and lower the Anus by a few centimetres.

Below the walls of the pelvic diaphragm, virtually in the "basement" of the pelvis, lies the **perineal region** (Regio perinealis): Tracing the urethra (Urethra) one reaches the **anterior perineum,** the urogenital triangle (Regio urogenitalis). The roots of the cavernous bodies of the Penis, which bears the male Urethra, originate in and protrude from this region. This region also encompasses the cavernous bodies of the Clitoris enclosing the opening of the short female Urethra. The posterior perineum, the anal triangle (Regio analis), is located below the pelvic diaphragm to the right or left side of the Rectum. It contains large, adipose-filled pits called Fossae ischioanales. They resemble cranially pointing pyramids with their bases directed caudally with respect to the Rectum. Major nerves and blood vessels are traceable in the Fossae ischioanales, supplying the organs of the perineal region (i.e. Penis, Clitoris, Labia majora and minora, Vestibulum vaginae, and Anus).

View of the Retroperitoneal Situs

Removal of the parietal peritoneum and the underlying adipose tissue first reveals the inferior vena cava (V. cava inferior, slightly to the right side of the vertebral column) and the abdominal aorta (Aorta abdominalis, immediately to the left side). Both are reminiscent of an "upside-down Y", bifurcating at the level of the lower lumbar vertebrae into the Aa. and Vv. iliacae communes, i.e. the iliac arteries and veins. The **V. cava inferior** has several tributaries; in the upper third especially the two renal veins (Vv. renales) and the short hepatic veins (Vv. hepaticae) are remarkable. The **Aorta abdominalis** has likewise many branches. The large vessels are densely covered with lymph nodes and lymph vessels that rise as paired **Trunci lumbales** from the pelvis. At the level of the branching renal vessels, the Trunci lumbales merge in the Cisterna chyli, which also receives the lymph of the intestines, to form the thoracic duct (Ductus thoracicus).

The **kidneys** (Renes) and the adrenal glands are located bilaterally in a perirenal fat capsule (Capsula adiposa) just below the diaphragmatic dome. Dorsal to the upper pole of each kidney lies rib XII. Medially, the Vasa renalia enter the kidneys at the hilum. The **Ureter** exits at the hilum descending into the pelvis along with the vessels of the gonads. The vessels of the gonads arise from the Aorta and enter – in a fascinating asymmetrical fashion (and therefore popular as an exam question) – the left renal vein and the V. cava inferior. Above and medial to the upper pole of the kidneys are the **adrenal (suprarenal) glands** (Glandulae suprarenales) which constitute endocrine glands that produce steroid hormones (e.g. cortisol) and catecholamines (adrenaline [epinephrine]).

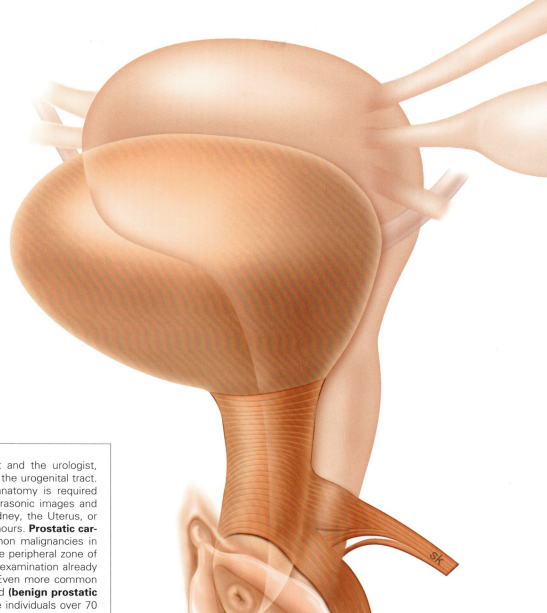

Clinical Remarks

Two medical specialists, the gynaecologist and the urologist, are involved in the treatment of diseases of the urogenital tract. Detailed knowledge of the topographical anatomy is required for the interpretation of radiological and ultrasonic images and during surgery, such as resection of the kidney, the Uterus, or the prostate gland in cases of malignant tumours. **Prostatic carcinomas** are among the three most common malignancies in men. Because they usually develop from the peripheral zone of the prostate gland, the simple digital rectal examination already provides important diagnostic information. Even more common are the benign tumours of the prostate gland **(benign prostatic hyperplasia)** which occur in almost all male individuals over 70 years of age. Since the hyperplasia occurs in the transitional zone of the gland surrounding the Urethra, problems with micturition are early symptoms. In women, **inflammatory processes of the uterine (FALLOPIAN) tube and the ovary** need to be considered in addition to an appendicitis as potential causes of pain in the right lower abdomen. These examples demonstrate the clinical relevance of topographical anatomy of the pelvis.

→ *Dissection Link*

It is useful to dissect the pelvis from the outside and from the inside in order to trace pathways that emerge from the pelvis. The Regio glutealis, the Regio perinealis with the Fossa ischioanalis, and the perineal cavities including all pathways are dissected **from the outside. From the inside,** the parietal peritoneum is removed together with the perirenal fat capsule including the anterior fascia up to the lesser pelvis. Kidneys and adrenal glands are exposed from the Capsula adiposa; the Ureter and the retroperitoneal neurovascular struckutres with their branches are traced. For proper dissection of the pelvis, it is useful to perform a midsagittal cut in order to split the pelvis into two equal parts. The urinary bladder and the Rectum are mobilised from the connective tissue of the subperitoneal space but remain attached to the blood vessels. The branches of the A. iliaca interna are to be presented as a whole. Some branches exit the pelvis via the Foramina suprapiriforme and infrapiriforme and enter the Regio glutealis and the Regio perinealis. At last, the pelvic floor with its muscle layers is exposed.

EXAM CHECK LIST

• Development: kidney, internal and external genitalia (major steps) • topography: positional relationships of the organs in the retroperitoneal space and the pelvis, composition of the pelvic floor, organisation of the Regio perinealis, sectional imaging with CT • organs: all organs with neurovascular pathways including the lymphatic drainage (in particular Testis and Ovarium), Anus (including zones) and continence organ, organisation of the Ureter and Urethra with constrictions, Uterus and ligaments, Corpora cavernosa penis with erection, male accessory sex glands with excretory ducts • vascular pathways: Aorta with branches, V. cava inferior with tributaries, Ductus thoracicus with lymphatic trunks, Plexus lumbosacralis with individual nerves and autonomic nerve plexuses around the Aorta

7 Pelvis and Retroperitoneal Space

Kidney and adrenal gland →

Organisation of the urinary system

Fig. 7.1 and Fig. 7.2 Organisation of the male (→ Fig. 7.1) and the female (→ Fig. 7.2) urinary system; lateral view from the left side.
The urinary system comprises the paired kidneys (Ren [Nephros]), producing the urine, and the efferent urinary tracts. These consist of:
- renal pelvis (Pelvis renalis)
- Ureter
- urinary bladder (Vesica urinaria)
- Urethra

Except for the Urethra, the urinary system is constructed identically in both sexes. The Urethra within the male penis provides the exit of urine as well as semen. Thus, the male Urethra also belongs to the external male genitalia.

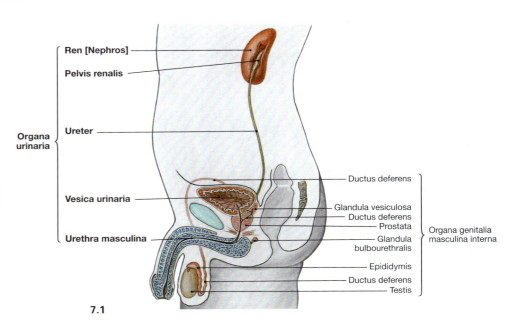

7.1

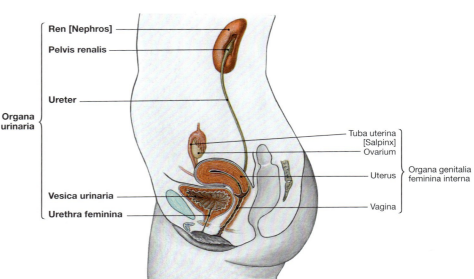

7.2

Figs. 7.3a and b Male and female endocrine organs; ventral view.
The adrenal gland (Glandula suprarenalis) does not belong to the urinary organs but to the endocrine glands. Several vital steroid hormones such as aldosterone (mineralocorticoid) and cortisol (glucocorticoid), as well as catecholamines (epinephrine and norepinephrine) are produced in the cortex and medulla, respectively, and released into the blood.
Since the adrenal glands are adjacent to the kidneys and are, in part, supplied by the same neurovascular structures, the adrenal gland is discussed here, too.

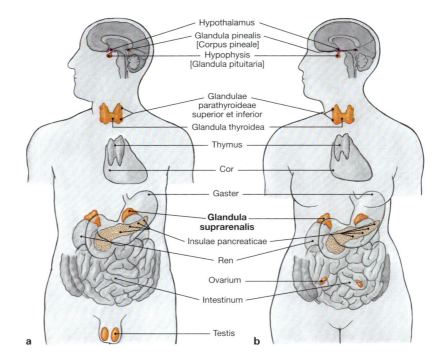

Efferent urinary system → Genitalia → Rectum and anal canal → Topography → Sections

Projection of kidney and adrenal gland

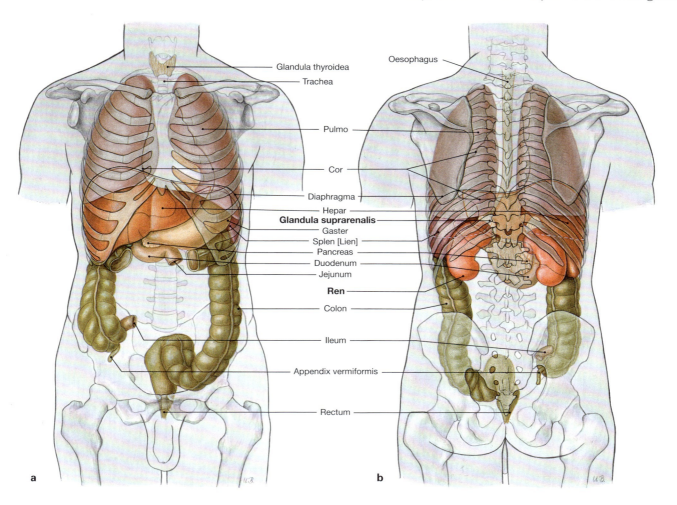

Figs. 7.4a and b Projection of the viscera onto the body surface; ventral (**a**) and dorsal (**b**) views.
Kidneys and adrenal glands are located in a **retroperitoneal position**. The adrenal glands are adjacent to the superior pole of the kidneys and are embedded in the common adipose capsule (Capsula adiposa), which is further enclosed in a sheath of connective tissue (Fascia renalis, GEROTA's fascia).

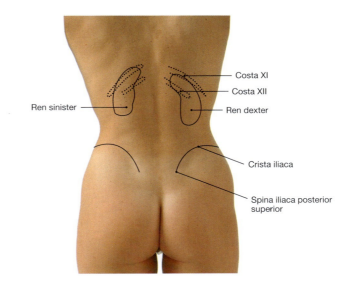

Fig. 7.5 Projection of the kidney onto the dorsal body wall.
- superior pole: 12th thoracic vertebra, rib XI
- hilum: 2nd lumbar vertebra
- inferior pole: 3rd lumbar vertebra

These positions only apply for the left kidney.
Due to the size of the liver, the right kidney is located about half a vertebra further down. The superior pole is thus positioned just below rib XI
Because of the proximity of the diaphragm, the position of both kidneys changes during respiration and moves about 3 cm lower during inspiration. The adrenal glands project onto the heads of ribs XI and XII.

Clinical Remarks

During physical examination a first step in assessing the pain sensitivity of the kidneys may be a well-dosed punch into the region of the kidneys in the flanks just below the inferior margin of the rib cage. However, the patients must not be warned in advance to prevent tension of the back muscles which would result in a cushioning of the impact. In the case of an inflammation of the renal pelvis (pyelonephritis), the patient will wince and report considerable pain in response to the punch. Even if carried out correctly, this examination can challenge the relationship between patient and physician.

7 Pelvis and Retroperitoneal Space

Kidney and adrenal gland →

Development of the kidney

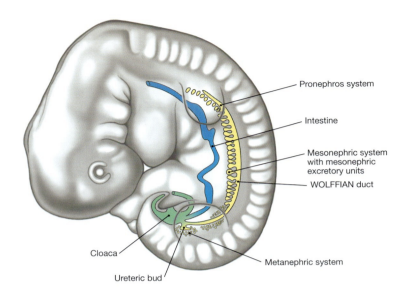

Fig. 7.6 Development of the kidneys in week 5. (according to [1])
The kidneys and the efferent urinary tract derive from the mesoderm which, next to the somites, forms **nephrogenic** cell clusters referred to as nephrotomes. These successively give rise to **three kidney generations** which are from cranial to caudal:
- **pronephros:** first generation of a rudimentary kidney which completely regresses.
- **mesonephros:** temporary excretory tubules are formed, but with the exception of the mesonephric duct (WOLFFIAN duct) the mesonephros also regresses. Its distal part contributes to the formation of the efferent ductules between Testis and Epididymis.
- **metanephros:** beginning in week 5, the ureteric bud from the WOLFFIAN duct induces the development of the parenchyma of the permanent kidney (nephrons) in the metanephric mesoderm. The collecting ducts and the proximal parts of the efferent urinary tract (renal pelvis and Ureter) develop from the ureteric bud.

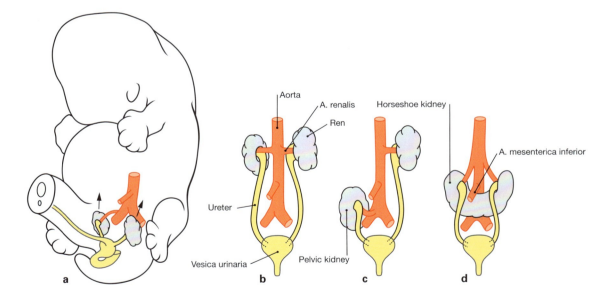

Figs. 7.7a to d Ascensus of the kidneys. (according to [1])
The metanephros develops at the level of the 1st to 4th sacral vertebrae and ascends during weeks 6 to 9 of development. In fact, this is a relative ascensus since the part of the developing body caudal to the inferior pole of the kidney grows faster (**a** and **b**). If the kidneys fail to ascend, a pelvic kidney (**c**) is present. A horseshoe kidney develops if both inferior renal poles position in close proximity to each other and fuse (**d**). The horseshoe kidney does not fully ascend because the root of the A. mesenterica inferior presents an obstacle.

Clinical Remarks

Pelvic kidneys and **horseshoe kidneys** are usually accidental findings and have no clinical relevance if the Ureter is not compromised. However, displacements of the Ureter may cause an urine stasis with resulting hydronephrosis and potential ascending urinary tract infections. These may cause damage to the kidney.

Efferent urinary system → Genitalia → Rectum and anal canal → Topography → Sections

Development of the urogenital organs

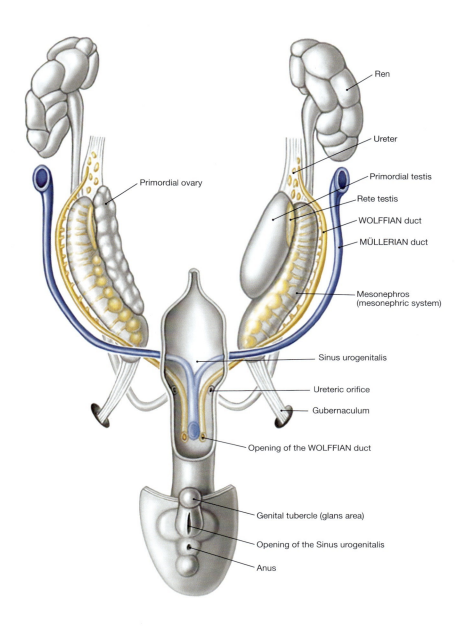

Fig. 7.8 Development of the urinary organs and early development of the internal genital organs in both sexes during week 8. (according to [1])
The kidneys develop from the metanephros and the ureteric bud which arises from the WOLFFIAN duct. The ureteric bud gives rise to the proximal efferent urinary tract (renal pelvis and Ureter) whereas the urinary bladder and the Urethra develop from the Sinus urogenitalis (ventral part of the cloaca of the hindgut).
Until week 7, the internal genitalia develop in a similar manner in men and women (sexually indifferent stage). Besides the indifferent gonads, two parallel duct systems exist: the Ductus mesonephricus or **WOLFFIAN duct** and the Ductus paramesonephricus or **MÜLLERIAN duct**. In contrast to the WOLFFIAN duct, the distal ends of the MÜLLERIAN duct fuse prior to entering the Sinus urogenitalis. At the end of week 7 the indifferent gonad develops into the Testis and into the ovary, respectively. The hormones toproduced in the Testis (testosterone and anti-MÜLLERIAN hormone) induce the differentiation of the WOLFFIAN duct to the male internal genitalia (→ Fig. 7.43) and the suppression of the further development of the MÜLLERIAN duct. If both hormones are not present, female internal genitalia develop (→ Fig. 7.73).

Pelvis and Retroperitoneal Space

Kidney and adrenal gland →

Topography of the kidney and adrenal gland

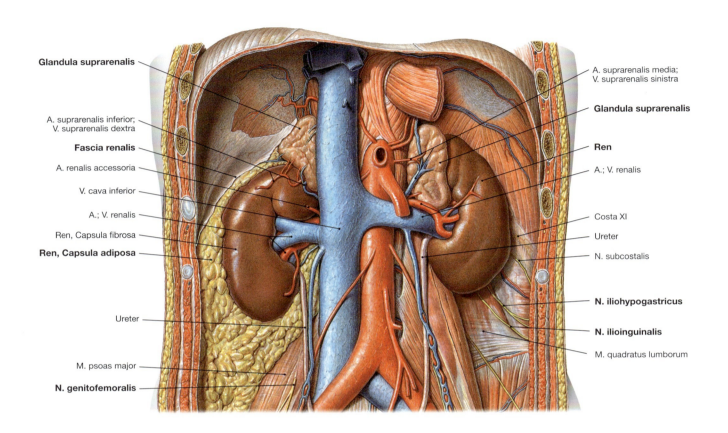

Fig. 7.9 Position of the kidney, Ren [Nephros], and adrenal gland, Glandula suprarenalis, in the retroperitoneal space; ventral view.
Kidney and adrenal gland are located in the retroperitoneal space ventrally of the M. psoas and the M. quadratus lumborum.
Fascial systems: The surface of the kidney is covered by an organ capsule of dense connective tissue (Capsula fibrosa). Together with the adrenal gland, the kidney is covered by a capsule of perinephric fat (Capsula adiposa). The perinephritic adipose tissue is surrounded by a connective tissue sheath (Fascia renalis). Medially and inferiorly, the renal fascia remains open for the passage of the Ureter and the blood vessels. The anterior lamina of the renal fascia is referred to by clinicians as GEROTA's fascia.

Proximity to the nerves of the Plexus lumbalis: Between the renal fascia in the area of the inferior renal pole and the muscles of the dorsal abdominal wall, the N. iliohypogastricus and the N. ilioinguinalis from the Plexus lumbosacralis descend. They provide sensory innervation to the skin of the inguinal region. The N. genitofemoralis courses further caudally and therefore has no contact to the kidney, but to the Ureter. Further cranially, the 11th and 12th intercostal nerves (12th intercostal nerve = N. subcostalis) course beneath the lower ribs along the posterior side of the kidney.

Clinical Remarks

The fascial systems and the topographical relationships of the kidneys are clinically relevant. In cases of **malignant tumours**, the kidney is always removed together with the adrenal gland and including the GEROTA's fascia (nephrectomy).

The close proximity of the kidney to the N. iliohypogastricus and N. ilioinguinalis explains why certain diseases of the kidney such as inflammation of the renal pelvis (pyelonephritis) or concrements in the renal pelvis (nephrolithiasis) may cause **radiating pain into the inguinal region.**

Segments and topographical relationships of the kidney

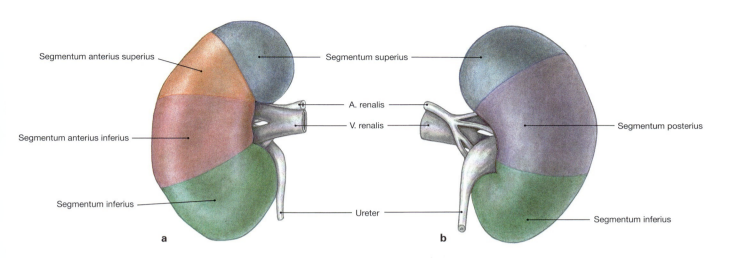

Figs. 7.10a and b Renal segments, Segmenta renalia, right side; ventral (**a**) and dorsal (**b**) views.
The renal artery (A. renalis) divides at the hilum of the kidney into a R. principalis anterior, which supplies the superior, the two anterior and the inferior renal segments with several branches, and the R. principalis posterior for the posterior segment. In the case of occlusion of one of the branches of the A. renalis, the extent of **renal infarction** correlates to the area of the affected renal segments. However, the branching patterns are highly variable among individuals.

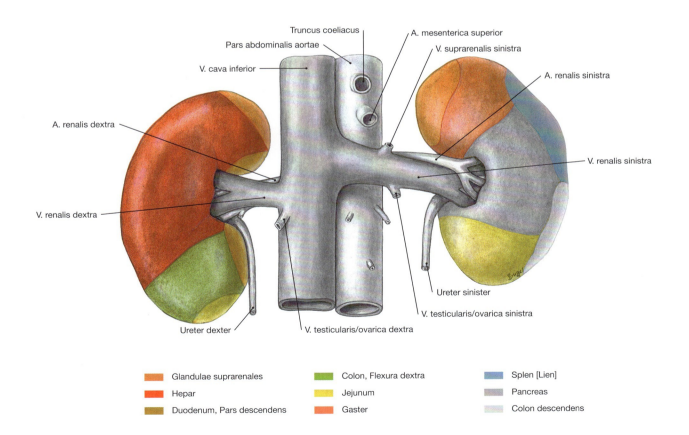

Fig. 7.11 Contact areas of the kidney, Ren [Nephros], with adjacent organs; ventral view.
The dorsal side of the kidney is adjacent to the dorsal abdominal wall. The anterior side has contact to several other organs. Together with the adrenal glands, the kidneys are separated from the other abdominal organs by the parietal peritoneum, the renal fascia, and the adipose capsule. Thus, the anterior contact areas have no clinical relevance.

Pelvis and Retroperitoneal Space

Organisation of the kidney

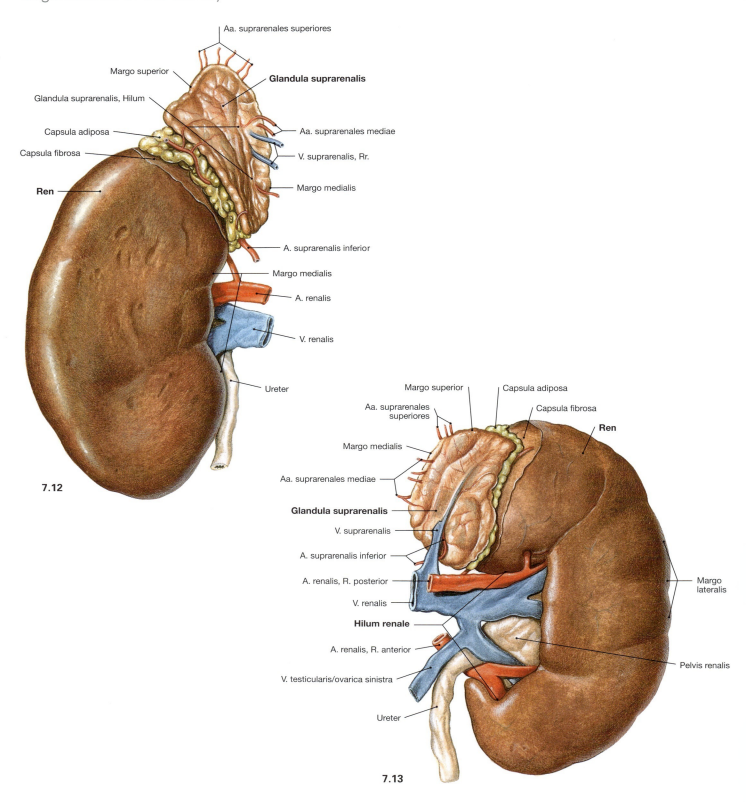

Fig. 7.12 and Fig. 7.13 Kidney, Ren [Nephros], and adrenal gland, Glandula suprarenalis, right side (→ Fig. 7.12) and left side (→ Fig. 7.13); ventral view.

The bean-shaped kidney has a superior and an inferior pole. Located between the poles and oriented medially is the hilum of the kidney (Hilum renale) which connects to the inner space of the kidney (Sinus renalis) and contains the renal blood vessels and the Ureter. The adrenal gland is adjacent to the superior pole of the kidney. The entrance of the blood vessels at the medial margin is sometimes also referred to as the hilum.

Efferent urinary system → Genitalia → Rectum and anal canal → Topography → Sections

Organisation of the kidney

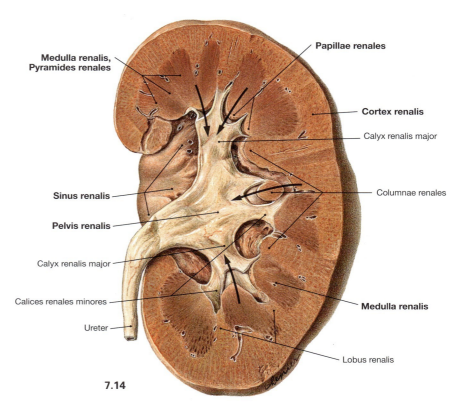

7.14

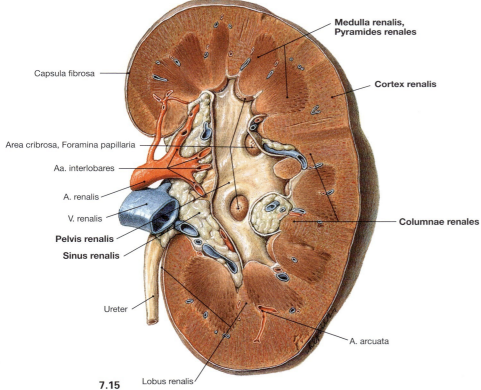

7.15

Fig. 7.14 and Fig. 7.15 Kidney, Ren [Nephros], left side; ventral view; after vertical bisection (→ Fig. 7.14) and opening of the renal pelvis (→ Fig. 7.15).

The kidney consists of a **cortex** (Cortex renalis) and a **medulla** (Medulla renalis). The medulla is subdivided into several parts which, according to their shape, are referred to as renal **pyramids** (Pyramides renales). Located between these renal pyramids are the renal columns (Columnae renales). One pyramid and its adjacent cortical area is called a **renal lobe** (Lobus renalis). The border between the 14 lobes is not visible at the surface of an adult human kidney. The tips of the pyramids (Papillae renales) enter the **renal calyces** (Calices renales majores and minores) to release the urine (arrows). Together with adipose tissue and the renal blood vessels, the **renal pelvis** (Pelvis renalis) is located in a medial recess of the parenchyma of the kidney (Sinus renalis).

167

Pelvis and Retroperitoneal Space

Organisation of the kidney

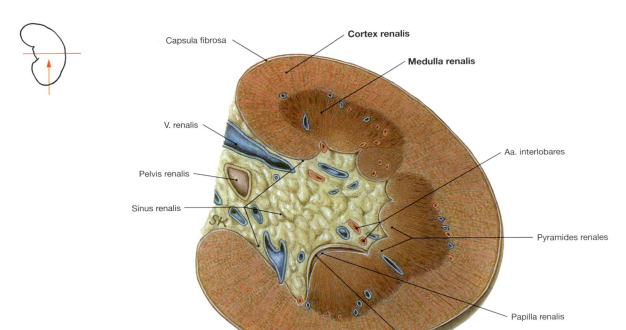

Fig. 7.16 Kidney, Ren [Nephros]; transverse section through the renal sinus (Sinus renalis); caudal view.

The parenchyma of the kidney is composed of a cortex (Cortex renalis) and a medulla (Medulla renalis).

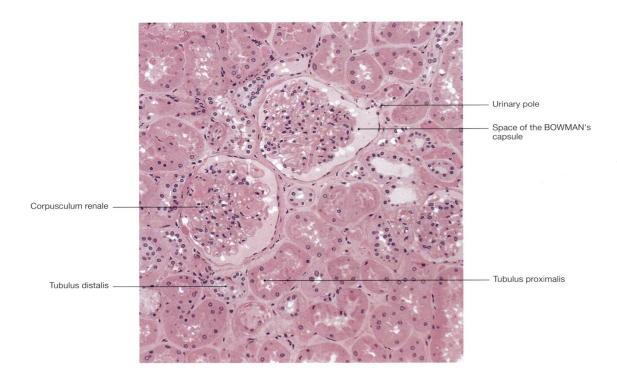

Fig. 7.17 Renal cortex (Cortex renalis); microscopic section, 100-fold. [26]

The entire parenchyma of the kidney consists of nephrons and collecting ducts. Nephrons comprise renal corpuscles and a tubular system. Renal corpuscles (Corpuscula renalia) are located in the renal cortex, but not in the renal medulla. In the renal corpuscles, water and low molecular weight constituents from the plasma are filtered into the space of the BOWMAN's capsule (primary urine, 170 l/day). From the urinary pole of the BOWMAN's capsule, the primary urine enters the proximal tubule (Tubulus proximalis). In the tubular system and the collecting ducts the major part of the primary urine is reabsorbed and the urine composition is altered by secretion before the final urine is released into the renal papillae and the renal pelvis (1.7 l/day).

Organisation of the kidney

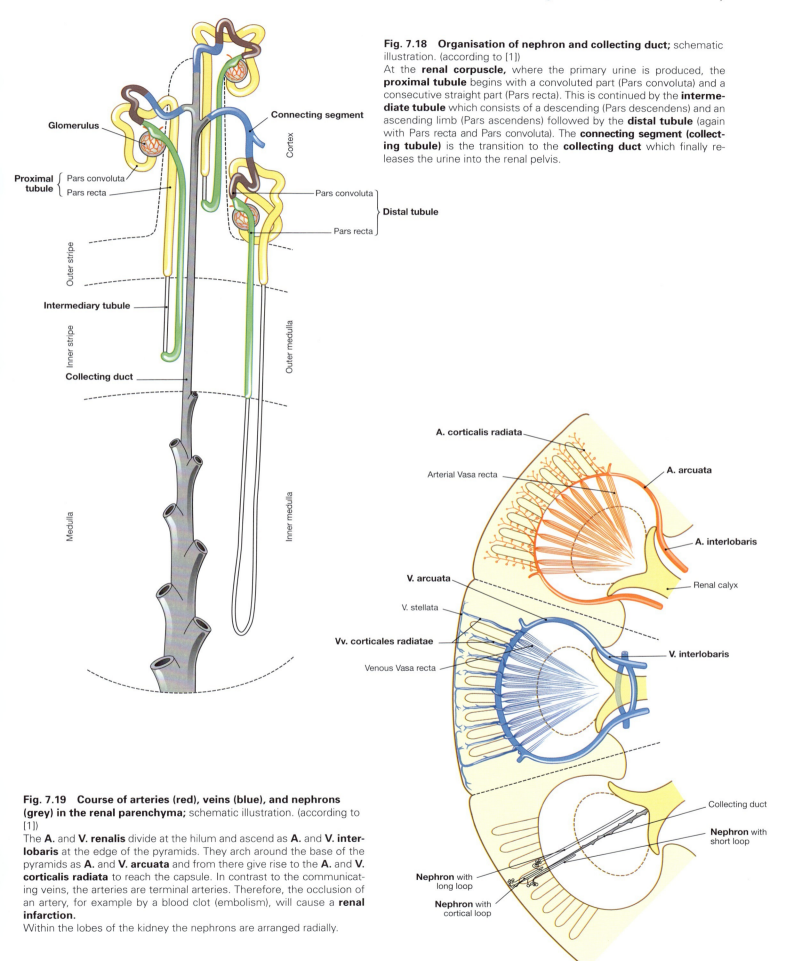

Fig. 7.18 Organisation of nephron and collecting duct; schematic illustration. (according to [1])
At the **renal corpuscle,** where the primary urine is produced, the **proximal tubule** begins with a convoluted part (Pars convoluta) and a consecutive straight part (Pars recta). This is continued by the **intermediate tubule** which consists of a descending (Pars descendens) and an ascending limb (Pars ascendens) followed by the **distal tubule** (again with Pars recta and Pars convoluta). The **connecting segment (collecting tubule)** is the transition to the **collecting duct** which finally releases the urine into the renal pelvis.

Fig. 7.19 Course of arteries (red), veins (blue), and nephrons (grey) in the renal parenchyma; schematic illustration. (according to [1])
The **A.** and **V. renalis** divide at the hilum and ascend as **A.** and **V. interlobaris** at the edge of the pyramids. They arch around the base of the pyramids as **A.** and **V. arcuata** and from there give rise to the **A.** and **V. corticalis radiata** to reach the capsule. In contrast to the communicating veins, the arteries are terminal arteries. Therefore, the occlusion of an artery, for example by a blood clot (embolism), will cause a **renal infarction.**
Within the lobes of the kidney the nephrons are arranged radially.

Pelvis and Retroperitoneal Space

Kidney and adrenal gland →

Organisation of the adrenal gland

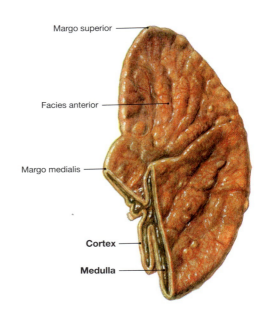

Fig. 7.20 Adrenal gland, Glandula suprarenalis, right side; ventral view.
The adrenal gland consists of cortex and medulla. Both have different developmental origins and functions. The cortex develops from the mesoderm of the dorsal abdominal cavity (intra-embryonic coeloma), the medulla, however, derives from neural crest cells and is equivalent to a modified sympathetic ganglion.

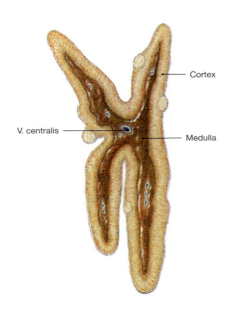

Fig. 7.21 Adrenal gland, Glandula suprarenalis, right side; sagittal section; lateral view.
The adrenal gland is a vital endocrine gland. The **cortex** produces **steroid hormones** (mineralocorticoids, glucocorticoids, androgens), the **medulla** produces **catecholamines** (epinephrine and norepinephrine) for the regulation of metabolism and blood pressure.

Clinical Remarks

If both adrenal glands have to be removed due to disease, the substitution with mineralocorticoids and glucocorticoids is essential to prevent **life-threatening conditions** such as hypoglycaemic shock or severely low blood pressure (arterial hypotension). Adrenocortical insufficiency (ADDISON's disease) may cause the same symptoms.

Efferent Urinary system → genitalia → Rectum and anal canal → Topography → Sections

Blood vessels of the kidney

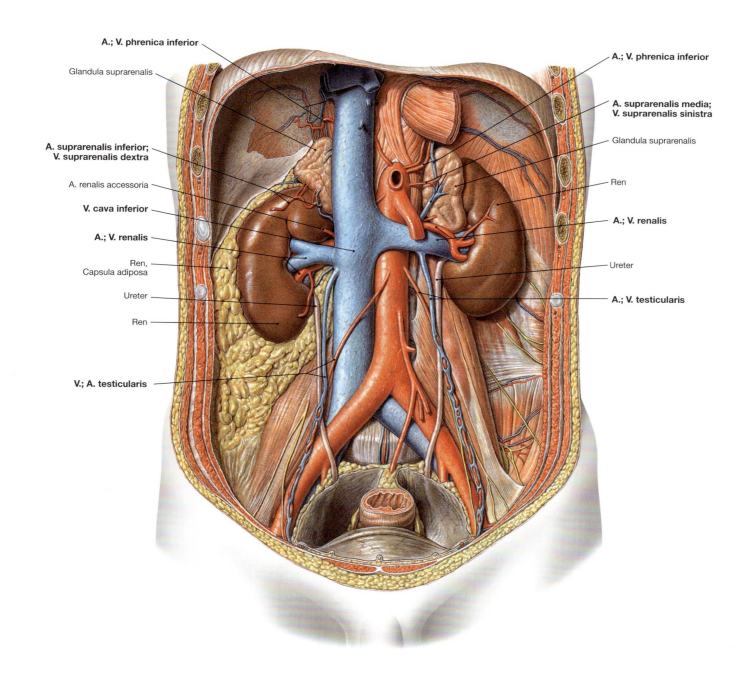

Fig. 7.22 Course of the A. and V. renalis; ventral view.
The paired **Aa. renales** arise from the abdominal aorta and course dorsal to the veins to the hilum of the kidney. The right A. renalis crosses the V. cava inferior posteriorly. At the hilum, they divide into several branches.
The **Vv. renales** drain into the V. cava inferior on both sides. The **left** V. renalis receives blood from three tributaries, whereas on the right side these veins enter the V. cava inferior directly:
- V. suprarenalis sinistra
- V. testicularis/ovarica sinistra
- V. phrenica inferior sinistra

The **regional lymph nodes** of the kidney are the Nodi lymphoidei lumbales around the aorta and the V. cava inferior.
The postganglionic **sympathetic nerves** to the kidney derive from the Ganglion aorticorenale and form the Plexus renalis around the A. renalis.

Clinical Remarks

Renal cell carcinoma frequently obstruct the renal veins and may, in case of a tumour on the left side, cause a venous blood stasis in the left testicular vein resulting in the dilation of testicular veins (**varicocele**) in the left Scrotum. Therefore, a varicocele on the left side always requires the exclusion of a renal cell carcinoma!

Pelvis and Retroperitoneal Space

Kidney and adrenal gland →

Blood vessels of kidney and adrenal gland

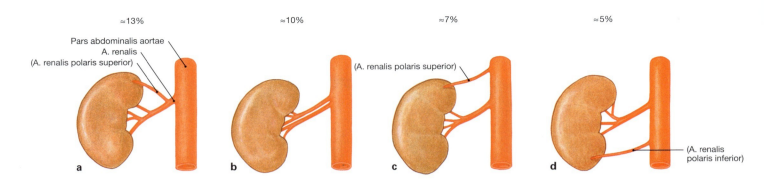

Figs. 7.23a to d Variations of the arterial supply of the kidney; ventral view.
Polar arteries do not enter the kidney at the hilum, but reach the renal parenchyma directly. **Accessory arteries** independently arise from the Aorta.

a A. renalis with a branch as superior polar artery
b two Aa. renales to the hilum of the kidney
c accessory superior polar artery
d accessory inferior polar artery

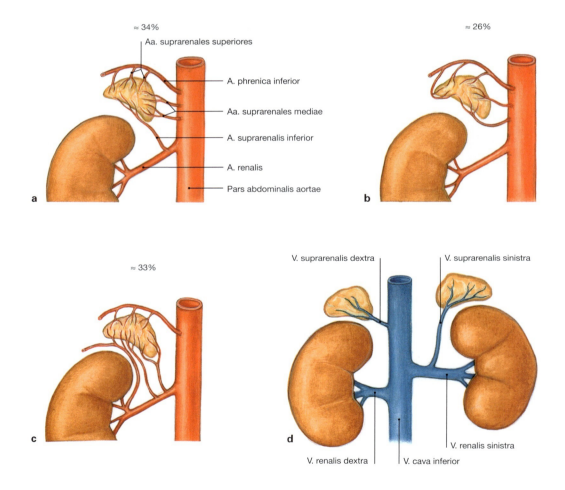

Fig. 7.24a to d Suprarenal arteries, Aa. suprarenales, and suprarenal vein, V. suprarenalis; ventral view.
Usually there are three arteries to the adrenal gland:
- A. suprarenalis superior: derives from the A. phrenica inferior
- A. suprarenalis media: arises directly from the Aorta
- A. suprarenalis inferior: branch of the A. renalis

This "luxurious" arterial supply prevents infarctions of the vital adrenal gland.
Variations of the arteries to the adrenal gland:
a arterial supply via three arteries (textbook case)
b arterial supply without tributary from the A. renalis
c arterial supply without a direct branch of the Aorta

In contrast, **only one suprarenal vein** exists for each adrenal gland. The V. suprarenalis collects the blood from the adrenal gland and drains into the V. cava inferior on the right side, and into the V. renalis sinistra on the left side (**d**).
The **regional lymph nodes** of the adrenal gland are the Nodi lymphoidei lumbales around the aorta and V. cava inferior.
The **autonomic innervation** derives from preganglionic (!) sympathetic nerve fibres from the Nn. splanchnici (the adrenal medulla represents a sympathetic paraganglion).

Kidney, imaging

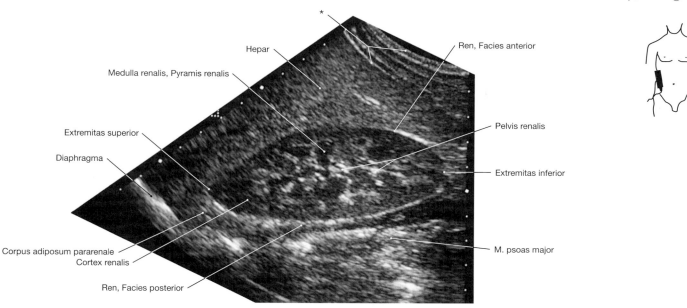

Fig. 7.25 Kidney, Ren [Nephros], right side; ultrasound image; lateral view; transducer positioned almost vertically.

* abdominal wall

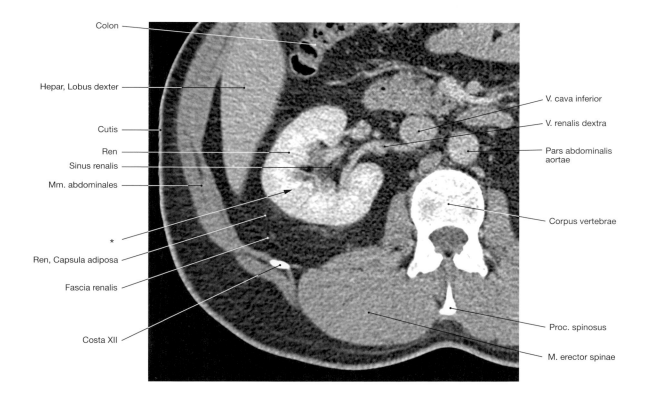

Fig. 7.26 Kidney, Ren [Nephros]; right side; computed tomographic transverse section (CT); caudal view.
CT-guided renal biopsies are performed to obtain tissue specimens for diagnostic purposes in cases of obscure dysfunctions of the kidney.

* direction of the needle for renal biopsy, also named fine needle aspiration biopsy (FNAB).

Clinical Remarks

Ultrasound (sonography) is a suitable imaging technique to visualise the kidneys. It enables the detection of solid or cystic tumours.
CT-imaging is performed in cases of undefined ultrasound findings, or to assess lymph node metastases or the invasion of tumours into the renal veins.

7 Pelvis and Retroperitoneal Space

Kidney and adrenal gland →

Renal pelvis and ureter

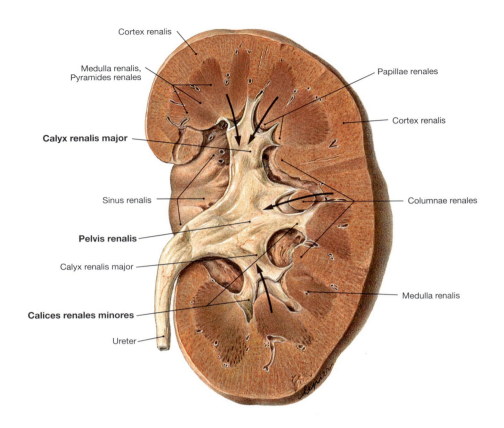

Fig. 7.27 Renal pelvis, Pelvis renalis, left side; ventral view. Urine is released from the renal pyramids to the renal calyces (Calices renales; arrows).

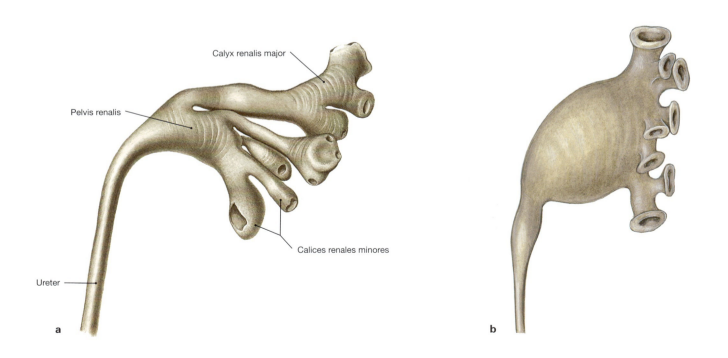

Figs. 7.28a and b Renal pelvis, Pelvis renalis, left side; mould preparation; ventral view.

According to the width and the length of the renal calyces, a dendritic (**a**) and an ampullary (**b**) type of renal pelvis are distinguished.

Ureter

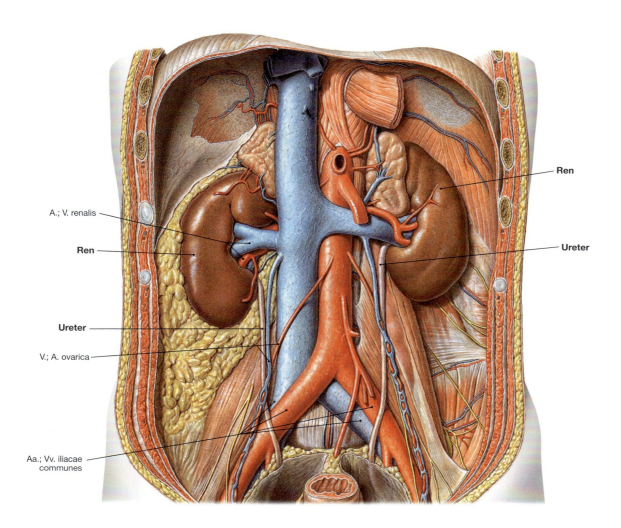

Fig. 7.29 Parts, constrictions, and course of the ureter; ventral view.

Parts:
- Pars abdominalis: in the retroperitoneal space
- Pars pelvica: in the lesser pelvis
- Pars intramuralis: traverses the wall of the urinary bladder

Constrictions:
- at the exit from the renal pelvis
- at the crossing of the A. iliaca communis or A. iliaca externa
- at the passage through the wall of the urinary bladder (most narrow part)

Course:
the ureter first crosses **over** the N. genitofemoralis, courses **under** the A. and V. testicularis/ovarica, crosses **over** the A. and V. iliaca and then crosses **under** and passes beneath the Ductus deferens in men and the A. uterina in women.

Clinical Remarks

Renal concrements may dislodge, descend in the ureter and get stuck at the ureteric constrictions. This causes intense, colic-like pain (ureteral colic).

The close proximity of the ureter to the uterine artery has to be considered in **hysterectomies** to avoid ligation of the ureter during surgery. The resulting urine stasis would irreversibly damage the affected kidney.

7 Pelvis and Retroperitoneal Space

Kidney and adrenal gland →

Renal pelvis and ureter, imaging

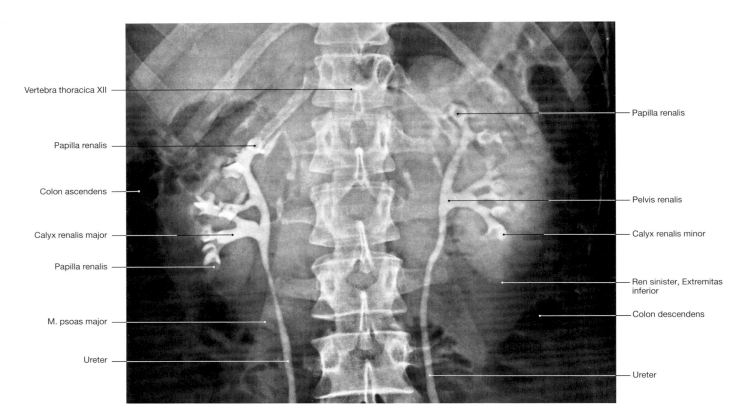

Fig. 7.30 Renal pelvis, Pelvis renalis, and ureter, Ureter; radiograph in anteroposterior (AP) beam projection after retrograde injection of contrast medium via both ureters; ventral view.

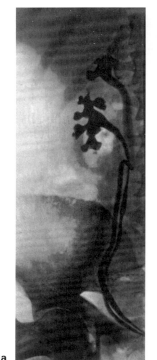
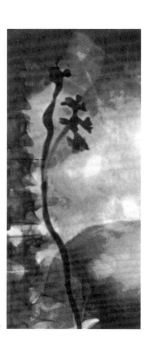

Figs. 7.31a and b Common variations of the ureter, Ureter; radiographs in anteroposterior (AP) beam projection after retrograde injection of contrast medium via both ureters; ventral view. [18]
a double ureter (Ureter duplex)
b split ureter (Ureter fissus)
In both cases two renal pelvises are present.

Clinical Remarks

The **Ureter fissus** often is an accidental finding and has no clinical relevance. In contrast, cases of an **Ureter duplex** are frequently accompanied with malformations of the ureteric opening into the urinary bladder, a condition potentially causing reflux of urine or incontinence. Frequently, both ureters cross each other (MEYER-WEIGERT rule). As a rule, the Ureter from the superior renal pelvis enters the urinary bladder more inferiorly or even directly enters the Urethra resulting in urinary incontinence. The Ureter from the lower renal pelvis often has a much shorter intramural part within the wall of the urinary bladder, facilitating reflux of urine. Urine reflux promotes ascending urinary tract infections potentially resulting in permanent damage to the kidney parenchyma.

Structure of the urinary bladder

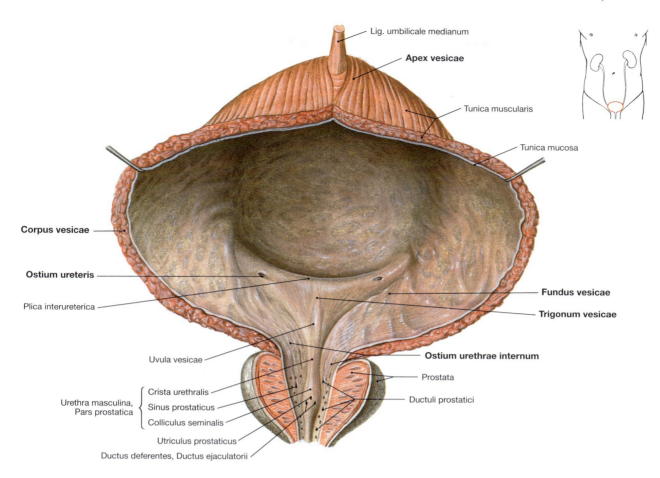

Fig. 7.32 Urinary bladder, Vesica urinaria, and opening into the male urethra, Urethra; ventral view.
The urinary bladder is located in the **subperitoneal space** and is composed of a body (Corpus vesicae), apex (Apex vesicae), and an inferior fundus (Fundus vesicae). At the fundus, the internal urethral orifice (Ostium urethrae internum) and the two ureteric orifices (Ostium ureteris) form the **trigone of the bladder** (Trigonum vesicae). The urinary bladder holds about 500–1500 ml of urine, although the urge to urinate starts when a volume of 250–500 ml is reached. The wall consists of the internal mucosal layer (Tunica mucosa) followed by three layers of smooth muscles with parasympathetic innervation (Tunica muscularis = M. detrusor vesicae), and the external Tunica adventitia or the cranial Tunica serosa (peritoneum), respectively.
The urinary bladder is surrounded by paravesical adipose tissue and stabilised by several **ligaments.** At the apex, the Lig. umbilicale medianum (contains the urachus, a remnant of the embryonic connection of the allantois) connects to the Umbilicus. In women, the bilateral Lig. pubovesicale (→ Fig. 7.116) and in men the bilateral Lig. puboprostaticum (→ Fig. 7.115) anchor the bladder to the bony pelvis. In men, the prostate gland is located directly beneath the fundus of the bladder and is traversed by the Urethra.

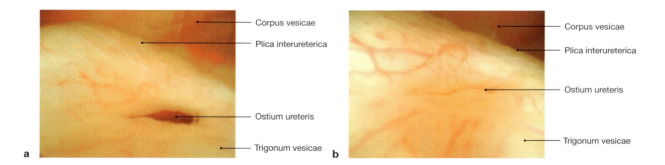

Figs. 7.33 a and b Ureteric orifice, Ostium ureteris; cystoscopy.
a opened ureteric orifice, a peristaltic wave has released urine into the bladder
b closed ureteric orifice

The valve-like shape of the ureteric orifice contributes substantially to the prevention of urine backflow which may endanger the kidneys via ascending urinary tract infections.

Pelvis and Retroperitoneal Space

Kidney and adrenal gland →

Urinary bladder and urethra in men

Fig. 7.34 Urinary bladder, Vesica urinaria, vas deferens, Ductus deferentes, seminal vesicle, Glandula vesiculosa, and prostate gland, Prostata; dorsal view.
In men, the following paired anatomical structures are positioned posterior and adjacent to the bladder, from **medial to lateral**:
- dilated part of the vas deferens (Ampulla ductus deferentis)
- seminal vesicle (Glandula vesiculosa)
- Ureter

The urinary bladder is positioned directly superior to the prostate gland.

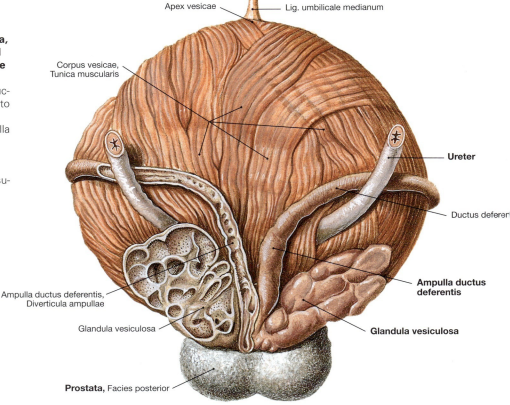

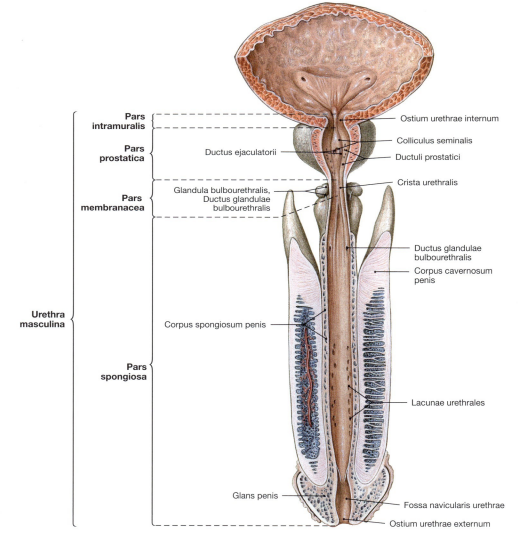

Fig. 7.35 Urinary bladder, Vesica urinaria, and male urethra, Urethra masculina; ventral view; urinary bladder and Urethra opened ventrally.

Parts of the Urethra:
- **Pars intramuralis** (1 cm): within the wall of the urinary bladder
- **Pars prostatica** (3.5 cm): traverses the prostate gland. Here the following ducts enter the Urethra: Ductus ejaculatorii (common duct of vas deferens and seminal vesicle) on the Colliculus seminalis and the prostatic ducts on both sides.
- **Pars membranacea** (1–2 cm): traverses the pelvic floor.
- **Pars spongiosa** (15 cm): embedded in the Corpus spongiosum of the Penis, runs to the external urethral orifice (Ostium urethrae externum). COWPER's glands (Glandulae bulbourethrales) and LITTRÉ's glands (Glandulae urethrales) enter here. The terminal part is dilated to form the Fossa navicularis.

The Urethra has the following **constrictions**:
- Ostium urethrae internum
- Pars membranaceae
- Ostium urethrae externum

Urethra in men

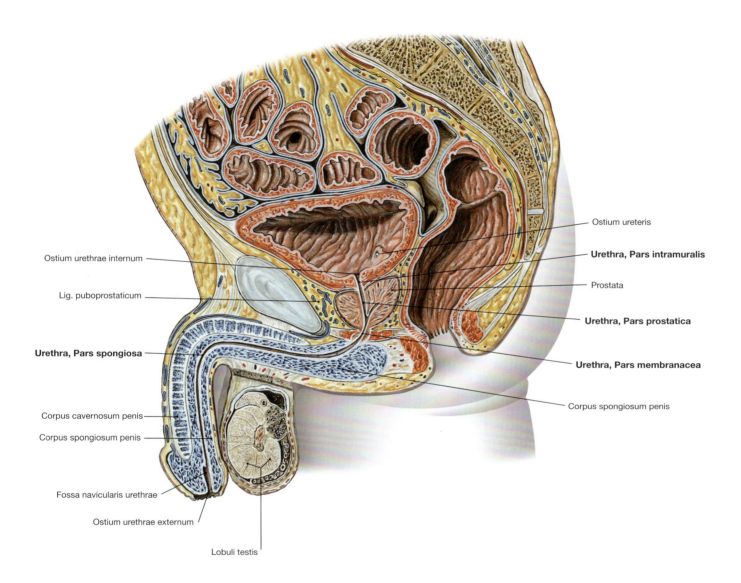

Fig. 7.36 Male pelvis, Pelvis; median section; view from the left side.
The illustration shows the course and the parts of the male Urethra (Urethra masculina):
- **Pars intramuralis:** within the wall of the urinary bladder
- **Pars prostatica:** traverses the prostate gland
- **Pars membranacea:** penetrates the pelvic floor
- **Pars spongiosa:** embedded in the Corpus spongiosum of the Penis, exits at the Glans penis

The Urethra has two **bends:**
- at the transition from Pars membranacea to Pars spongiosa
- in the middle part of the Pars spongiosa

Pelvis and Retroperitoneal Space

Urethra in women

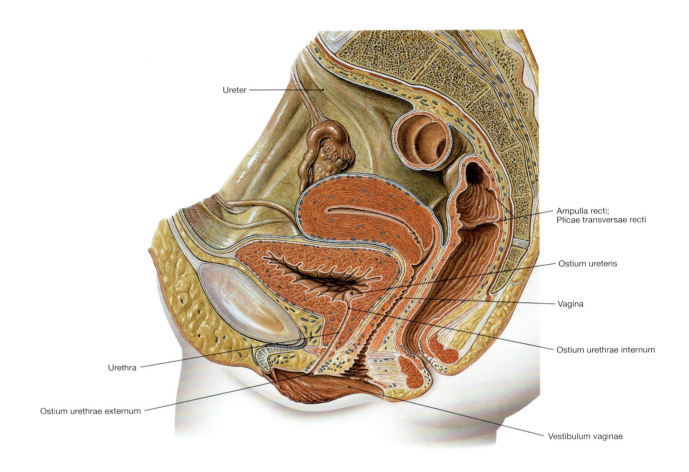

Fig. 7.37 Female pelvis, Pelvis; median section; view from the left side.
The illustration shows the course and the external orifice of the female urethra. The female urethra is 3–5 cm long and enters directly in front of the Vagina in the vestibule (Vestibulum vaginae).

Clinical Remarks

Because of the shorter length of the female Urethra, ascending infections of the urinary bladder **(cystitis)** are more common in women than in men.
Positioning of a **transurethral catheter** is easier in women due to the straight course of the shorter Urethra. However, it has to be considered that the urethral orifice in the vestibule is located **ventral** to the Vagina.

In men, the bends of the Urethra have to be straightened prior to inserting a catheter to avoid painful perforations in the area of the Pars membranacea or the Pars prostatica with consecutive profuse bleedings. First, the Penis is straightened to compensate for the kink in the Pars spongiosa of the penile Urethra, then the catheter is inserted until the resistance from the second bend in the Pars membranacea is noticed. To straighten it, the Penis is positioned downwards between the thighs before the catheter is carefully advanced further into the bladder.

Sphincter mechanisms of the urinary bladder

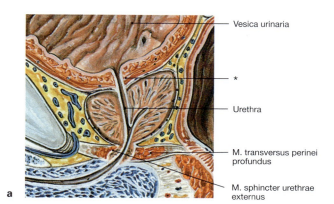
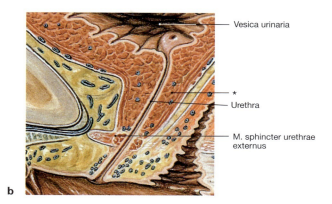

Figs. 7.38a and b   Sphincter mechanisms of urinary bladder, Vesica urinaria, and urethra, Urethra, in men (a) and in women (b); median section; view from the left side.
Contributing to the sphincter mechanisms are not only smooth muscle fibres in the wall of the urinary bladder but also striated muscles of the perineum:
- **smooth muscles** of the circular muscle layer of the Urethra ("M. sphincter urethrae internus"): morphologically, a true sphincter muscle is not identified.
- **M. sphincter urethrae externus:** in men a separation of the M. transversus perinei profundus which often does not exist in women.

In addition, the shape of the pelvic floor (Diaphragma pelvis) is important in supporting the urinary bladder, and thus ensuring urinary continence.
During urination (micturition) the smooth muscles of the wall of the bladder (M. detrusor vesicae) contract following parasympathetic activation. At the same time, the striated muscles of the pelvic floor relax allowing the bladder to descend, the sphincter muscles to relax, and urination to occur.

*   smooth muscles of the Urethra

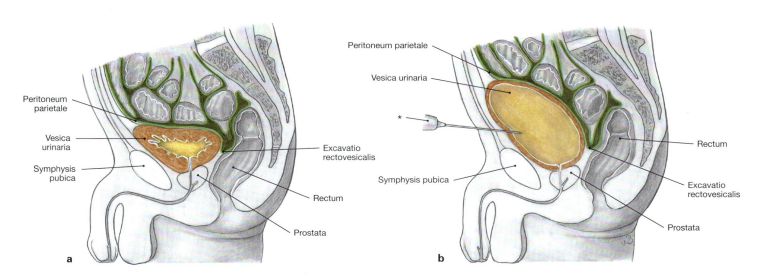

Figs. 7.39a and b   Urinary bladder, Vesica urinaria, empty (a) and urine-filled (b); schematic median section; view from the left.
The urinary bladder is located in the subperitoneal space and is covered by parietal peritoneum on its upper surface. The empty bladder is positioned behind the pubic symphysis (Symphysis pubica). When filled, the bladder rises above the pubic sumphysis and can be accessed without opening the peritoneal cavity (suprapubic cystostomy) for cystoscopy or insertion of a suprapubic catheter.

*   puncture needle

7 Pelvis and Retroperitoneal Space

Kidney and adrenal gland →

External male genitalia

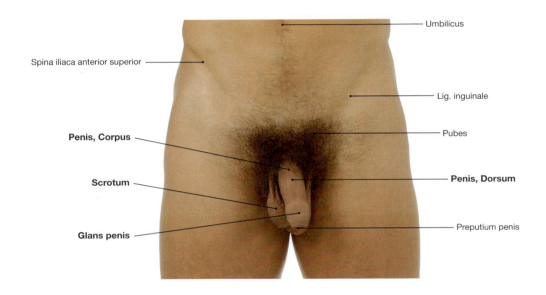

Fig. 7.40 External male genitalia, Organa genitalia masculina externa; ventral view.
The male genitalia are categorised as external genitalia (Organa genitalia masculina externa) and internal genitalia (Organa genitalia masculina interna → Fig. 7.41).
The **external male genitalia** comprise:
- Penis
- Urethra masculina
- Scrotum

The external genitalia are the **sexual organs**. The Penis serves intercourse.
The Urethra is described with the efferent urinary system (→ pp. 178 and 179).

Internal male genitalia

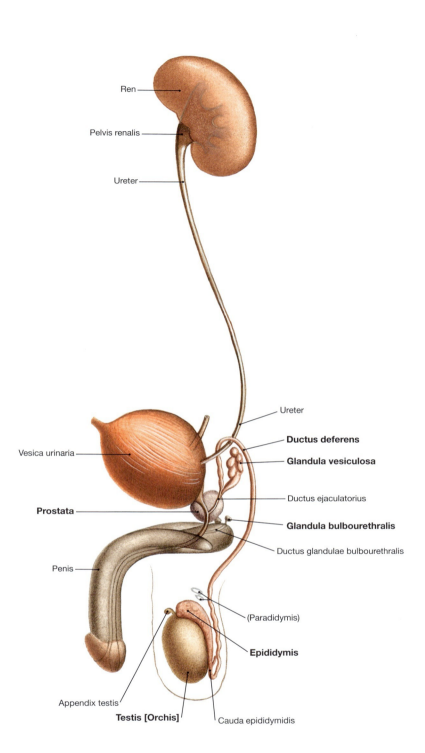

Fig. 7.41 Male urinary and sex organs, Organa urogenitalia masculina; view from the right side.
The **inner male genitalia** comprise:
- Testis
- Epididymis
- Ductus deferens
- Funiculus spermaticus
- accessory sex glands:
  - prostate gland (Prostata)
  - seminal vesicle (Glandula vesiculosa)
  - COWPER's glands (Glandula bulbourethralis), paired

Testis and Epididymis belong to the internal genitalia because during development they were relocated from the intra-abdominal cavity into the Scrotum together with a peritoneal covering (forming the Cavitas serosa scroti).

The internal genitalia are **reproductive organs** and serve the production, maturation, and transport of spermatozoa and the production of seminal fluid. The testes also produce male sex hormones (testosterone).

Pelvis and Retroperitoneal Space

Development of the external male genitalia

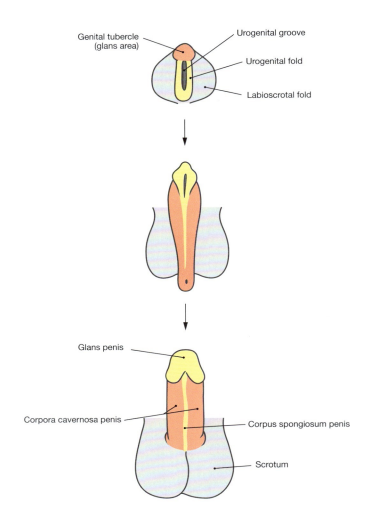

Fig. 7.42 Development of the external male genitalia, Organa genitalia masculina externa.
The external genitalia develop from the caudal part of the Sinus urogenitals. The Sinus urogenitalis develops from the cloaca of the hindgut and gives rise to the urinary bladder and parts of the Urethra (→ Fig. 7.8). Also contributing are the ectoderm and the connective tissue (mesenchyme) beneath. The first part in the development of the external genitalia is identical in both sexes (indifferent gonad). The anterior wall of the Sinus urogenitalis indents to form the **urethral groove** which is bordered on both sides by the **urethral folds**. Lateral to those the **labioscrotal folds** are located and anterior to the groove lie the **genital tubercles**. Subsequently, in men the genital tubercle develops into the **Penis** (Corpora cavernosa) due to the influence of the male sex hormone testosterone which is produced in the Testes. The genital folds merge above the urethral groove to form the Corpus spongiosum and the Glans penis. This way, simultaneously the Pars spongiosa of the **Urethra** develops. The Pars prostatica and the Pars membranacea of the Urethra derive further proximally from the Sinus urogenitalis. The labioscrotal folds enlarge and fuse to form the **Scrotum.**

Clinical Remarks

If incomplete fusions of the urethral folds occur, the opening of the Urethra is not located at the tip of the Glans penis but further proximally. In **hypospadiasis**, the Urethra exits at the inferior side of the Penis between the Scrotum and the glans.

In **epispadias**, the Urethra opens into a ridge at the dorsal side of the Penis. In addition to problems with urination, this condition may involve a distortion in the penile body requiring surgical correction within the first years of life.

Efferent urinary system → **Genitalia** → Rectum and anal canal → Topography → Sections

Development of the internal male genitalia

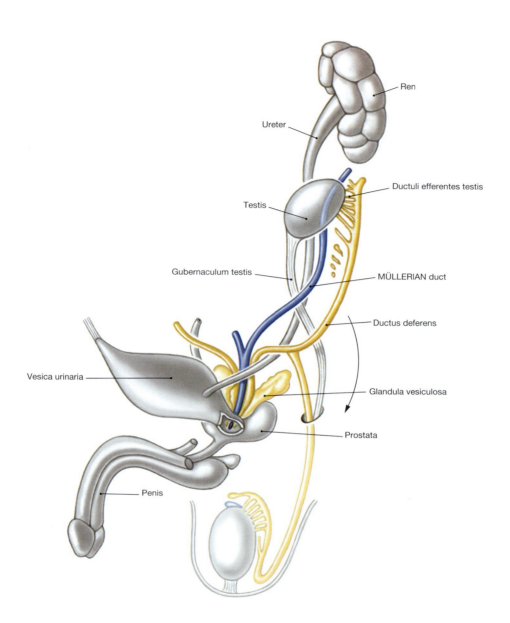

Fig. 7.43 Development of the internal male genitalia, Organa genitalia masculina interna. (according to [1])
Up to week 7, development of the internal genitalia is identical in both sexes (sexual indifferent stage, → Fig. 7.8). In the male, the primordium of the primitive gonad then develops into the Testis. The Testis develops in the lumbar region at the level of the mesonephros which contributes several canaliculi as a connection between the Testis and the Epididymis. Due to the longitudinal growth of the body the Testis is then relocated caudally **(Descensus testis)** but remains connected to its vascular structures. Along the inferior mesenchymal gubernaculum (Gubernaculum testis) a peritoneal pouch is formed (Proc. vaginalis peritonei) which reaches down to the future Scrotum and serves in guiding the descent of the Testis, a process normally completed at birth. At birth, the Proc. vaginalis peritonei closes and obliterates in the area of the Funiculus spermaticus. The distal part of the Proc. vaginalis remains and forms a part of the testicular coverings (Tunica vaginalis testis).
The sex hormones of the Testis (mainly testosterone) induce the **final differentiation of the WOLFFIAN duct** to the internal male genitalia (Epididymis, Ductus deferens), the seminal vesicles, and other accessory sex glands (prostate gland, COWPER's glands) from the Sinus urogenitalis. The anti-MÜLLERIAN hormone suppresses the differentiation of the MÜLLERIAN ducts into female genitalia.

Clinical Remarks

The descent of the Testis explains why the testicular blood vessels arise at the level of the kidneys and why the regional lymph nodes of the Testis are positioned at this level in the retroperitoneal space. Thus, lymph node metastases from **testicular cancer** are to be expected in the lumbar peri-aortal region, not in the inguinal region. Persistent incomplete testicular descent within the first years of life **(cryptorchidism)** may result in infertility and increases the risk of testicular cancer. Recent research indicates that a timely hormonal or surgical therapy of cryptorchidism within the first year of life may prevent infertility. However, this treatment does not influence the risk of testicular cancer. If the Proc. vaginalis peritonei fails to obliterate, accumulation of fluids may occur (even in adulthood) in the Scrotum **(hydrocele testis)** or abdominal organs may prolapse into the Scrotum **(congenital inguinal hernia)**.

7 Pelvis and Retroperitoneal Space

Kidney and adrenal gland →

Penis

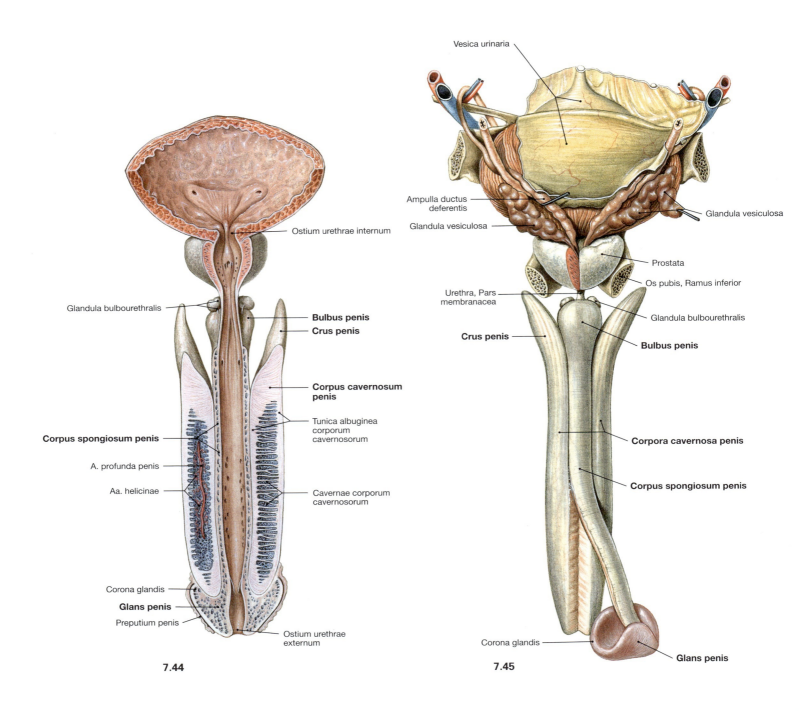

Fig. 7.44 and **Fig. 7.45** Urinary bladder, Vesica urinaria, prostate gland, Prostata, and penis, Penis, with exposed cavernous bodies; ventral view, urinary bladder and Urethra opened (→ Fig. 7.44) and dorsal view (→ Fig. 7.45).

In a flaccid state, the Penis is usually about 10 cm long and divided into the body (Corpus penis), glans (Glans penis), and base or root (Radix penis). It consists of the paired Corpora cavernosa which are enclosed in a dense fibrous covering (Tunica albuginea) and separated by a Septum penis. The other component is the Corpus spongiosum surrounding the Urethra. The proximal parts (Crura penis) of the Corpora cavernosa are fixed to the inferior pubic rami. The proximal and distal parts of the Corpus spongiosum are dilated to form the Bulbus penis and the Glans penis, respectively. All cavernous bodies together are ensheathed by the fascia of the Penis (Fascia penis), which was removed in this illustration.

For the different parts of the male Urethra (Urethra masculina) → Figs. 7.35 and 7.36.

Clinical Remarks

If the prepuce is very narrow (**phimosis**) and cannot be retracted, problems in micturition and infections may occur. In this case, the removal of the prepuce by circumcision is required.

Efferent urinary system → **Genitalia** → Rectum and anal canal → Topography → Sections

Penis and scrotum

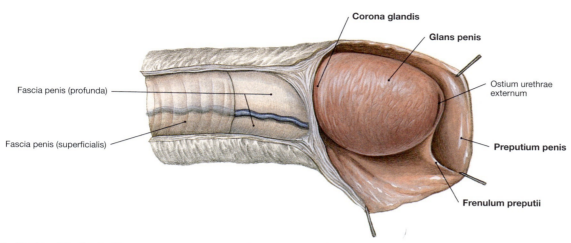

Fig. 7.46 Penis with glans, Glans penis, and prepuce, Preputium penis; view from the right side.

The distal end of the Penis is enlarged to form the Glans penis and shows a ridge (Corona glandis) at its base. In the flaccid state, the glans is covered by the prepuce (Preputium penis). At its underside, the prepuce is connected by a small ligament (Frenulum preputii).

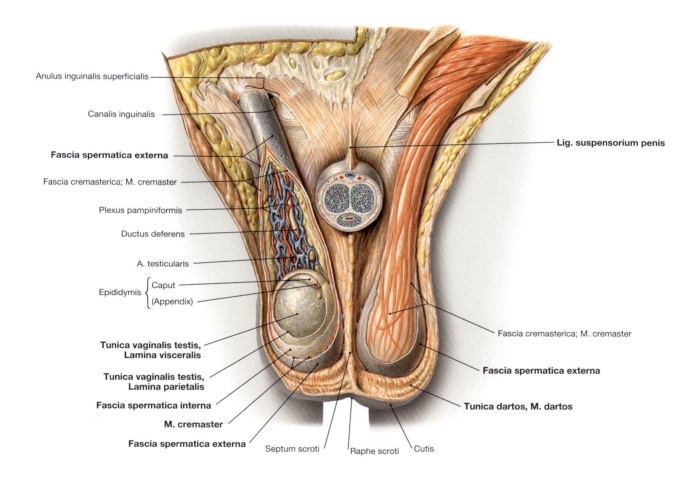

Fig. 7.47 Scrotum, Scrotum; ventral view; the Scrotum opened and the Penis sectioned in the front.
The root of the Penis is attached to the anterior body wall by the superficial Lig. fundiforme penis and the deep Lig. suspensorium penis. The Scrotum is divided internally by a septum which at the outside corresponds to the Raphe scrotum of the skin.

Testis and **Funiculus spermaticus** have the following **coverings:**
* skin of the Scrotum
* Tunica dartos: subcutaneous layer with smooth muscles
* Fascia spermatica externa: continuation of the superficial body fascia (Fascia abdominalis superficialis)
* M. cremaster with Fascia cremasterica
* Fascia spermatica interna: continuation of the Fascia transversalis

In addition, the testis is covered with the Tunica vaginalis testis which consists of an external Lamina parietalis (periorchium) and an inner Lamina visceralis (epiorchium). Both are connected by the mesorchium and create between them the Cavitas serosa scroti.

→ dissection link 187

Pelvis and Retroperitoneal Space

Testis and epididymis

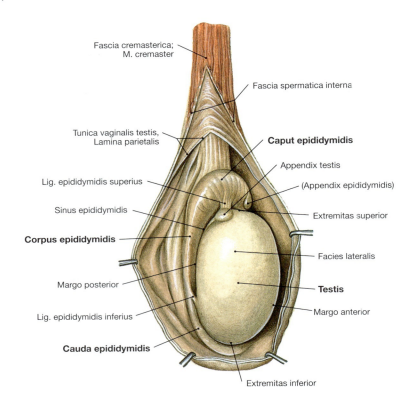

Fig. 7.48 Testis, Testis [Orchis], and epididymis, Epididymis; view from the right side.
The Testis is egg-shaped and 4 × 3 cm in size (20–30 g). It has a **superior** and an **inferior pole** (Extremitas superior and inferior). The **Epididymis** is located adjacent to the superior and dorsal aspect of the Testis and is attached to it by a superior and an inferior ligament (Ligg. epididymidis superius and inferius). The Epididymis has the following parts: head (Caput), body (Corpus), and tail (Cauda) which continues as vas deferens.

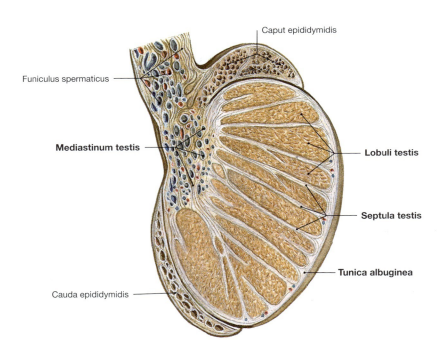

Fig. 7.49 Testis, Testis [Orchis], and epididymis, Epididymis; sagittal section; view from the right side.
The dense Tunica albuginea surrounding the Testis sends septa into the parenchyma of the Testis and, thus, subdivides the parenchyma into 370 **lobules** (Lobuli testis). The **seminiferous tubules** within these lobules are the site of sperm production. The interstitial tissue between the seminiferous tubules harbours the testosterone producing testicular LEYDIG's cells. At the Mediastinum testis neurovascular structures enter and exit the testis and here the seminiferous tubules are connected to the head of the Epididymis.

Testis and epididymis

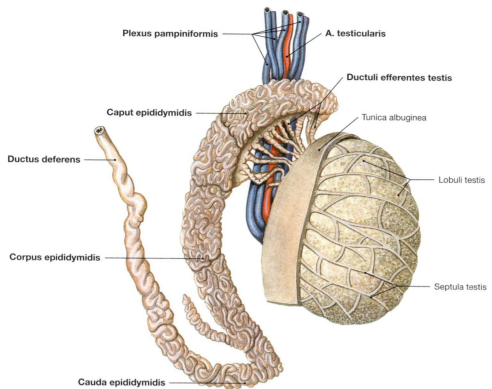

Fig. 7.50 Testis, Testis [Orchis], and epididymis, Epididymis, with blood vessels; view from the right side.
The testis is connected to the head of the Epididymis (Caput epididymis) via tiny tubules (Ductuli efferentes testis). The Epididymis itself consists of a 6 m long convoluted duct which continues as vas deferens (Ductus deferens) at the tail of the Epididymis. With a length of 35–40 cm and a thickness of 3 mm, the vas deferens is located within the spermatic cord and courses through the inguinal canal to the dorsal aspect of the urinary bladder. The terminal part of the vas deferens combines with the excretory duct of the seminal vesicle to form the Ductus ejaculatorius, which enters the Pars prostatica of the male Urethra. Testis and Epididymis are supplied by the **A. testicularis** and a plexus of veins **(Plexus pampiniformis)**.

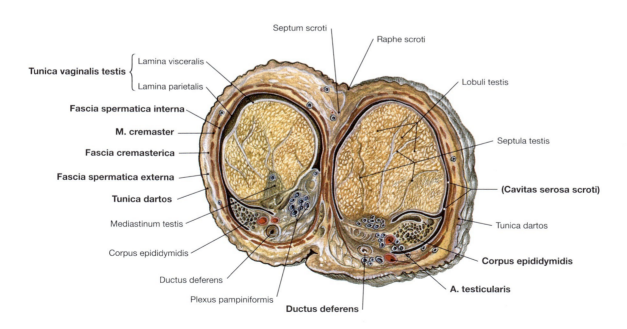

Fig. 7.51 Testis, Testis [Orchis], and epididymis, Epididymis; transverse section; cranial view.
In addition to the testicular coverings (→ Fig. 7.55), the vascular structures and the vas deferens (Ductus deferens) are sectioned.

7 Pelvis and Retroperitoneal Space

Kidney and adrenal gland →

Accessory sex glands in the male

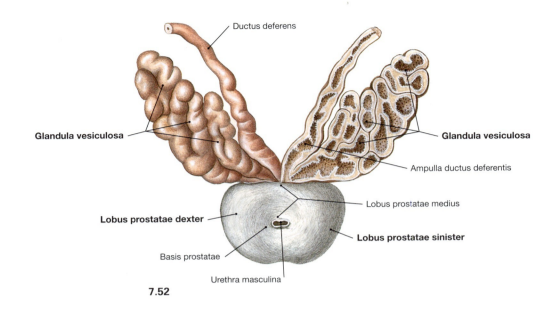

7.52

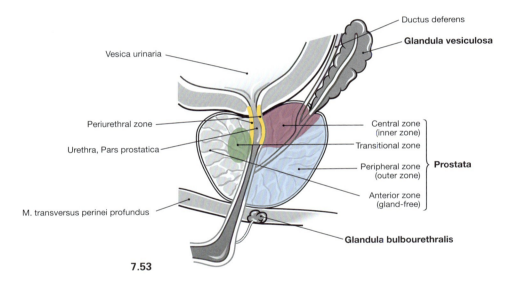

7.53

Fig. 7.52 and Fig. 7.53   Seminal vesicles, Glandulae vesiculosae, and prostate gland, Prostata; cranial view (→ Fig. 7.52) and view from the left side; median section (→ Fig. 7.53).
The **accessory sex glands** consist of:
- **prostate gland:** unpaired gland beneath the base of the bladder. The prostate gland measures 4 × 3 × 2 cm (20 g) and has a superior base and an inferior apex. It consists of a right lobe and a left lobe (Lobus dexter and Lobus sinister), demarcated by a small groove, and a middle lobe (Lobus medius). The prostate gland discharges its secretions into the centrally traversing Urethra (Pars prostatica).
- **seminal vesicle** (Glandula vesiculosa): paired gland at the dorsal aspect of the urinary bladder (→ Fig. 7.34). The seminal vesicles are elongated oval glands (5 × 1 × 1 cm). Their excretory ducts combine with the Ductus deferens to form the Ductus ejaculatorius and enter the Pars prostatica of the Urethra.
- **COWPER's gland** (Glandula bulbourethralis): paired gland located within the perineal muscles (→ Fig. 7.35). The excretory ducts of the lentil-sized COWPER's glands enter the Pars spongiosa of the Urethra.

Seminal vesicles and prostate gland produce the liquid component of the ejaculate which nurtures the spermatozoa. The secretion of the COWPER's glands enters the Urethra prior to ejaculation and functions in lubrication.

Clinical Remarks

Prostatic carcinoma is one of the three most common malignant tumours in men. It usually develops from the microscopically distinct peripheral zone of the gland. Therefore, symptoms related to micturition are only caused at advanced stages. Due to the fact that the prostate gland is separated from the Rectum only by the thin rectoprostatic fascia (DENONVILLIER's fascia; → Fig. 7.115) prostatic carcinomas are usually palpable through the Rectum. The digital rectal examination (DRE) is therefore part of a complete physical examination in men over 50 years of age. The **benign prostatic hypertrophy** (**BPH;** hyperplasia) is a benign tumour of the prostate gland, causing it to enlarge up to a weight of 100 g. BPH is a condition usually present in various degrees in all men over 70 years of age. Since BPH develops from the central zone of the gland, constriction of the Urethra and resulting micturition difficulties are early signs of this condition.

Spermatic cord

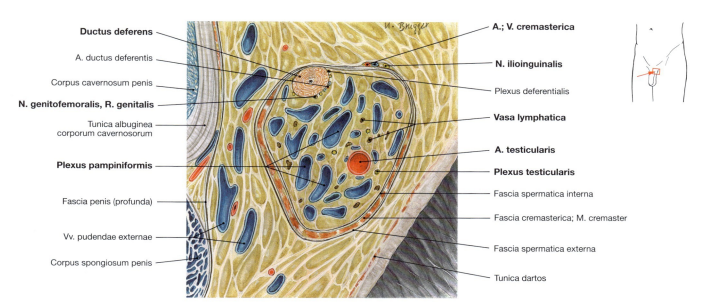

Fig. 7.54 Spermatic cord, Funiculus spermaticus, left side; frontal section; ventral view, magnification 2,5-fold.
The spermatic cord contains the following structures:
- vas deferens (Ductus deferens) with A. ductus deferentis (from the A. umbilicalis)
- A. testicularis from the abdominal aorta and the Plexus pampiniformis as accompanying veins
- N. genitofemoralis, R. genitalis (→ Fig. 7.56)
- lymph vessels (Vasa lymphatica) to the lumbar lymph nodes
- autonomic nerve fibres (Plexus testicularis) from the aortic plexus

Externally, the N. ilioinguinalis and the A. and V. cremasterica are adjacent to the spermatic cord (→ Figs. 7.55 and 7.56).

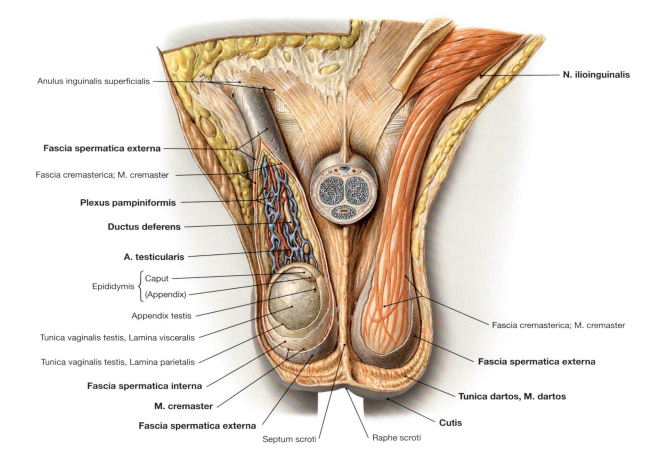

Fig. 7.55 Coverings of the spermatic cord, Funiculus spermaticus, and the testis, Testis; ventral view; Scrotum opened.
Testis and **spermatic cord** have the following **coverings:**
- scrotal skin (Cutis)
- Tunica dartos: Subcutis with smooth muscle cells
- Fascia spermatica externa: continuation of the superficial body fascia (Fascia abdominalis superficialis)
- M. cremaster with Fascia cremasterica
- Fascia spermatica interna: continuation of the Fascia transversalis

Pelvis and Retroperitoneal Space

Blood vessels and nerves of the penis

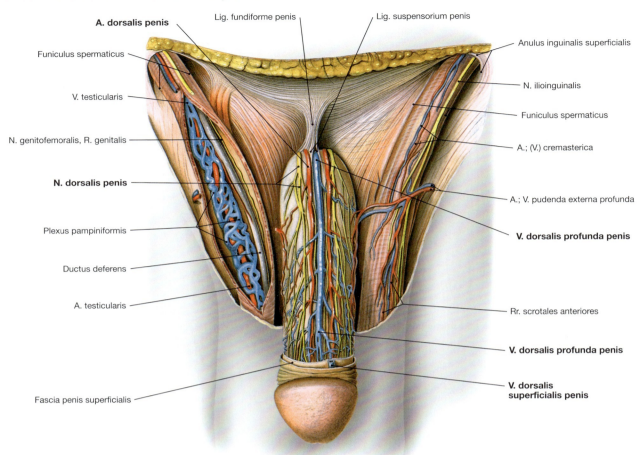

Fig. 7.56 External male genitalia, Organa genitalia masculina externa, with neurovascular structures; ventral view; after removal of the fascia of the Penis.
The Penis receives its arterial blood supply from **three paired arteries** arising from the A. pudenda interna:
- A. dorsalis penis: subfascial course, supplies the skin of the Penis and the glans penis
- A. profunda penis: located within the Corpora cavernosa; regulates the filling of the corpora cavernosa
- A. bulbi penis: enters the Bulbus penis, supplies the Glandula bulbourethralis and as A. urethralis it supplies the Urethra and the Corpus spongiosum

The venous blood is collected by **three venous systems**:
- V. dorsalis superficialis penis: paired or unpaired, epifascial course, drains blood from the penile skin to the V. pudenda externa
- V. dorsalis profunda penis: unpaired, subfascial course, drains blood from the Corpora cavernosa to the Plexus venosus prostaticus
- V. bulbi penis: paired, drains blood from the Bulbus penis to the V. dorsalis profunda penis

Innervation:
- sensory: N. dorsalis penis (from the N. pudendus)
- autonomic: Nn. cavernosi penis (from the Plexus hypogastricus inferior) penetrate the pelvic floor and course adjacent to the N. dorsalis penis (sympathetic stimulation causes vasoconstriction; parasympathetic stimulation causes vasodilation and consecutive erection).

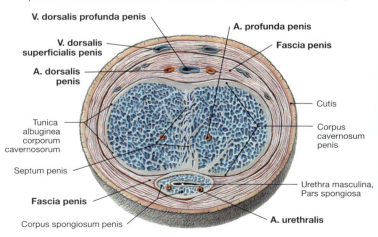

Fig. 7.57 Penis, Penis; cross-section at the midlevel of the penile body; ventral view.
The location of the blood vessels is important for the erection of the Penis. Following parasympathetic innervation, dilation of the A. profunda penis causes the filling of the Corpora cavernosa. These compress the V. dorsalis profunda penis beneath the tough Fascia penis and prevent venous drainage. Supported by the contraction of the Mm. ischiocavernosi (innervated by the N. pudendus), this results in penile erection.

Clinical Remarks

Parasympathetic stimulation induces elevated levels of nitric monoxide (NO). In turn, this increases the concentration of the second messenger cGMP in the smooth muscle cells of the arterial walls with resulting smooth muscle relaxation. **Inhibitors of the enzyme phosphodiesterase** (such as Viagra®, Cialis®) delay the metabolism of cGMP and improve **erection**.

Efferent urinary system → **Genitalia** → Rectum and anal canal → Topography → Sections

Blood vessels of testis and epididymis

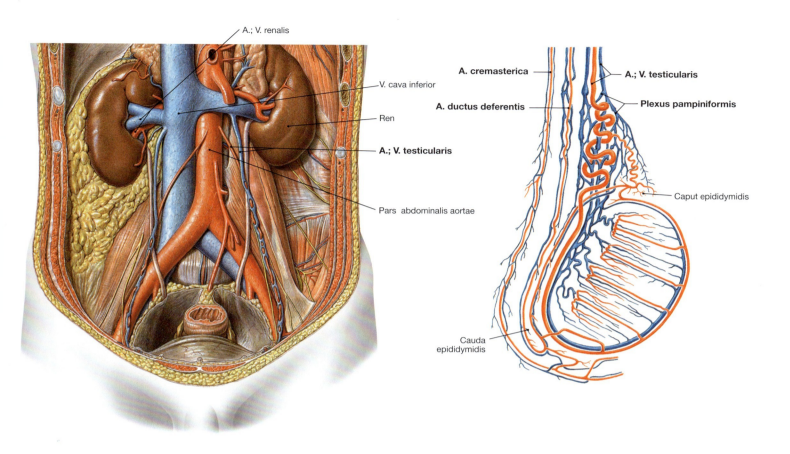

Fig. 7.58 Course of the A. and V. testicularis; ventral view.

Fig. 7.59 Blood vessels of the internal male genitalia; view from the right side.

Blood Vessels of the Internal Genitalia		
	Organ	**Blood Vessel**
Arteries	Testis and Epididymis	A. testicularis (from the Aorta abdominalis)
	vas deferens	A. ductus deferentis (usually from the A. umbilicalis)
	spermatic cord (M. cremaster)	A. cremasterica (from the A. epigastrica inferior)
	accessory sex glands	A. vesicalis inferior and A. rectalis media (from the A. iliaca interna)
Veins	Testis, Epididymis, Ductus deferens, spermatic cord	Plexus pampiniformis: plexus of veins that merge to form the V. testicularis which drains into the V. cava inferior on the right side and the V. renalis sinistra on the left side
	accessory sex glands	Plexus venosi vesicalis and prostaticus with outflow into the V. iliaca interna

Clinical Remarks

Obstruction of the venous drainage into the left V. renalis or **renal cell carcinomas** growing into the renal vein may cause a congestion of blood as revealed by a palpable and visible dilation of the veins in the left Plexus pampiniformis **(varicocele)**. A left-sided varicocele requires the exclusion of a renal cell carcinoma as a possible cause. A persistent varicocele may cause infertility.

Pelvis and Retroperitoneal Space

Kidney and adrenal gland →

Innervation of the male genitalia

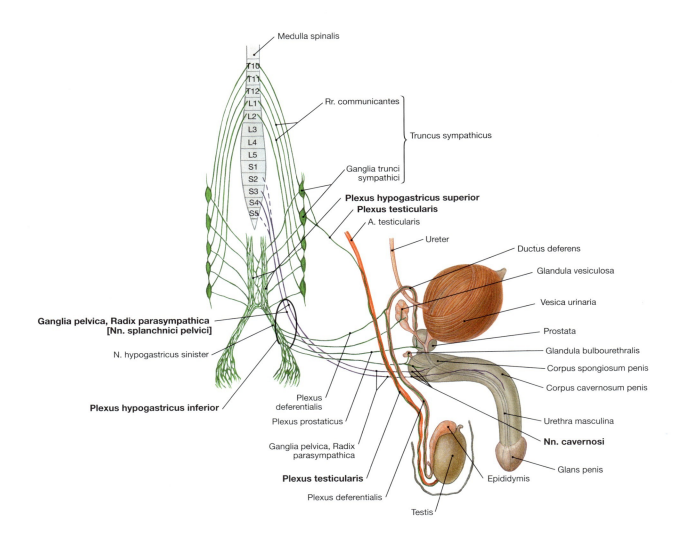

Fig. 7.60 Innervation of the male genitalia; ventral and lateral view; schematic illustration. The Plexus hypogastricus inferior contains sympathetic (green) and parasympathetic (purple) nerve fibres.

The preganglionic **sympathetic fibres** (T10–L2) descend from the Plexus aorticus abdominalis via the Plexus hypogastricus superior and from the sacral ganglia of the sympathetic trunk (Truncus sympathicus) via the Nn. splanchnici sacrales. They are predominantly synapsed to postganglionic sympathetic neurons in the Plexus hypogastricus inferior. These postganglionic fibres reach the pelvic viscera, including the accessory sex glands. Sympathetic fibres to the vas deferens (Plexus deferentialis) activate smooth muscle contractions for the **emission** of spermatozoa into the Urethra. Some fibres also join the Nn. cavernosi and penetrate the pelvic floor to reach the Corpora cavernosa of the Penis. The (mostly) postganglionic sympathetic fibres to the Testis and Epididymis course in the Plexus testicularis alongside the A. testicularis after being already synapsed in the Ganglia aorticorenalia or the Plexus hypogastricus superior.

Preganglionic **parasympathetic fibres** derive from the sacral division of the parasympathetic nervous system (S2–S4) via the Nn. splanchnici pelvici and reach the ganglia of the Plexus hypogastricus inferior. They are synapsed either here or in the vicinity of the pelvic organs (Ganglia pelvica) to postganglionic neurons for the accessory glands. The Nn. cavernosi penetrate the pelvic floor and course to the Corpora cavernosa (partly adjacent to the N. dorsalis penis) to induce **erection** upon parasympathetic stimulation.
Somatic innervation via the **N. pudendus** conveys sensory innervation to the Penis via the N. dorsalis penis and aids in **ejaculation** of spermatozoa through the motor innervation to the M. bulbospongiosus and M. ischiocavernosus via the Nn. perineales in the perineum.
Parasympathetic stimulation induces **erection**, while **sympathetic** fibres initiate the **emission,** and the **N. pudendus** is involved in **ejaculation.**

Clinical Remarks

During surgical resection of para-aortal lymph nodes, as required with testicular or colorectal carcinomas, and surgical procedures involving the abdominal aorta or the larger pelvic arteries, sympathetic fibres may be damaged and emission as well as subsequent ejaculation may be compromised resulting in **impotence**. Surgical procedures on the prostate gland or the rectum as required in prostatic or rectal carcinoma may injure the parasympathetic fibres to the Penis causing **erectile dysfunction**.

Efferent urinary system → **Genitalia** → Rectum and anal canal → Topography → Sections

Lymph vessels of the male genitalia

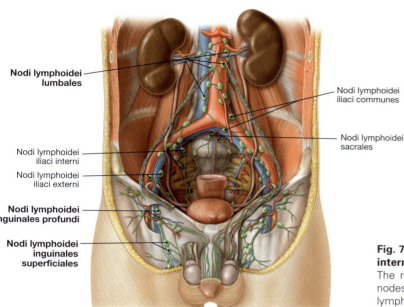

Fig. 7.61 Lymph vessels and lymph nodes of the external and internal male genitalia; ventral view.
The regional lymph nodes for the external genitalia are the inguinal nodes **(Nodi lymphoidei inguinales)**. In contrast, the first regional lymph nodes for the Testes and Epididymis are located in the retroperitoneal space at the level of the kidneys **(Nodi lymphoidei lumbales)**.

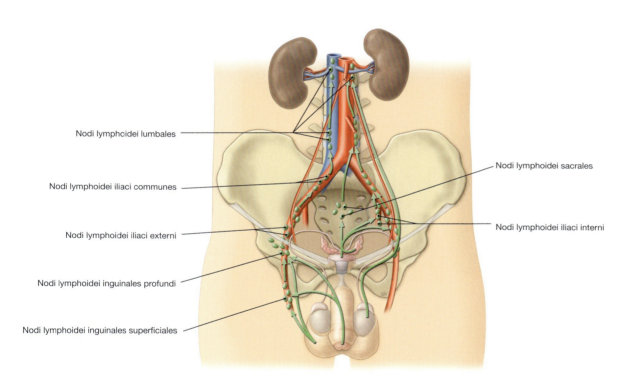

Fig. 7.62 Lymphatic drainage pathways of the external and internal male genitalia; ventral view.
In men, external and internal genitalia have completely different lymphatic drainage pathways.
External genitalia:
- Penis and Scrotum: Nodi lymphoidei inguinales

Internal genitalia:
- Testes and Epididymis: Nodi lymphoidei lumbales at the level of the kidneys
- vas deferens, spermatic cord, and accessory sex glands: Nodi lymphoidei iliaci interni/externi and Nodi lymphoidei sacrales

---

Clinical Remarks

The different lymphatic drainage pathways explain why **lymphatic metastases** of penile carcinoma first appear in the inguinal region, whereas those of testicular carcinoma manifest in the retroperitoneal space. Because the lymphatic drainage pathways of the external and internal genitalia do not communicate, **no transscrotal testicular biopsy** should be performed when suspecting **testicular carcinoma** since this may cause the dissemination of malignant cells into the inguinal lymph nodes. In these cases, biopsies must be taken from the inguinal canal.

Pelvis and Retroperitoneal Space

Pelvic floor in men

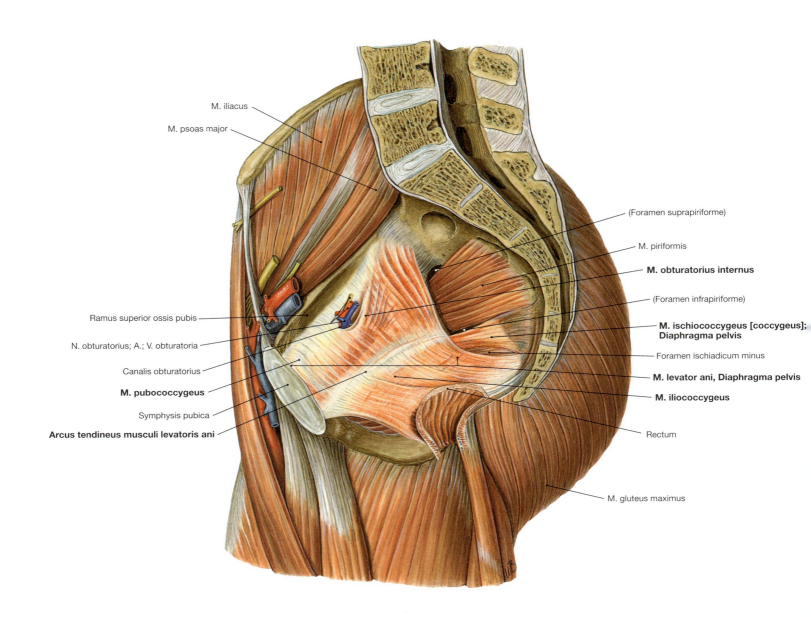

Fig. 7.63 Muscles of the pelvic floor, Diaphragma pelvis, thigh and hip in men; view from the left side.
The pelvic floor closes the pelvic cavity caudally.
Organisation:
- M. levator ani, comprising M. pubococcygeus, M. iliococcygeus, and M. puborectalis
- M. ischiococcygeus

In contrast to the M. pubococcygeus and the M. ischiococcygeus, the M. iliococcygeus does not originate from the Os coxae but from the Arcus tendineus musculi levatoris ani, a reinforcement of the fascia of the M. obturatorius internus.
The muscles of both sides spare the levator hiatus between them (Hiatus levatorius) (→ Fig. 7.87). This muscular gap is divided by the connective tissue of the Corpus perineale (Centrum perinei) into the anterior **Hiatus urogenitalis** and the posterior **Hiatus analis** for the passage of Urethra and Rectum, respectively.
The pelvic floor is innervated by direct branches of the Plexus sacralis (S3–S4).
Function: The pelvic floor stabilises the position of the pelvic viscera and, thus, is essential for urinary and fecal continence. Pelvic floor insufficiency with resulting incontinence is rare in men since potential injuries due to repetitive strain during childbirth is lacking.

→ T 20a

Perineal muscles in men

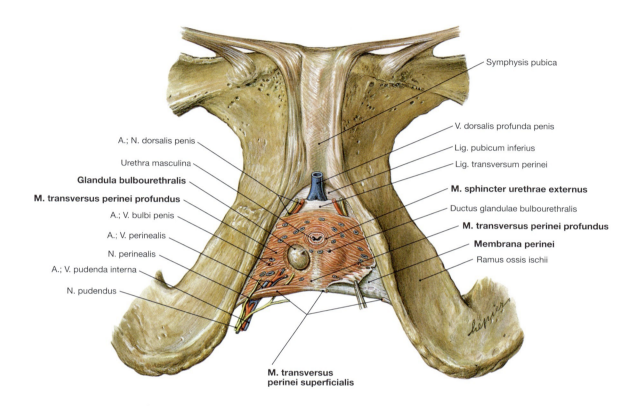

Fig. 7.64 Perineal muscles in men; caudal view; after removal of all other muscles.

In men, the muscular gap of the levator hiatus (Hiatus levatorius) is almost entirely closed by the perineal muscles beneath which leave only the passage for the Urethra masculina.

The perineal muscles in men comprise the strong **M. transversus perinei profundus** and the thin **M. transversus perinei superficialis** located at its posterior margin. These muscles have formerly been referred to as "Diaphragma urogenitale" analogous to the Diaphragma pelvis. Since a true diaphragm does not exist and because a similar muscular plate is missing in women, this term is not used any more. The voluntary sphincter muscle of the urinary bladder, the M. sphincter urethrae externus, is a part of the M. transversus perinei profundus. The M. transversus perinei profundus is covered by a fascia on both sides. The stronger inferior fascia is referred to as perineal membrane **(Membrana perinei)**.

The space between both fascias is the **deep perineal space** (Spatium profundum perinei) and is entirely occupied by the M. transversus perinei profundus. This space also contains the Urethra and the COWPER's glands (Glandulae bulbourethrales) and is traversed by deep branches of the N. pudendus as well as the A. and V. pudenda interna before they reach the Radix penis.

The **superficial perineal space** (Spatium superficiale perinei) lies caudal to the perineal membrane and contains amongst others the M. transversus perinei superficialis.

→ T 20b

Pelvis and Retroperitoneal Space

Kidney and adrenal gland →

Pelvic floor and perineal muscles in men

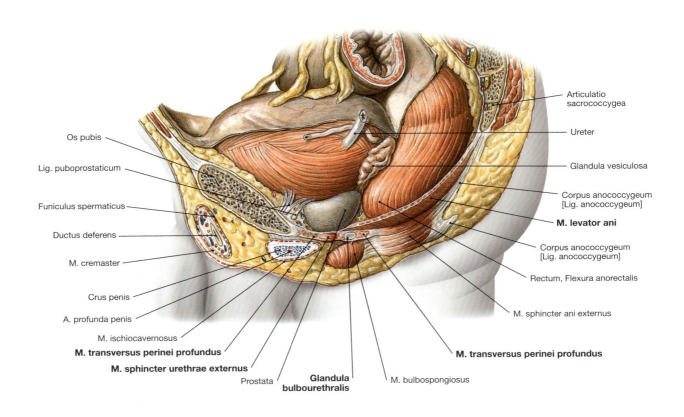

Fig. 7.65 Pelvic floor, Diaphragma pelvis, and perineal muscles in men; view from the left side.
At its anterior and posterior aspect, the pelvic floor consists of the M. levator ani and the M. ischiococcygeus, respectively. Located beneath the pelvic floor is the deep perineal muscle (M. transversus perinei profundus). A partition of the latter, the M. sphincter urethrae externus, functions as sphincter of the urinary bladder. Embedded within the M. transversus perinei profundus are the COWPER's glands.

→ T 20

→ dissection link

Perineal region in men

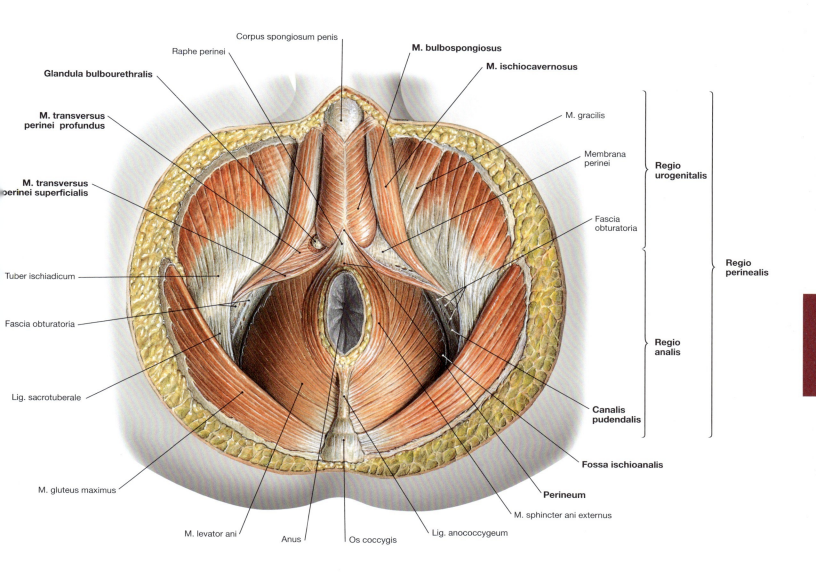

Fig. 7.66 Perineal region, Regio perinealis, in men; caudal view; after removal of all neurovascular structures.

The **perineal region** extends from the inferior margin of the pubic symphysis (Symphysis pubica) to the tip of the coccyx (Os coccygis). The term **perineum** in men, however, exclusively describes the small connective tissue bridge between the Radix penis and the Anus. The perineal region is subdivided into the **anterior Regio urogenitalis** (urogenital triangle), containing the external genitalia and the Urethra, and the **posterior Regio analis** (anal triangle) around the Anus. The following spaces can be found within these triangles:

- The Regio analis contains the **Fossa ischioanalis** (→ Table), which constitutes a pyramid-shaped space on both sides of the Anus. The cranial border is the M. levator ani of the pelvic floor. The lateral wall encloses the fascial duplicature of the M. obturatorius internus (Fascia obturatoria), and the pudendal canal (ALCOCK's canal). The pudendal canal contains the A. and V. pudenda interna, and the N. pudendus after their passage from the gluteal region through the Foramen ischiadicum minus.

The Regio urogenitalis has two **perineal spaces:**
- The **deep perineal space** (Spatium profundum perinei) comprises the M. transversus perinei profundus and the COWPER's glands (Glandulae bulbourethrales).
- The **superficial perineal space** (Spatium superficiale perinei) comprises the M. transversus perinei superficialis, the M. bulbospongiosus, and the M. ischiocavernosus, which stabilise the cavernous bodies of the Radix penis and enable ejaculation.

Borders of the Fossa ischioanalis	
Medial and cranial	M. sphincter ani externus and M. levator ani
Lateral	M. obturatorius externus
Dorsal	M. gluteus maximus and Lig. sacrotuberale
Ventral	posterior margin of the superficial and the deep perineal spaces; anterior recess reaches the pubic symphysis
Caudal	fascia and skin of the perineum

7 Pelvis and Retroperitoneal Space

Kidney and adrenal gland →

Perineal region in men

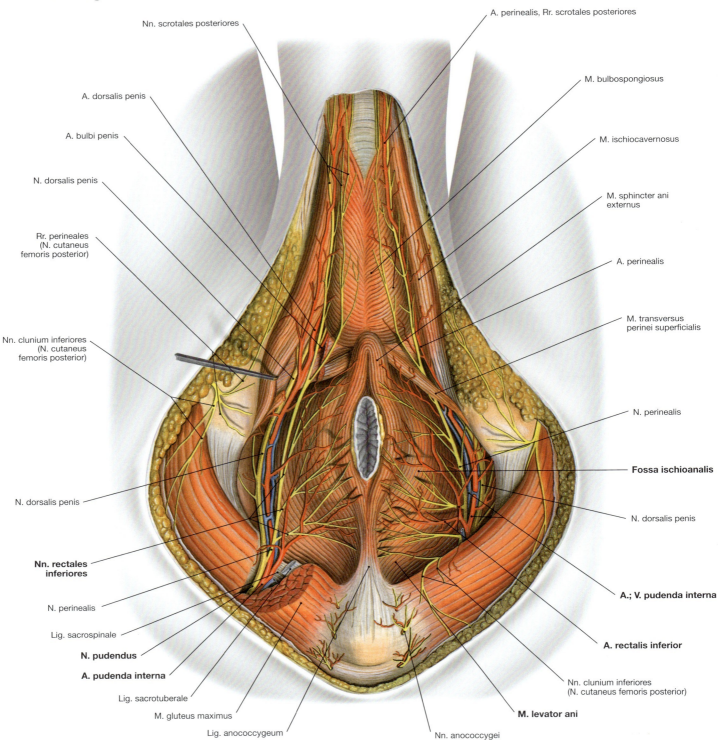

Fig. 7.67 Blood vessels and nerves of the perineal region, Regio perinealis, in men; caudal view.
Covered by a fascial duplicature of the M. obturatorius internus, the Canalis pudendalis (ALCOCK's canal), the neurovascular structures enter the **Fossa ischioanalis** from a dorsolateral direction. The pyramid-shaped fossa is filled with adipose tissue. Branches to the Anus and the anal canal come off first and cross the ischio-anal fossa to reach the anus. The neurovascular structures then continue ventrally to the Radix penis and the two perineal spaces.

Contents of the Fossa ischioanalis:
- A. and V. pudenda interna and N. pudendus: in the Canalis pudendalis (ALCOCK's canal)
- A., V., and N. rectalis inferior: to the anal canal

Clinical Remarks

The Fossa ischioanalis is of great clinical relevance because of its expansion to both sides of the anus. **Collection of pus** (abscesses), e.g. fistulas from the anal canal, may expand within the entire ischio-anal fossa, including its anterior recess and even extend to the pubic symphysis. These abscesses not only generate non-specific inflammatory signs but also cause intense pain in the perineal region.

Efferent urinary system → **Genitalia** → Rectum and anal canal → Topography → Sections

Perineal spaces in men

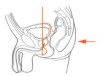

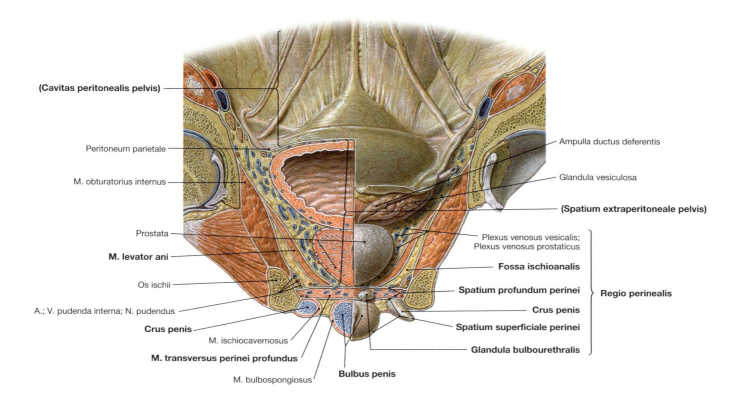

Fig. 7.68 Perineal spaces in men; left side; frontal section at the level of the femoral head; dorsal view.

The frontal section shows **three levels** of the male pelvis:
- peritoneal cavity of the pelvis (Cavitas peritonealis pelvis), caudally bordered by the parietal peritoneum
- subperitoneal space (Spatium extraperitoneale pelvis), caudally bordered by the M. levator ani of the pelvic floor
- perineal region (Regio perinealis) inferior to the pelvic floor. The anterior portion contains the two perineal spaces, and includes the variably expanded anterior recess of the ischio-anal fossa (illustrated here in different ways for the right side and the left side).

The **deep perineal space** (Spatium profundum perinei) consists of the M. transversus perinei profundus. It also contains the COWPER's glands (Glandulae bulbourethrales) and the passage of the Urethra (Urethra masculina). It is traversed by the deep branches of the N. pudendus (N. dorsalis penis), and the A. and V. pudenda interna (A. bulbi penis, A. dorsalis penis, A. profunda penis) before reaching the Radix penis. The Nn. cavernosi penis pierce the perineum and enter the Corpora cavernosa of the Penis.

The **superficial perineal space** (Spatium superficiale perinei) is located between the perineal membrane (Membrana perinei) at the underside of the M. transversus perinei profundus and the body fascia (Fascia perinei). It contains the M. transversus perinei superficialis and the proximal parts of the Corpora cavernosa of the Penis. The Bulbus penis is ensheathed by the M. bulbospongiosus, the Crura penis by the M. ischiocavernosus. The superficial branches of the N. pudendus (N. perinealis with Nn. scrotales posteriores) and the A. and V. pudenda interna (A. perinealis with Rr. scrotales posteriores) also traverse this space to reach the Scrotum.

Pelvis and Retroperitoneal Space

External female genitalia

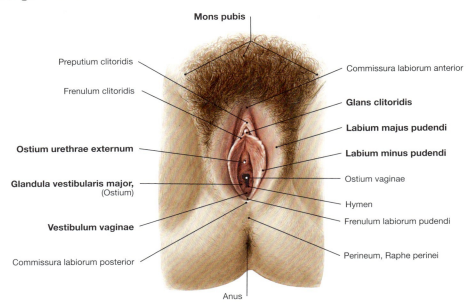

Fig. 7.69 External female genitalia, Organa genitalia feminina externa; caudal view.
The female genitalia can be categorised into external genitalia (Organa genitalia feminina externa) and internal genitalia (Organa genitalia feminina interna → Fig. 7.71).
The **external genitalia** are referred to as **Vulva** and comprise:
- Mons pubis
- Labia majora pudendi
- Labia minora pudendi
- Clitoris
- vestibule (Vestibulum vaginae)
- Glandulae vestibulares majores (BARTHOLIN's glands), and minores

The vestibule extends to the hymen at the vaginal orifice (Ostium vaginae). Ventral thereof is the external urethral orifice (Ostium urethrae externum).
The external genitalia are the **sex organs** and serve for intercourse.

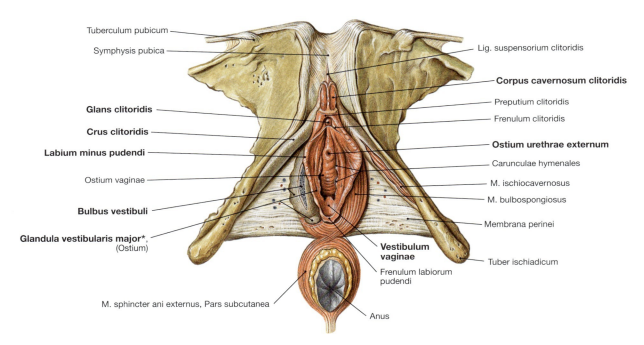

Fig. 7.70 External female genitalia, Organa genitalia feminina externa; caudal view; after removal of body fascia and neurovascular structures.
The Labia majora pudendi are removed in this illustration. They contain the cavernous body of the **vestibule** (Bulbus vestibuli). The Labia minora pudendi surround the vestibule (Vestibulum vaginae) and continue anteriorly as Frenulum clitoridis to the glans of the clitoris (Glans clitoridis). The vestibular glands (Glandulae vestibulares majores [BARTHOLIN's glands] and minores) enter the vestibule from lateral. The **Clitoris** is the sensory organ for sexual arousal. The Corpora cavernosa clitoridis form a short body (Corpus clitoridis) with the glans at the inferior end. The crura of the clitoris (Crura clitoridis) are attached to the inferior ischiopubic rami and covered by the M. ischiocavernosus on both sides. The M. bulbospongiosus stabilises the bulb of the vestibule.
Developmentally, the organisation of the Penis and the Clitoris is similar including the presence of the prepuce (Preputium clitoridis). The filling mechanisms of the cavernous bodies and the process of erection are also similar in both sexes.

* clinical term: BARTHOLIN's gland

Efferent urinary system → **Genitalia** → Rectum and anal canal → Topography → Sections

Internal female genitalia

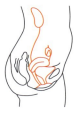

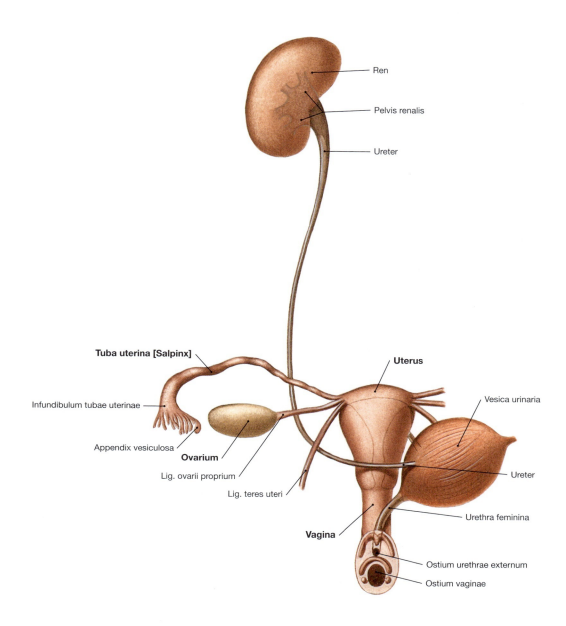

Fig. 7.71 Female urinary and genital organs, Organa urogenitalia feminina; ventral view.
The **internal genitalia** comprise:
- vagina (Vagina)
- uterus (Uterus)
- uterine tube (Tuba uterina)
- ovary (Ovarium)

Uterine tube and ovary are paired organs and are collectively referred to as uterine **adnexa**.

The internal genitalia in women are **reproductive** and **sex organs**. Functionally, the ovary serves for the maturation of follicles (and ova) and the production of female sex hormones (oestrogens and progesterone). The uterine tube provides the place for the fertilisation of ova and transports the zygote to the Uterus where the embryo/fetus develops and grows during pregnancy. The Vagina serves the sexual intercourse and is part of the birth canal.

Pelvis and Retroperitoneal Space

Development of the external female genitalia

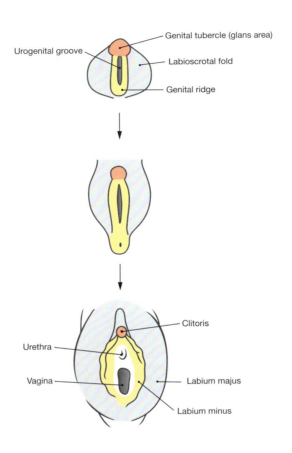

Fig. 7.72 Development of the external female genitalia, Organa genitalia feminina externa.
The external genitalia develop from the caudal part of the Sinus urogenitalis. The Sinus urogenitalis develops from the cloaca of the hindgut and gives rise to the urinary bladder and parts of the Urethra (→ Fig. 7.6). Contributing to these structures are also the ectoderm and the connective tissue (mesenchyme) located beneath the Sinus urogenitalis. First, the external genitalia develop identically in both sexes (indifferent gonad). The anterior wall of the Sinus urogenitalis indents to form the **urethral groove**, and is bordered on both sides by the **urethral folds**. Lateral of those are the **labioscrotal folds** and anterior the **genital tubercle**. Subsequently, the genital tubercle develops into the **Clitoris** (Corpora cavernosa) under the influence of the female sex hormone oestrogen which is produced in the ovary. In contrast to the development in men, the genital folds and the labioscrotal folds do not merge. The genital folds develop into the **Labia minora** and the labioscrotal folds into the **Labia majora.** The short female Urethra and the BARTHOLIN's glands develop from the Sinus urogenitalis.

Clinical Remarks

The common developmental stages of the external genitalia in both sexes explains the development of penis-like hyperplasias of the Clitoris in cases of excessive production of male sex hormones such as in **adrenogenital syndrome** (production of androgens in the cortex of the adrenal glands).

Efferent urinary system → **Genitalia** → Rectum and anal canal → Topography → Sections

Development of the internal female genitalia

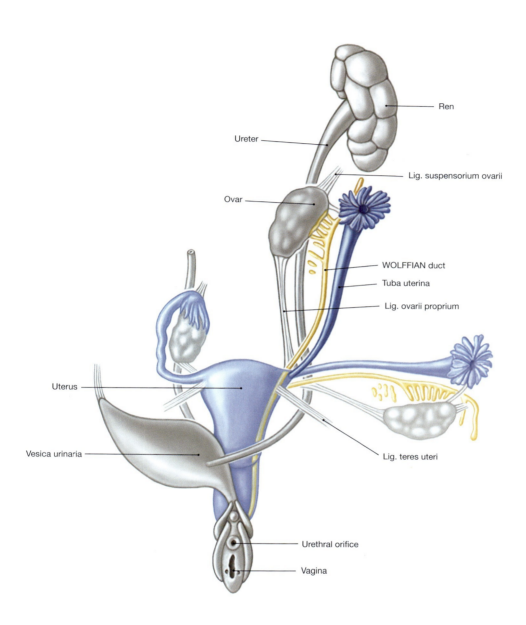

Fig. 7.73 Development of the internal female genitalia, Organa genitalia feminina interna. (according to [1])
The internal genitalia develop identically in both sexes up to week 7 (sexual indifferent stage, → Fig. 7.8). In the female, the primordium of the primitive gonad then develops into the ovary. Similar to the Testis, the ovary also develops in the lumbar region at the level of the mesonephros. Due to the longitudinal growth of the body the ovary is then relocated caudally to the lesser pelvis without leaving the peritoneal cavity. Thus, ovary and uterine tube have an **intraperitoneal** position.

Without the suppressing effects of the anti-MÜLLERIAN hormone from the Testis, the MÜLLERIAN ducts differentiate into female genitalia. Beginning in week 12, the MÜLLERIAN ducts form the uterine tube. Their distal portions merge and give rise to the Uterus and the upper Vagina. The lower Vagina develops from the Sinus urogenitalis. If the MÜLLERIAN ducts fail to fuse, a **septate uterus** (Uterus septus or subseptus) or a **double uterus** (Uterus duplex, Uterus didelphys) may result.

Pelvis and Retroperitoneal Space

Uterus, uterine tube and ovary

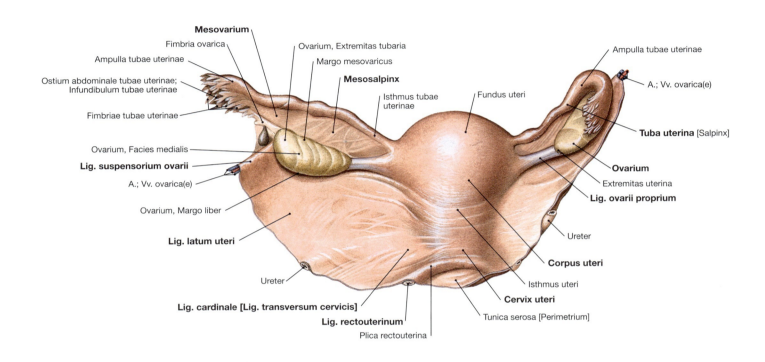

Fig. 7.74 Uterus, Uterus, ovary, Ovarium, and uterine tube, Tuba uterina, with peritoneal duplications; dorsal view.

The **Uterus** (Metra) is 8 cm long, 5 cm wide and 2–3 cm thick. It consists of the body (Corpus uteri) with a superior fundus (Fundus uteri) and a neck (Cervix uteri). A constriction (Isthmus uteri) marks the transition between body and neck of the Uterus. The uterine tube (Tuba uterina) extends on both sides from the uterine body to connect to the ovaries.

The **uterine tube** (Tuba uterina) is 10 – 14 cm long and has several parts:
- Infundibulum tubae uterinae: 1 – 2 cm long, contains the opening to the peritoneal cavity (Ostium abdominale tubae uterinae) and the fimbriae (Fimbriae tubae uterinae) for the collection of ovulated ova.
- Ampulla tubae uterinae: 7 – 8 cm long, crescent-shaped around the ovary
- Isthmus tubae uterinae: 3 – 6 cm long, constriction at the transition to the Uterus
- intramural part (Pars uterina tubae), enters the Uterus (Ostium uterinum)

The **ovary** (Ovarium) is 3 × 1.5 × 1 cm in size and oval. A tubal extremity (Extremitas tubaria) and an uterine extremity (Extremitas uterina) are distinguished. The mesovarium is attached to the anterior margin (Margo mesovaricus), but the posterior margin is loose (Margo liber).

Uterus, uterine tube, and ovary have an **intraperitoneal** position and thus, have individual **peritoneal duplicatures** covered by a Tunica serosa. The following **ligaments** and attachments are relevant for gynaecological surgical procedures:
- Lig. latum uteri: broad ligament as frontal peritoneal fold
- Mesovar and Mesosalpinx: peritoneal duplicatures of ovary and uterine tube, respectively, connected to the Lig. latum
- Lig. cardinale (Lig. transversum cervicis): connective tissue connecting the Cervix to the lateral pelvic wall
- Lig. rectouterinum (clinical term: Lig. sacrouterinum): connective tissue attaching the Cervix dorsally
- Lig. teres uteri (clinical term: Lig. rotundum): the round ligament coursing from the uterotubal junction through the inguinal canal to the Labia majora
- Lig. ovarii proprium: the ovarian ligament connects ovary and Uterus
- Lig. suspensorium ovarii (clinical term: Lig. infundibulopelvicum): connects ovary and lateral pelvic wall, carries the A. and V. ovarica

Efferent urinary system → **Genitalia** → Rectum and anal canal → Topography → Sections

Uterus and vagina

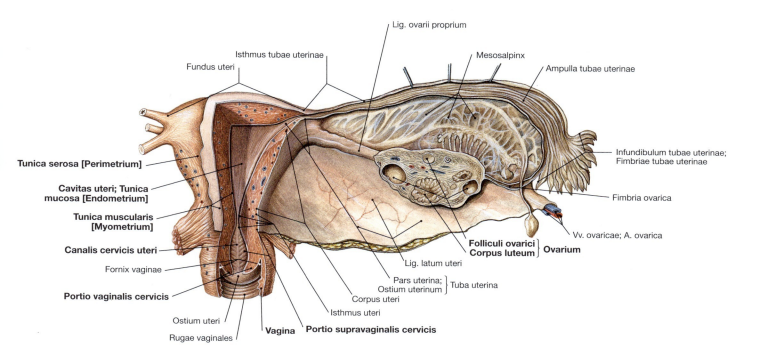

Fig. 7.75 Uterus, Uterus, vagina, Vagina, ovary, Ovarium, and uterine tube, Tuba uterina; frontal section; dorsal view.
The space inside the **Uterus** is divided into the Cavitas uteri in the body and the Canalis cervicis uteri in the uterine cervix. The lower portion of the Cervix enters the **Vagina** and is referred to as Portio vaginalis cervicis. The upper portion is the Portio supravaginalis cervicis. The **Vagina** is a hollow muscular organ of about 10 cm length in a **subperitoneal** location. The Fornix vaginae surrounds the Portio vaginalis cervicis. At the inner surface, both the anterior and posterior walls (Paries anterior and Paries posterior) of the Vagina reveal transverse mucosal folds (Rugae vaginales).

The frontal section also shows the **structure of the uterine wall**: the internal mucosal layer (Tunica mucosa; endometrium), then the strong muscular layer (Tunica muscularis; myometrium) of smooth muscles, and the outermost peritoneal lining (Tunica serosa; perimetrium).
Embedded in the stroma of the **ovary** are the ovarian follicles (Folliculi ovarici) which contain the ova and develop into the Corpus luteum following ovulation. Follicles and Corpora lutea produce the female sex hormones (oestrogens and progesterone) which regulate the cycle-dependent differentiation of the endometrium.

Pelvis and Retroperitoneal Space

Position of the uterus and adnexa

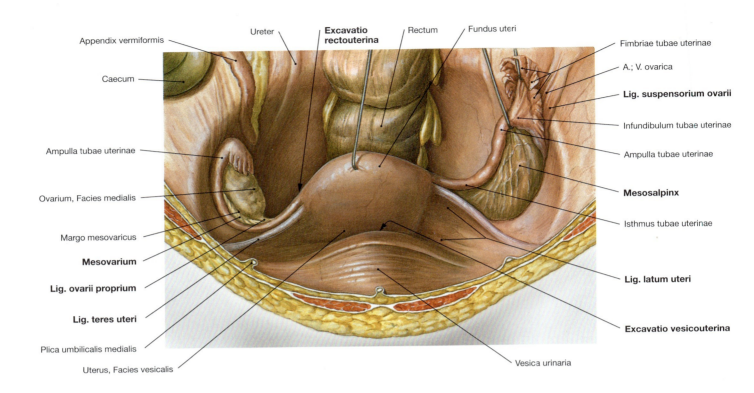

Fig. 7.76 Uterus, Uterus, ovary, Ovarium, and uterine tube, Tuba uterina, with peritoneal duplicatures; ventral view.
Uterus, uterine tubes, and ovary have an **intraperitoneal** position. Their **peritoneal duplicatures** (Lig. latum uteri, Mesosalpinx, Mesovarium) form a transverse fold in the lesser pelvis. The Lig. teres uteri reaches ventral from the uterotubal junction to the lateral wall of the lesser pelvis and traverses the inguinal canal to merge with the connective tissue of the Labia majora. The Lig. ovarii proprium connects Uterus and ovary. The Lig. suspensorium ovarii connects ovary and lateral pelvic wall and contains the A. and V. ovarica.

The close topographical relationship between the adnexa (ovary and uterine tube) and the Appendix vermiformis of the Colon explain why inflammations of the appendix (appendicitis) as well as those of the uterine tube (salpingitis) may cause similar pain in the right lower abdominal quadrant. The peritoneal pouch between the Uterus and the urinary bladder is called **Excavatio vesicouterina**. The **Excavatio rectouterina** (pouch of DOUGLAS) behind the Uterus is the most caudal extension of the peritoneal cavity in women and may collect fluids and pus in cases of inflammatory processes in the lower abdomen.

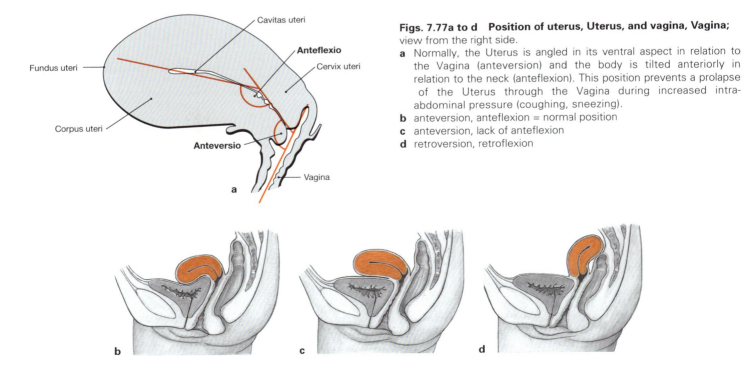

Figs. 7.77a to d   Position of uterus, Uterus, and vagina, Vagina; view from the right side.
a Normally, the Uterus is angled in its ventral aspect in relation to the Vagina (anteversion) and the body is tilted anteriorly in relation to the neck (anteflexion). This position prevents a prolapse of the Uterus through the Vagina during increased intra-abdominal pressure (coughing, sneezing).
b anteversion, anteflexion = normal position
c anteversion, lack of anteflexion
d retroversion, retroflexion

Position of the uterus and connective tissue spaces

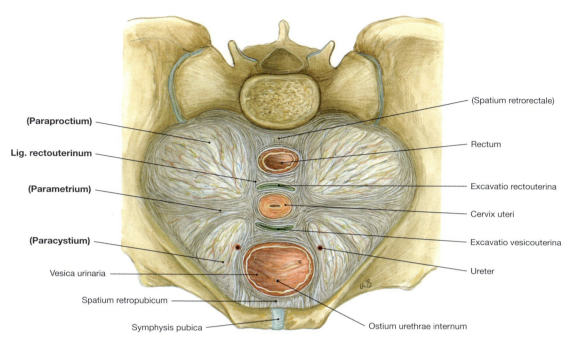

Fig. 7.78 Ligaments and connective tissue spaces of the uterus, Uterus; transverse section at the level of the Cervix uteri; caudal view; semischematic illustration.
The connective tissue in the lesser pelvis is categorised according to the relation to adjacent organs. Some of the connective tissue strands are referred to as ligaments in clinical terms although an anatomical demarcation is not possible.

- **parametrium:** connective tissue from the cervix to the pelvic wall (Lig. cardinale)
- **paraproctium:** connective tissue around the Rectum
- **paracystium:** connective tissue around the urinary bladder
- **paracolpium:** connective tissue around the Vagina

The **Lig. rectouterinum** between the Cervix uteri and the dorsal pelvic wall is the only separable ligament and is preserved during gynaecological surgery to protect the autonomic nerves of the Plexus hypogastricus inferior.

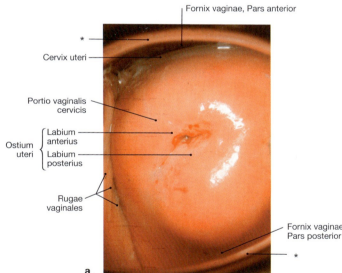
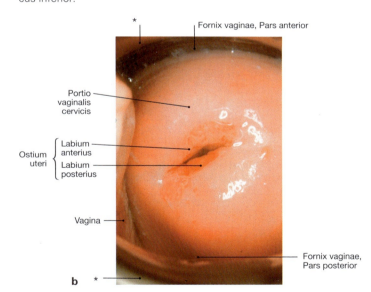

Figs. 7.79 a and b Uterine neck, Portio vaginalis cervicis; caudal view.
a uterine neck of a young woman who has not yet delivered a child (nullipara)
b uterine neck of a young woman who has delivered two children

For the inspection of the Portio vaginalis cervicis the Vagina is distended by two specula.

* speculum

Clinical Remarks

Inspection and cervical swabs (PAPANICOLAOU smear) are routinely performed for **gynaecological screening examinations** and the costs are covered by the public health system for women above the age of 20 years. This examination should be performed annually to detect precancerous lesions indicative of the development of cer**vical carcinoma** and to enable early curative surgery. Cervical carcinoma is among the most common malignancies in women below the age of 40 years. It is caused by infections with viruses of the human papilloma virus (HPV) group. A vaccine was developed and vaccination is recommended for girls during puberty to prevent infections. However, due to the low experience with this vaccine and the lack of evidence that vaccination can prevent cervical carcinoma, the benefit of this vaccine is currently disputed.

Pelvis and Retroperitoneal Space

Uterus in pregnancy

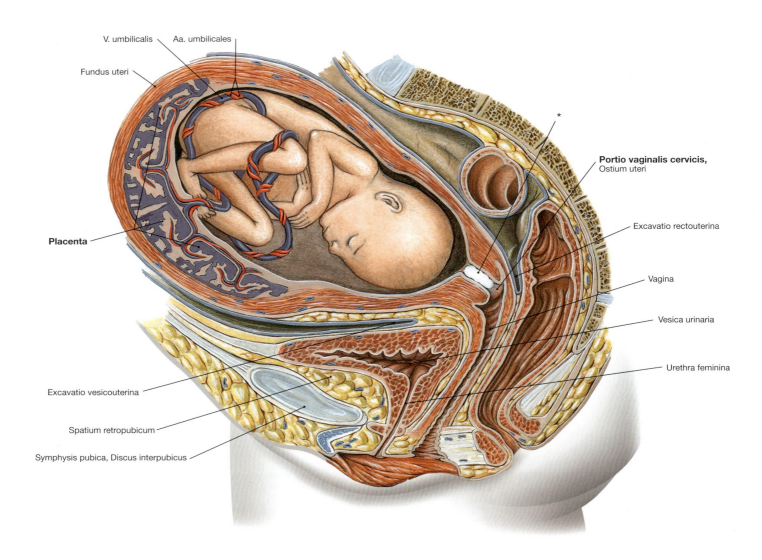

Fig. 7.80 Uterus, Uterus with placenta, Placenta, and fetus; median section of the pelvis except for the fetus; view from the left side.

The developing child in the Uterus is nourished via the Placenta which develops from maternal and fetal tissues after implantation. The Cervix uteri is closed during pregnancy by the KRISTELLER's mucous plug (*).

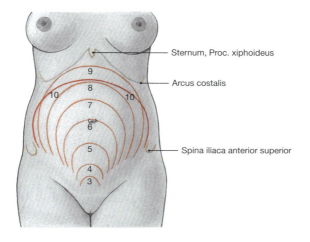

Fig. 7.81 Level of the Fundus uteri during pregnancy; ventral view.
The numbers represent the end of the respective month of pregnancy. In the 6th month (week 24) the Fundus uteri is at the level of the umbilical region, in the 9th month (week 36) at the costal margin. Up to parturition, the uterine volume increases 800 – 1200 times and the uterine weight increases from 30 – 120 g to 1000 – 1500 g.

Efferent urinary system → **Genitalia** → Rectum and anal canal → Topography → Sections

Arteries of the internal female genitalia

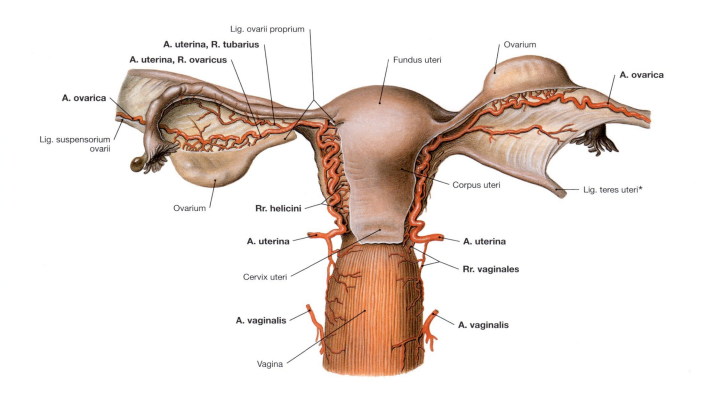

Fig. 7.82 Arteries of the internal female genitalia; dorsal view.
The internal female genitalia are supplied by **three paired arteries:**
- **Uterus:** A. uterina (from the A. iliaca interna) with Rr. helicini
- **Ovarium:** A. ovarica (from the abdominal aorta) and A. uterina with R. ovaricus
- **Tuba uterina:** A. uterina with R. tubarius and A. ovarica
- **Vagina:** A. vaginalis (from the A. iliaca interna) and A. uterina with Rr. vaginales

The venous drainage occurs via **two venous systems:**
- venous plexus in the lesser pelvis (Plexus venosi uterinus and vaginalis) with drainage into the V. iliaca interna
- V. ovarica; drains into the V. cava inferior on the right side and the V. renalis sinistra on the left side.

* clinical term: Lig. rotundum

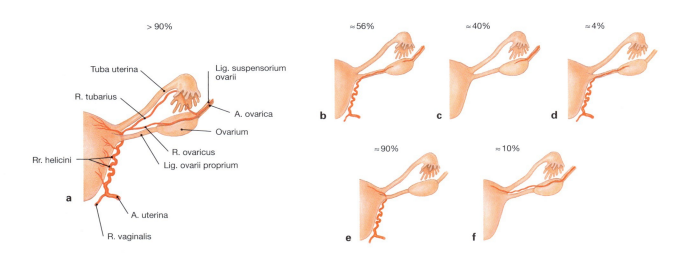

Figs. 7.83 a to f Variations of the arterial supply of the internal female genitalia; dorsal view.

- **a** arterial supply of the Uterus (textbook case)
- **c** and **d** arterial supply of the ovary (**b** textbook case)
- **e** and **f** arterial supply of the Fundus uteri (**e** textbook case)

Innervation of the female genitalia

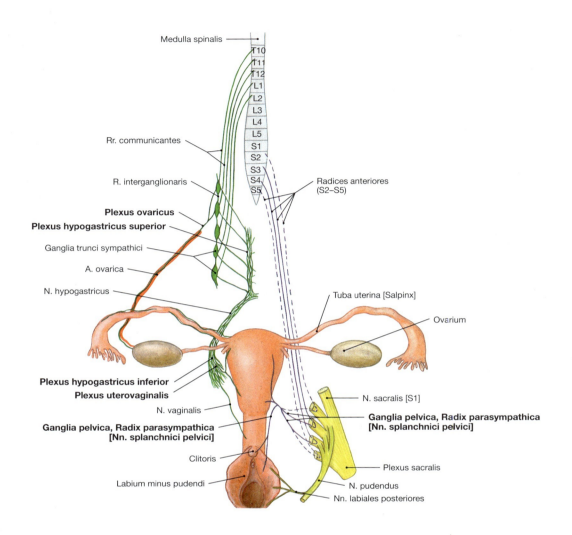

Fig. 7.84 Innervation of the female genitalia; ventral view; schematic illustration. Plexus hypogastricus inferior and Plexus uterovaginalis contain sympathetic (green) and parasympathetic (purple) nerve fibres.

Preganglionic **sympathetic nerve fibres** (T10 – L2) descend from the Plexus aorticus abdominalis via the Plexus hypogastricus superior and from the sacral ganglia of the sympathetic trunk (Truncus sympathicus) via the Nn. splanchnici sacrales to be synapsed to postganglionic neurons in the ganglia of the Plexus hypogastricus inferior. Axons of the postganglionic neurons continue to the pelvic target organs and reach the Plexus uterovaginalis (FRANKENHÄUSER's plexus) for the innervation of Uterus, Tuba uterina, and Vagina. The (predominantly) postganglionic sympathetic nerve fibres to the ovary have already been synapsed in the Ganglia aorticorenalia or in the Plexus hypogastricus superior and descend within the Plexus ovaricus alongside the A. ovarica.

Preganglionic **parasympathetic nerve fibres** derive from the sacral parasympathetic division (S2–S4) and reach the ganglia of the Plexus hypogastricus inferior via the Nn. splanchnici pelvici. They are synapsed to postganglionic neurons either here or in close vicinity to the pelvic viscera (Ganglia pelvica) to innervate the Uterus, Tuba uterina and Vagina.

Somatic innervation by the N. pudendus conveys sensory innervation to the lower part of the Vagina and the Labia minora and majora via the Rr. labiales posteriores and to the Clitoris via the N. dorsalis clitoridis.

Efferent urinary system → **Genitalia** → Rectum and anal canal → Topography → Sections

Lymph vessels of the female genitalia

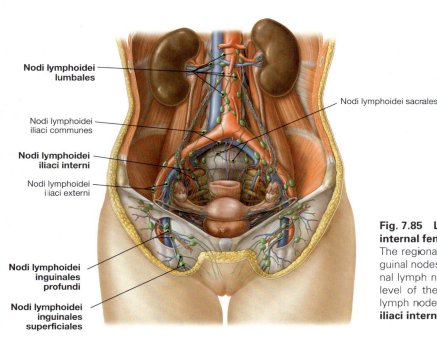

Fig. 7.85 Lymph vessels and lymph nodes of the external and internal female genitalia; ventral view.
The regional lymph nodes for the external female genitalia are the inguinal nodes (**Nodi lymphoidei inguinales**). In contrast, the first regional lymph node station of the ovary is located retroperitoneally at the level of the kidneys (**Nodi lymphoidei lumbales**) and the regional lymph nodes of the Uterus are in the lesser pelvis (**Nodi lymphoidei iliaci interni**).

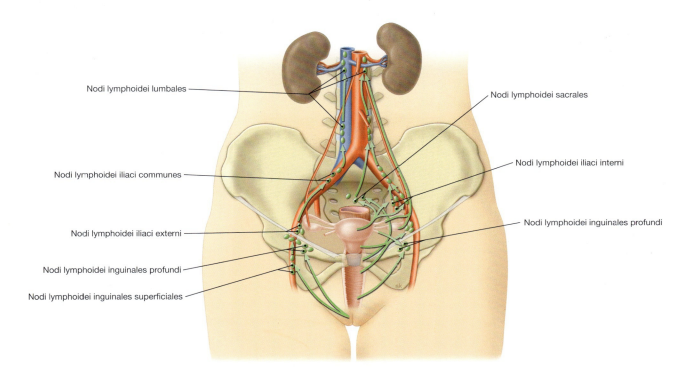

Fig. 7.86 Lymphatic drainage pathways of the external and internal female genitalia; ventral view.
Unlike the situation in men, the lymphatic drainage pathways of the external and internal female genitalia are not completely separate, and parts of the lymph of the internal genitalia also drain into the inguinal lymph nodes.

External genitalia:
- Nodi lymphoidei inguinales: Vulva

Internal genitalia:
- Nodi lymphoidei lumbales at the level of the kidneys: Ovarium, Tuba uterina, Uterus (uterotubal junction), lymphatic vessels within the Lig. suspensorium ovarii
- Nodi lymphoidei iliaci interni/externi and Nodi lymphoidei sacrales: Uterus, Vagina, Tuba uterina
- Nodi lymphoidei inguinales: lower Vagina, Uterus (uterotubal junction), lymph vessels within the Lig. teres uteri

Clinical Remarks

Due to the different lymphatic drainage pathways, the primary **lymph node metastases** are: with carcinoma of the Vulva the inguinal lymph nodes, with carcinoma of the Endometrium and the Cervix the lymph nodes in the lesser pelvis, and with ovarian carcinoma the retroperitoneal lymph nodes.

Pelvis and Retroperitoneal Space

Pelvic floor in women

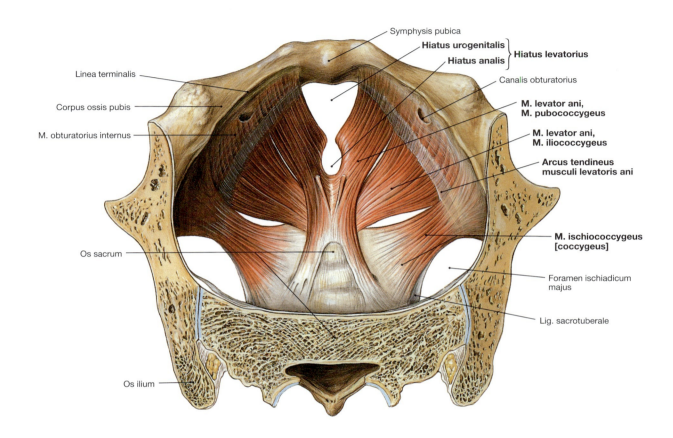

Fig. 7.87 Pelvic floor, Diaphragma pelvis, in women; cranial view. The organisation of the pelvic floor in women is similar to men. The pelvic floor closes the pelvic cavity caudally.

Organisation:
- M. levator ani, comprising the M. pubococcygeus, M. iliococcygeus, and M. puborectalis
- M. ischiococcygeus

In contrast to the M. pubococcygeus and M. ischiococcygeus, the M. iliococcygeus does not originate from the bone of the hip but from the Arcus tendineus musculi levatoris ani, a reinforcement of the fascia of the M. obturatorius internus.

The muscles of both sides spare the levator hiatus between them (Hiatus levatorius) This muscular gap is subdivided by the connective tissue of the perineum (Centrum perinei) into the anterior **Hiatus urogenitalis** for the passage of Urethra and Vagina and the posterior **Hiatus analis** for the passage of the Rectum.
The pelvic floor is innervated by direct branches of the Plexus sacralis (S3–S4).
Function: The pelvic floor stabilises the position of the pelvic viscera and, thus, is essential for urinary and faecal continence.

→ T 20a

Clinical Remarks

Women more frequently suffer from **pelvic floor insufficiency** due to the extensive dilation of the levator hiatus during vaginal deliveries. As a consequence, a lowering **(descensus)** or **prolapse** of Uterus and Vagina may occur. This condition is often combined with a prolapse of the bladder (cystocele) and the Rectum (rectocele) resulting in **urinary** and **faecal incontinence** because the Uterus is firmly connected to the posterior wall of the urinary bladder and the Vagina adheres to the anterior wall of the Rectum.

Efferent urinary system → **Genitalia** → Rectum and anal canal → Topography → Sections

Pelvic floor in women

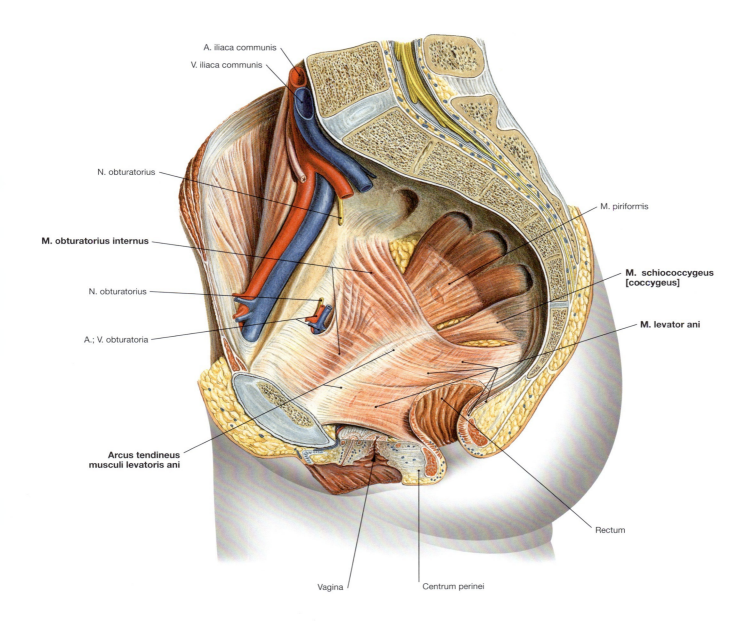

Fig. 7.88 Pelvic floor, Diaphragma pelvis, in women; view from the left side.
The pelvic floor consists of the **M. levator ani** and the **M. ischiococcygeus.** The M. iliococcygeus of the M. levator ani originates from the Arcus tendineus musculi levatoris ani. The latter is a reinforcement of the fascia of the M. obturatorius internus. One of the origins of the M. obturatorius internus is the superior pubic ramus where it is pierced by the Canalis obturatorius with the A. and V. obturatoria and the N. obturatorius. The M. obturatorius internus then exits the pelvis laterally through the Foramen ischiadicum minus. The M. levator ani extends to the sacrum and the coccyx and closes the pelvic cavity caudally.

→ T 20a

7 Pelvis and Retroperitoneal Space

Perineal muscles in women

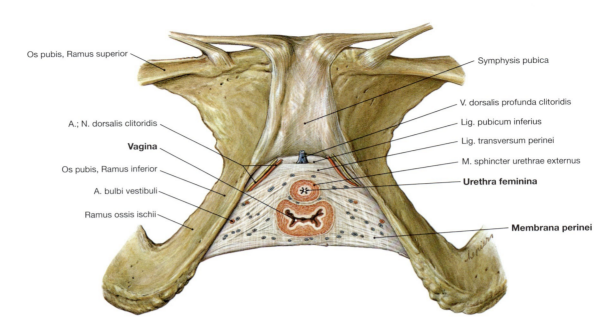

Fig. 7.89 Perineal muscles in women; caudal view; after removal of all other muscles.
In women, the muscular gap of the levator hiatus (Hiatus levatorius) is almost entirely closed by connective tissue which leaves only the passage for the Vagina and the Urethra feminina. Unlike in men, the perineal muscles in women are weak (→ Fig. 7.64). The weak **M. transversus perinei profundus,** which only consists of single muscle fibres embedded within connective tissue (→ Fig. 7.90), and the **M. transversus perinei superficialis** do **not form** a **muscular plate.** Therefore, the term "Diaphragma urogenitale" is not used anymore.
While in men the **deep perineal space** (Spatium profundum perinei) is filled with the M. transversus perinei profundus, the separation of the perineal spaces is more difficult in women. However, similar to men the female **deep perineal space** is confined inferiorly by the perineal membrane (**Membrana perinei**). In addition, it contains the Vagina and the Urethra and is traversed by deep branches of the N. pudendus and A. and V. pudenda interna before they reach the Vulva.
The **superficial perineal space** (Spatium superficiale perinei) is located caudal to the perineal membrane and, amongst others, contains the M. transversus perinei superficialis.

→ T 20b

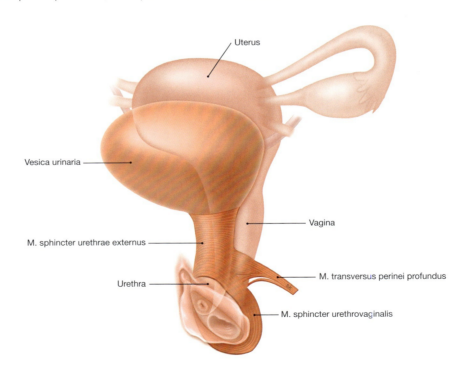

Fig. 7.90 Voluntary sphincter muscles of the urinary bladder.
The M. transversus perinei profundus in women does not form a continuous muscular plate. Instead, individual striated muscle fibres around the Urethra form the **M. sphincter urethrae externus** which constitutes the voluntary sphincter muscle of the urinary bladder (→ Fig. 7.89). Some distal fibres continue to surround the distal Vagina and are referred to as **M. sphincter urethrovaginalis.**

→ T 20b

Perineal region in women

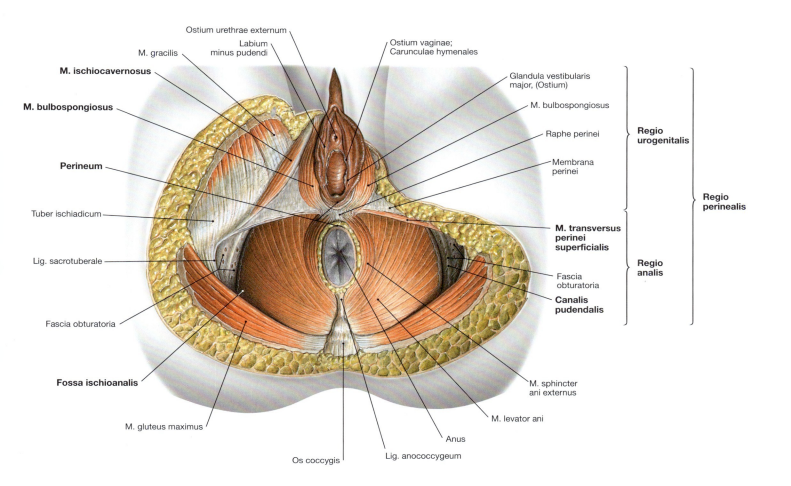

Fig. 7.91 Perineal region, Regio perinealis, in women; caudal view; after removal of all neurovascular structures.
The **perineal region** reaches from the inferior margin of the pubic symphysis (Symphysis pubica) to the tip of the coccyx (Os coccygis). The term **perineum** in women, however, describes exclusively the small connective tissue bridge between the posterior margin of the Labia majora and the Anus. The perineal region is subdivided into the **anterior Regio urogenitalis** (urogenital triangle) containing the external genitalia and the Urethra and the **posterior Regio analis** (anal triangle) around the Anus. The following spaces can be found within these triangles:
- The Regio analis contains the **Fossa ischioanalis** (→ Table) which constitutes a pyramid-shaped space on both sides of the Anus. The Fossa ischioanalis is similar in men and women. The lateral wall contains in a fascial duplicature of the M. obturatorius internus (Fascia obturatoria) the pudendal canal (ALCOCK's canal). The pudendal canal harbours the A. and V. pudenda interna, and the N. pudendus after their passage from the gluteal region through the Foramen ischiadicum minus.
- The Regio urogenitalis has two **perineal spaces:**
  – The **deep perineal space** (Spatium profundum perinei) is bordered inferiorly by the perineal membrane (Membrana perinei) and, in women, contains the weak M. transversus perinei profundus and the M. sphincter urethrae externus.
  – The **superficial perineal space** (Spatium superficiale perinei) between the Membrana perinei and the body fascia (Fascia perinei) contains the M. transversus perinei superficialis, the M. bulbospongiosus, and the M. ischiocavernosus. These three muscles stabilise the cavernous bodies of vestibule and Clitoris.

Borders of the Fossa ischioanalis	
Medial und cranial	M. sphincter ani externus and M. levator ani
Lateral	M. obturatorius externus
Dorsal	M. gluteus maximus and Lig. sacrotuberale
Ventral	posterior margin of the superficial and the deep perineal spaces; anterior recesses reach the pubic symphysis
Caudal	fascia and skin of the Perineum

Clinical Remarks

During vaginal delivery tears of the perineal skin and the perineal muscles, including the anal sphincter muscles, may occur **(perineal tears).** Selective incisions extending from the Vagina medially or laterally **(episiotomy)** are performed to prevent uncontrolled perineal tears.

Pelvis and Retroperitoneal Space

Perineal region in women

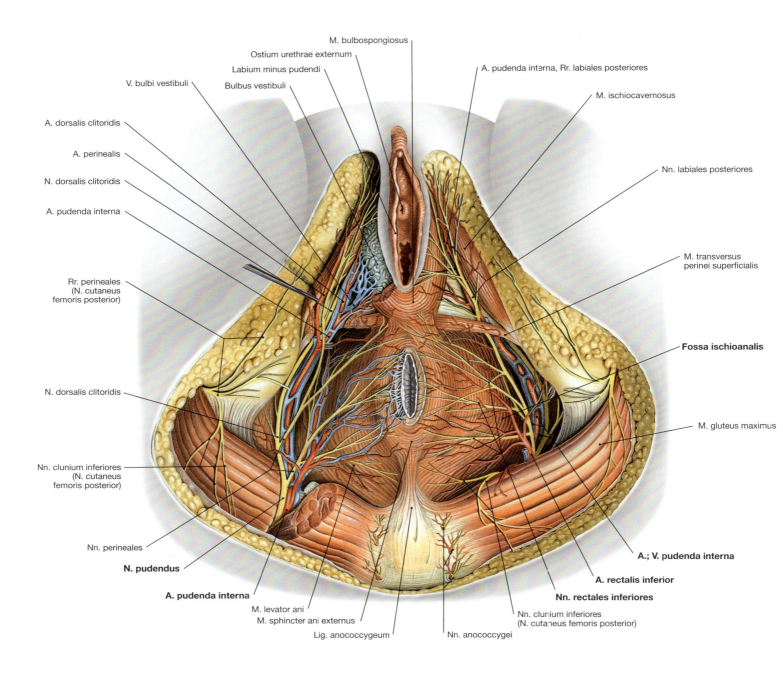

Fig. 7.92 Blood vessels and nerves of the perineal region, Regio perinealis, in women; caudal view.
The **Fossa ischioanalis** has a very similar anatomy in men and women. The pyramid-shaped fossa is filled with adipose tissue. Covered by a fascial duplicature of the M. obturatorius internus, the Canalis pudendalis (ALCOCK's canal), the neurovascular structures enter the Fossa ischioanalis from dorsolateral. At first branches to the Anus and the anal canal exit and cross the ischio-anal fossa to reach the Anus. The neurovascular structures then continue ventrally to the Vulva and the two perineal spaces.

Contents of the Fossa ischioanalis:
- A. and V. pudenda interna, and N. pudendus: in the Canalis pudendalis (ALCOCK's canal)
- A., V. and N. rectalis inferior: to the anal canal

Clinical Remarks

Similar to men, the Fossa ischioanalis is of great clinical relevance because of its expansion to both sides of the Anus. **Collections of pus** (abscesses), e.g. fistulas from the anal canal, may expand within the entire ischio-anal fossa, including its anterior recesses and even extend to the pubic symphysis. These abscesses not only cause non-specific inflammatory signs but also result in intense pain in the perineal region.

Perineal spaces in women

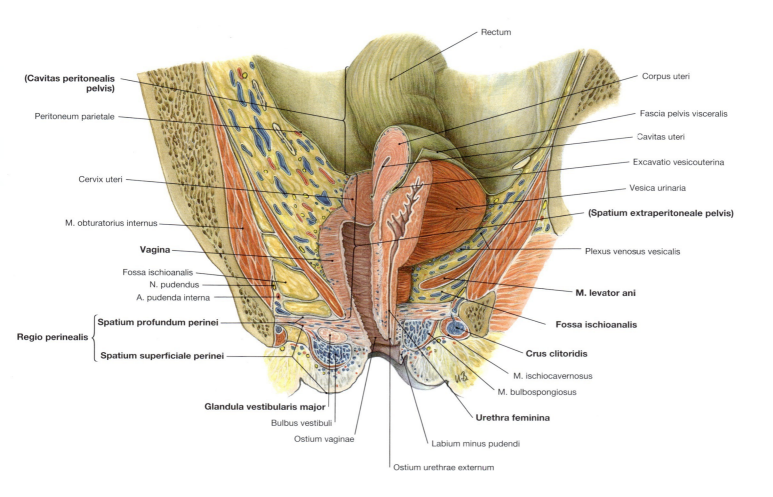

Fig. 7.93 Perineal spaces in women; median section, and frontal section on the right side; ventral view.
The frontal section shows **three levels** of the female pelvis:
- peritoneal cavity of the pelvis (Cavitas peritonealis pelvis) bordered caudally by the parietal peritoneum
- subperitoneal space (Spatium extraperitoneale pelvis), caudally bordered by the M. levator ani of the pelvic floor
- perineal region (Regio perinealis) inferior to the pelvic floor. The anterior portion contains the two perineal spaces, and includes the variably expanded anterior recesses of the ischio-anal fossa (illustrated here in two different ways for the right and left sides).

The **deep perineal space** (Spatium profundum perinei) consists of connective tissue and single muscle fibres of the M. transversus perinei profundus. It also contains the passage of the Vagina and the Urethra. The deep perineal space is traversed by the deep branches of the N. pudendus (N. dorsalis clitoridis), and the A. and V. pudenda interna (A. bulbi vestibuli, A. dorsalis clitoridis, A. profunda clitoridis) before they reach the Vulva. The Nn. cavernosi clitoridis pierce the Perineum and enter the Corpora cavernosa of the Clitoris.

The **superficial perineal space** (Spatium superficiale perinei) is located between the perineal membrane (Membrana perinei) and the body fascia (Fascia perinei). It contains the M. transversus perinei superficialis, the proximal parts of the Corpora cavernosa clitoridis, the Glandulae vestibulares majores (BARTHOLIN's glands), and the vestibular bulb (Bulbus vestibuli). The bulb of the vestibule is embraced by the M. bulbospongiosus, the Crura clitoridis by the M. ischiocavernosus on both sides. The superficial branches of the N. pudendus (N. perinealis with Nn. labiales posteriores), and of the A. and V. pudenda interna (A. perinealis with Rr. labiales posteriores) also traverse this space to reach the labia.

7 Pelvis and Retroperitoneal Space

Kidney and adrenal gland →

Projection of the rectum and anal canal

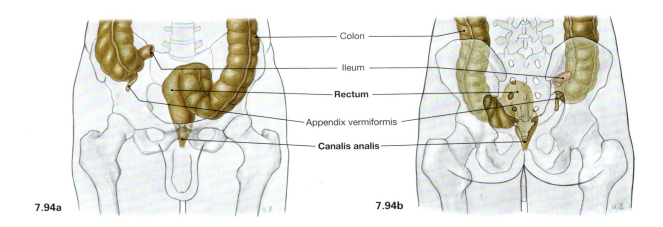

7.94a   7.94b

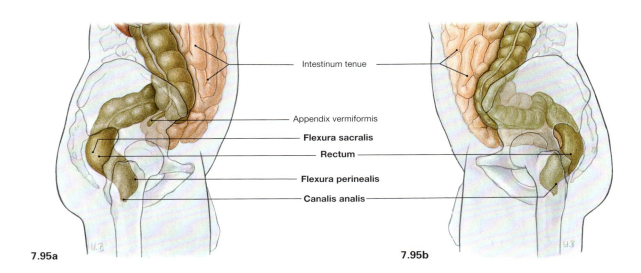

7.95a   7.95b

Fig. 7.94 and Fig. 7.95 Projection of the rectum, Rectum, and of the anal canal, Canalis analis, onto the body surface; ventral (→ Fig. 7.94a), dorsal (→ Fig. 7.94b), and lateral (→ Figs. 7.95a and b) views.
The Rectum begins at the level of the 2nd or 3rd sacral vertebrae and ends on the pelvic floor which is traversed by the anal canal. In the sagittal plane, the Rectum has two bends: the dorsally convex Flexura sacralis and the ventrally convex Flexura perinealis. The upper portion of the Rectum above the Flexura sacralis is a **secondarily retroperitoneal organ,** the distal portion and the anal canal have a **subperitoneal position.**

Position of the rectum

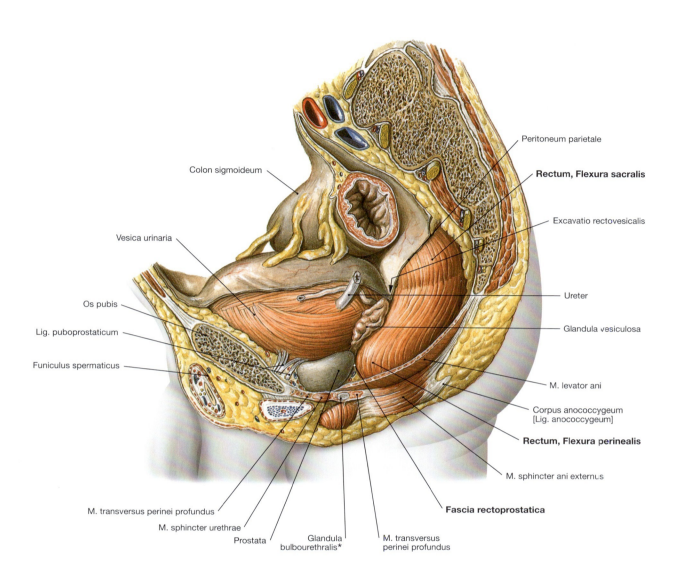

Fig. 7.96 Rectum, Rectum, in the male pelvis; view from the left side.
The illustration shows the two bends of the Rectum in the sagittal plane. In the upper secondary retroperitoneal portion, the Rectum adjusts to the curvature of the sacrum and displays the **dorsally convex Flexura sacralis**. Inferior to this part, the Rectum is not covered by parietal peritoneum, but has a subperitoneal position. The **ventrally convex Flexura perinealis** is at the level of the pelvic diaphragm. Inferior to the pelvic diaphragm, the Rectum continues as the anal canal in an inferior and dorsal direction. In men, the anterior aspect of the Rectum is adjacent to the posterior wall of the urinary bladder (Vesica urinaria) and the seminal vesicles (Glandulae vesiculosae) and further caudally to the prostate gland. Here, the Rectum is separated from the prostate gland only by the thin **Fascia rectoprostatica** (DENONVILLIER's fascia). In women, the Rectum is closely adjacent to the posterior aspect of the Vagina and only separated from the Vagina by the Fascia rectovaginalis (→ Fig. 7.116).

* clinical term: COWPER's glands

Clinical Remarks

Because the prostate gland is separated from the Rectum only by the thin Fascia rectoprostatica (DENONVILLIER's fascia), the prostate gland can be assessed by **digital rectal examination (DRE)**. Due to the high incidence of benign prostatic hyperplasia (BPH) and prostatic carcinoma, the digital rectal examination is part of a complete physical examination in men over 50 years of age.

Pelvis and Retroperitoneal Space

Kidney and adrenal gland →

Structure of the rectum

Fig. 7.97 Rectum, Rectum; view from the left side.
Cranially, the Rectum forms the dorsally convex Flexura sacralis and caudally, at the level of the passage through the pelvic floor, the ventrally convex Flexura perinealis.
Unlike the Colon, the muscular layer (Tunica muscularis) of the Rectum not only contains the circular layer (Stratum circulare) but also a continuous longitudinal layer (Stratum longitudinale).

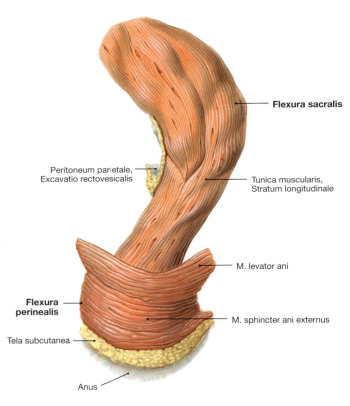

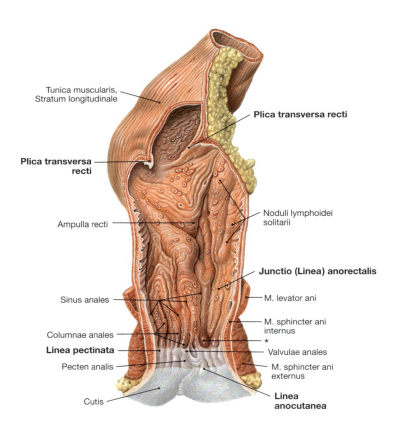

Fig. 7.98 Rectum, Rectum, and anal canal, Canalis analis; ventral view.
The inner relief of the Rectum shows transverse folds, so-called Plicae transversae recti. One of the three folds is palpable regularly at about 6–7 cm above the Anus (KOHLRAUSCH's fold). Below this fold, the Rectum is dilated to form the Ampulla recti. The Linea anorectalis marks the transition to the anal canal. This area is characterised by the change from the transverse folds of the Rectum to the longitudinal folds of the anal canal and represents a transitional zone between Rectum and anal canal (Junctio anorectalis).
The **anal canal** is divided into **three segments**:
- **Zona columnaris:** contains longitudinal folds (Columnae anales) formed by the underlying Corpus cavernosum recti
- **Pecten analis:** the stratified non-keratinised squamous epithelium creates a white zone in the mucosa (**Zona alba**); the superior border of this zone is referred to as **Linea pectinata** (clinical term: **Linea dentata**); here, the Valvulae anales and the white squamous epithelium meet.
- **Zona cutanea:** external skin, inconsistently limited by the Linea anocutanea

* haemorrhoidal knots

Efferent urinary system → Genitalia → **Rectum and anal canal** → Topography → Sections

Structure of the anal canal

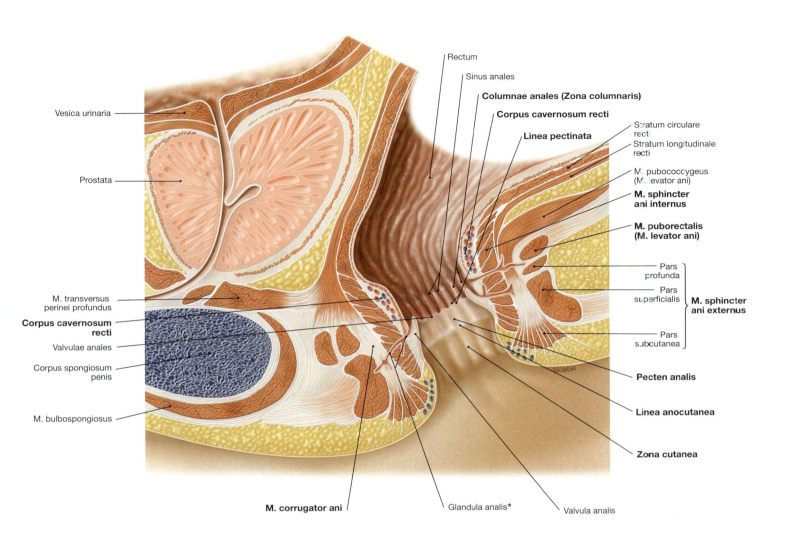

Fig. 7.99 Rectum, Rectum, and anal canal, Canalis analis, in men; median section; view from the left side. (according to [1])
This illustration demonstrates the segments of the anal canal and the organisation of the continence organ. The anal canal is divided into **three segments** (→ Fig. 7.98):
The pectinate line **(Linea pectinata)** is the developmental border between the hindgut and the proctodeum and marks the border between the Zona columnaris and the Pecten analis in the adult. Similar to the left colic flexure, the pectinate line represents the watershed for several neurovascular structures and serves as clinically important landmark in the anal canal.
The anal canal possesses a **continence organ** controlled by the CNS which is composed of the anus, sphincter muscles, and the Corpus cavernosum recti. Apart from defecation, the Anus is closed by the permanent contractions of the internal anal sphincter muscles. The Corpus cavernosum recti is supplied by the A. rectalis superior and this warrants a gas-tight closure of the anal canal.

The **sphincter muscles** comprise:
- **M. sphincter ani internus** (smooth muscles, involuntary sympathetic innervation): continuation of the circular muscular layer
- **M. corrugator ani** (smooth muscles): continuation of the longitudinal muscular layer
- **M. sphincter ani externus** (striated muscles, voluntary control via the N. pudendus): has different segments (Partes subcutanea, superficialis, profunda)
- **M. puborectalis** (striated muscles, voluntary control via the N. pudendus and direct branches of the sacral plexus): part of the M. levator ani; forms a loop behind the Rectum to pull it ventrally and create the Flexura perinealis. The resulting kink of the Rectum enables the storage of faeces in the rectal ampulla.

For lymphatic drainage → page 99.

* proctodeal gland

→ T 20

Clinical Remarks

Since the Rectum has transverse folds (Plicae transversae recti) and the anal canal has longitudinal folds (Columnae anales), inspection of the mucosa of a prolapse allows the visual discrimination between a **rectal** versus an **anal prolapse**. Both result in faecal incontinence. Due to the different neurovascular supply of the Anus, the Linea pectinata serves as clinically relevant landmark during **surgery of anal cancer**. Proximal tumours metastasise to the pelvic lymph nodes, distal carcinomas spread first to the inguinal lymph nodes. Nevertheless, the tumours are staged according to their proximity to the Linea anocutanea.

Dilations of the Corpus cavernosum recti are referred to as **haemorrhoids** (→ Figs. 7.104 and 7.105). Behind the Valvulae anales, the Sinus anales are located as depressions in which proctodeal glands (Glandulae anales) enter the anal canal. These glands may traverse the sphincter muscles and cause **fistulas** when inflamed and, thus, potentially facilitate the spread of the inflammation into the ischio-anal fossa.

Pelvis and Retroperitoneal Space

Arteries of the rectum and anal canal

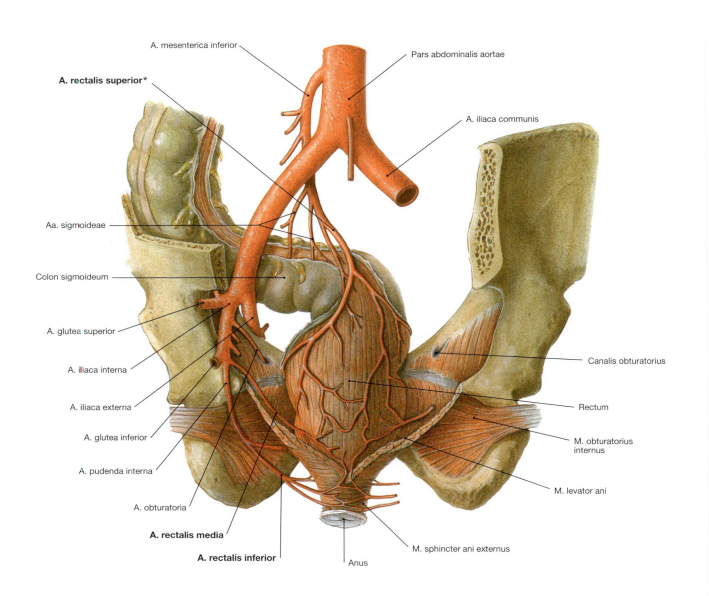

Fig. 7.100 Rectal arteries, Aa. rectales; dorsal view.
Rectum and anal canal are supplied by three arteries:
- **A. rectalis superior** (unpaired): from the A. mesenterica inferior
- **A. rectalis media** (paired): from the A. iliaca interna above the pelvic floor (M. levator ani)
- **A. rectalis inferior** (paired): from the A. pudenda interna beneath the pelvic floor

The border between the corresponding arterial supply from the A. mesenterica inferior and the A. iliaca interna is located at the Linea pectinata where numerous anastomoses between these arteries exist. The A. rectalis superior is the last branch of the A. mesenterica inferior and provides a branch for the anastomosis with the Aa. sigmoideae. From this point onwards (clinical term: SUDECK's point [*]), the A. rectalis superior is considered a terminal artery. The Corpus cavernosum recti is primarily supplied by the A. rectalis superior. Therefore, bleedings of haemorrhoids, which represent dilated rectal cavernous bodies, are arterial bleedings as shown by the bright red colour.

Veins of the rectum and anal canal

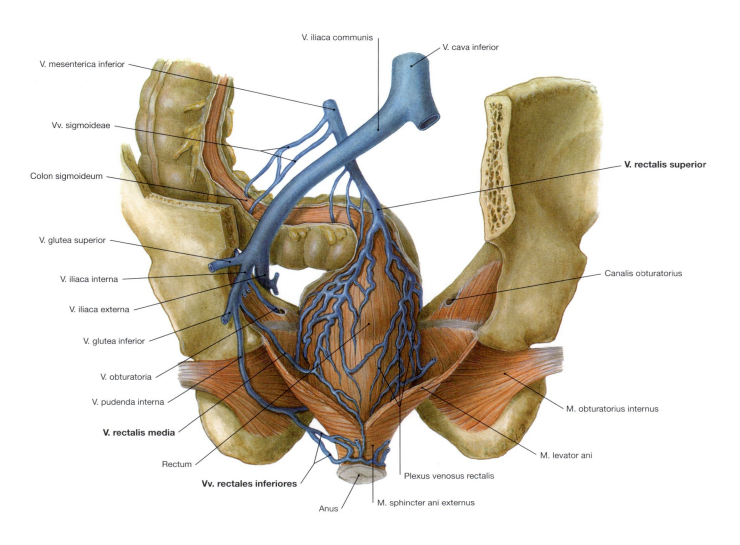

Fig. 7.101 Rectal veins, Vv. rectales; dorsal view.
Corresponding to the rectal arteries, the venous blood from the Rectum and the anal canal drains via three veins:
- **V. rectalis superior** (unpaired): access to the portal vein (V. portae hepatis) via the V. mesenterica inferior
- **V. rectalis media** (paired): access to the V. cava inferior via the V. iliaca interna
- **V. rectalis inferior** (paired): access to the V. cava inferior via the V. pudenda interna and the V. iliaca interna

The watershed between the venous drainage to the V. portae hepatis and the V. cava inferior is in the area of the Linea pectinata. There are numerous anastomoses.

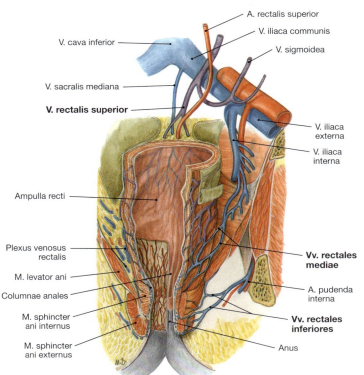

Fig. 7.102 Venous drainage of rectum, Rectum, and anal canal, Canalis analis; ventral view. Tributaries to the V. portae hepatis (purple) and to the V. cava inferior (blue).
This illustration demonstrates that the venous drainage pathways to the portal vein and to the inferior vena cava have numerous anastomoses. With increased blood pressure in the portal system **(portal hypertension),** e.g. in liver cirrhosis, these anastomoses are utilised for the drainage of blood to the V. cava inferior **(portocaval anastomoses).** Since they do not result in haemorrhoids, the anastomoses have no clinical relevance.

Pelvis and Retroperitoneal Space

Innervation of the rectum and anal canal

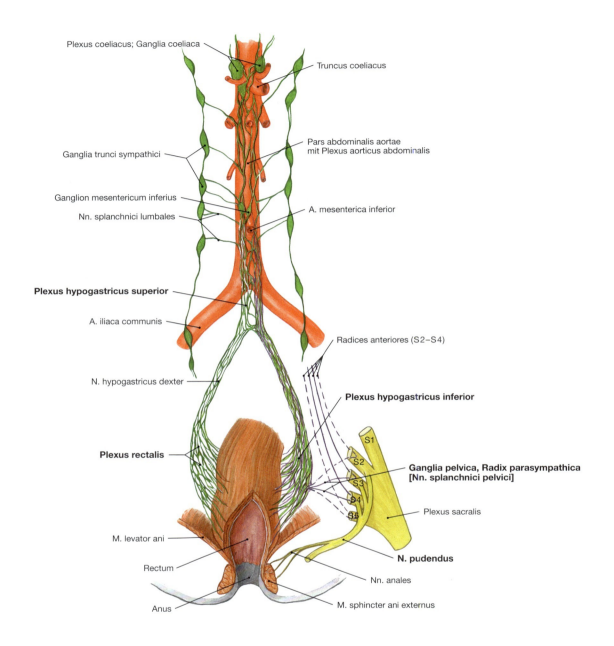

Fig. 7.103 **Innervation of the rectum, Rectum, and anal canal, Canalis analis;** ventral view; schematic illustration. The Plexus rectalis contains sympathetic (green) and parasympathetic (purple) nerve fibres.

The Plexus rectalis is a continuation of the Plexus hypogastricus inferior.

The preganglionic **sympathetic fibres** (T10–L2) descend from the Plexus aorticus abdominalis via the Plexus hypogastricus superior and from the sacral ganglia of the sympathetic trunk (Truncus sympathicus) via the Nn. splanchnici sacrales. They are predominantly synapsed to postganglionic sympathetic neurons in the Plexus hypogastricus inferior. These postganglionic fibres reach the Rectum and anal canal via the Plexus rectalis. Sympathetic fibres activate the sphincter muscles (M. sphincter ani internus).

Preganglionic **parasympathetic fibres** derive from the sacral division of the parasympathetic nervous system (S2–S4) via the Nn. splanchnici pelvici to the ganglia of the Plexus hypogastricus inferior. They are synapsed to postganglionic fibres either here or in the vicinity of the intestines for the stimulation of the peristalsis and the inhibition of the internal anal sphincter muscles (M. sphincter ani internus) to facilitate defaecation.

The autonomic innervation ends approximately in the area of the Linea pectinata. The inferior portion of the anal canal is innervated by the somatic **N. pudendus** to convey sensory innervation to the skin inferior to the pectinate line. Thus, anal carcinomas inferior to the pectinate line are extremely painful, whereas anal carcinomas located above this demarcation line are not. In addition, the N. pudendus conveys motor fibres to the M. sphincter ani externus and to the M. puborectalis and, thus, facilitates voluntary closure of the Anus.

Efferent urinary system → Genitalia → **Rectum and anal canal** → Topography → Sections

Haemorrhoids

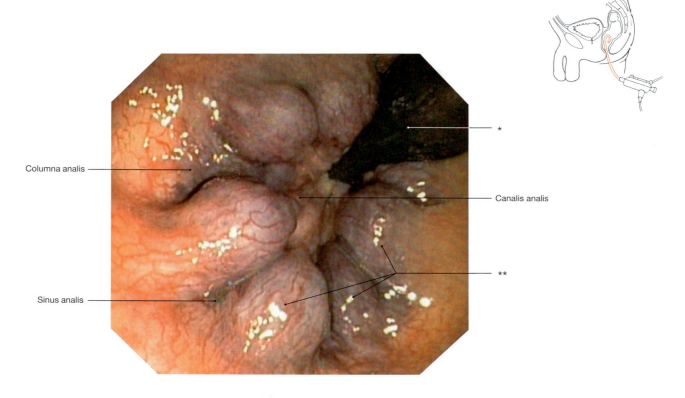

Fig. 7.104 Anal canal, Canalis analis; rectoscopy; cranial view. Clearly, six substantially enlarged knots of the Corpus cavernosum recti are visible (haemorrhoids).

* coloscope
** three haemorrhoidal knots

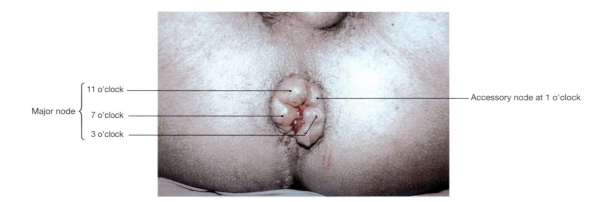

Fig. 7.105 Haemorrhoids grade IV; caudal view with the patient in supine position and the examiner facing the Perineum. [4]
The position of haemorrhoidal knots is documented according to the clock-face. Due to the major branching pattern of the A. rectalis superior in the Corpus cavernosus recti, major haemorrhoidal knots typically appear at 3, 7 and 11 o'clock. Minor knots may derive from the smaller arterial branches. A smaller knot is visible here at 1 o'clock.

Clinical Remarks

Haemorrhoids are frequently occuring pathological dilations of the Corpus cavernosum recti. The causes are not fully understood but the nutrition in industrialised countries (rich in fat, poor in fibres) may be a contributing factor. Haemorrhoids are categorised in different **grades**:
- grade I: only visible endoscopically
- grade II: protrude during bearing down for bowel movements; afterwards retract into the anal canal
- grade III: protrude spontaneously, can be reposited manually
- grade IV: cannot be reposited

Beginning at grade II, therapeutic intervention is recommended either by sclerotherapy, rubber band ligation, or surgical excision (haemorrhoidectomy; grade III and IV).

7 Pelvis and Retroperitoneal Space

Kidney and adrenal gland →

Blood vessels of the retroperitoneal space

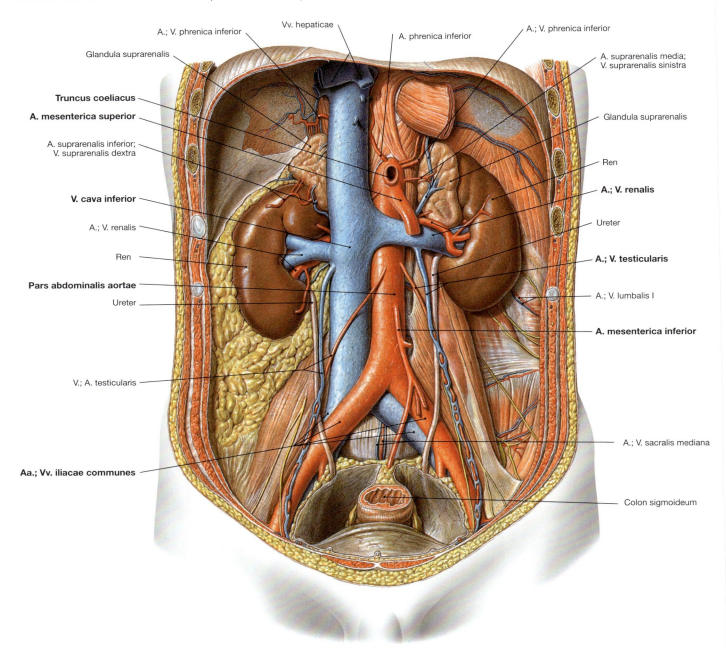

Fig. 7.106 Blood vessels in the retroperitoneal space; ventral view.

After its passage through the diaphragm, the Aorta continues as Pars abdominalis and is located in the retroperitoneal space at the left side of the V. cava inferior and anterior to the vertebral column. The branches of the **Pars abdominalis aortae** are listed in the table.

The **V. cava inferior** originates from the merging of the two Vv. iliacae communes and is located at the right side of the Aorta.

Tributaries of the V. cava inferior

- Vv. iliacae communes
- V. sacralis mediana
- Vv. lumbales
- V. phrenica inferior dextra, enters the V. renalis on the left side
- V. testicularis/ovarica dextra, enters the V. renalis on the left side
- V. suprarenalis dextra, enters the V. renalis on the left side
- Vv. renales dextra and sinistra
- three Vv. hepaticae (Vv. hepaticae dextra, intermedia and sinistra)

Branches of the Pars abdominalis aortae

Parietal branches to the body wall	• A. phrenica inferior: at the inferior side of the diaphragm, gives rise to the A. suprarenalis superior to the adrenal gland • Aa. lumbales: four pairs directly branching off the Aorta, the fifth pair derives from the A. sacralis mediana
Visceral branches to the viscera	• Truncus coeliacus: unpaired, originates directly beneath the Hiatus aorticus and supplies the viscera of the Epigastrium (→ Fig. 6.113) • A. suprarenalis media: supplies the adrenal gland • A. renalis: to the kidney, also gives rise to the A. suprarenalis inferior to the adrenal gland • A. mesenterica superior: unpaired, supplies parts of the Pancreas, the entire small intestines and the Colon up to the left colic flexure (→ Fig. 6.115) • A. testicularis/ovarica: supplies Testis and Epididymis in men and the ovary in women • A. mesenterica inferior: unpaired, supplies the Colon descendens and upper Rectum (→ Fig. 6.118)
Terminal branches	• A. iliaca communis: to the pelvis and the lower extremity • A. sacralis mediana: descends on the sacrum

→ dissection link

Lymph vessels of the retroperitoneal space

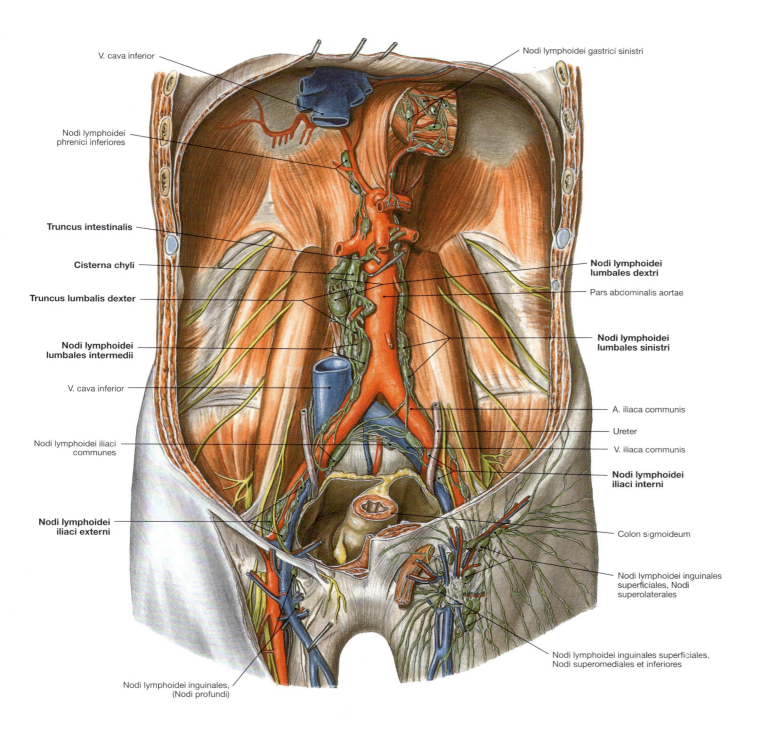

Fig. 7.107 Lymph vessels and lymph nodes of the retroperitoneal space; ventral view.
The lymph from the pelvis drains via the Nodi lymphoidei iliaci communes into the parietal lymph nodes of the retroperitoneal space which are collectively referred to as **Nodi lymphoidei lumbales.** These are positioned in three chains as Nodi lymphoidei lumbales sinistri around the Aorta, as Nodi lymphoidei lumbales dextri to both sides of the V. cava inferior, and as Nodi lymphoidei lumbales intermedii in between both blood vessels. The lumbar lymph nodes not only collect the lymph from the lower extremities, pelvic viscera, and the Colon descendens, but they also serve as regional lymph node stations for the kidney, the adrenal gland, and the testis/ovary.
The efferent lymph vessels from the lumbar lymph nodes form the bilateral **Trunci lumbales.** Both Trunci lumbales merge with the **Truncus intestinalis** (collects lymph from the visceral lymph nodes of the abdominal cavity) in the Cisterna chyli and continue as **Ductus thoracicus.** Thus, the Ductus thoracicus below the diaphragm drains the lymph from the entire lower half of the body.

Pelvis and Retroperitoneal Space

Kidney and adrenal gland →

Somatic nerves of the retroperitoneal space

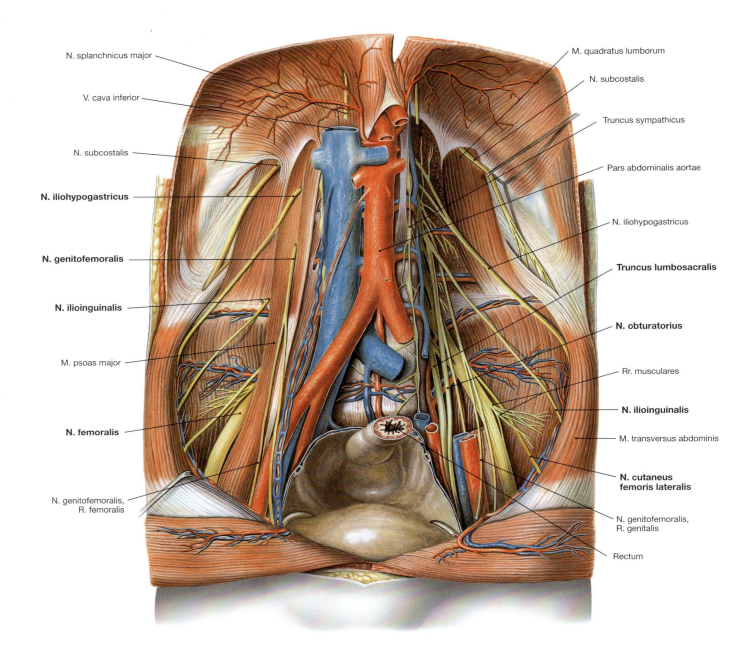

Fig. 7.108 Somatic nerves of the retroperitoneal space; ventral view.
In addition to the blood and lymph vessels, the nerves of the **Plexus lumbalis** for the innervation of the inguinal region and the anterior aspect of the thigh are also located in the retroperitoneal space (→ p. 330, Vol. 1). The Truncus lumbosacralis is the connection to the Plexus sacralis in the lesser pelvis. Thus, the Plexus lumbosacralis constitutes a continuous nerve plexus.

Branches of the Plexus lumbalis (T12–L4):
motor branches to the M. iliopsoas and M. quadratus lumborum (T12–L4)
- N. iliohypogastricus (T12, L1)
- N. ilioinguinalis (T12, L1)
- N. genitofemoralis (L1, L2)
- N. cutaneus femoris lateralis (L2, L3)
- N. femoralis (L2, L4)
- N. obturatorius (L2, L4)

→ T 40

Autonomic nerves of the retroperitoneal space

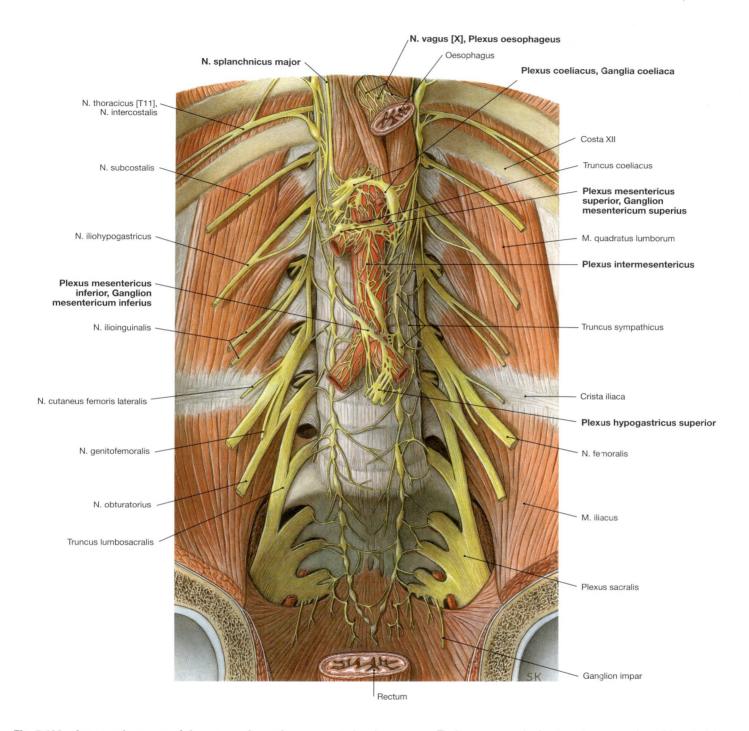

Fig. 7.109 Autonomic nerves of the retroperitoneal space; ventral view; after removal of the viscera.

The autonomic nerves of the sympathetic and the parasympathetic system form a plexus of nerve fibres on the anterior aspect of the Aorta (**Plexus aorticus abdominalis**). It contributes to additional nerve plexuses at the origins of the branches of the Aorta. The nerve fibres thereof accompany the arteries to their target organs. These plexuses include those at the three unpaired branches of the Aorta: the **Plexus coeliacus,** the **Plexus mesentericus superior** and **inferior** and the **Plexus intermesentericus** (→ Fig. 6.51). Farther caudal, the plexuses continue via the Plexus hypogastricus superior to the Plexus hypogastricus inferior in the lesser pelvis for the innervation of the pelvic viscera.

The preganglionic **sympathetic neurons** are located in the lateral column of the thoracic and upper lumbar spinal cord. They pass through the sympathetic trunk (Truncus sympathicus) without being synapsed and continue as Nn. splanchnici major and minor to the aortic plexuses. Here they synapse in different ganglia (Ganglia coeliaca, Ganglia mesenterica superius and inferius, Ganglia aorticorenalia) onto postganglionic neurons. Their axons reach the target organs alongside arterial branches.

The preganglionic **parasympathetic neurons** of the **Nn. vagi [X]** (→ p. 316, Vol. 3) descend along the Oesophagus as Trunci vagales anterior and posterior, traverse the diaphragm and travel within the autonomic nerve plexuses around the Aorta without synapsing to reach their target organs. The postganglionic parasympathetic neurons are located in the vicinity or within the wall of the target organs. The visceral innervation of the Nn. vagi [X] ends in the Plexus mesentericus superior and thus, in the area of the left colic flexure (CANNON-BOEHM's point).

The **Colon descendens** is innervated by the **sacral division of the parasympathetic nervous system.** The preganglionic neurons are located in the sacral spinal cord (S2–S4), exit the vertebral column together with the spinal nerves and travel as Nn. splanchnici pelvici to the Plexus hypogastricus inferior in the vicinity of the Rectum. After being synapsed, the postganglionic nerve fibres ascend to the Colon descendens and Colon sigmoideum.

Pelvis and Retroperitoneal Space

A. iliaca interna

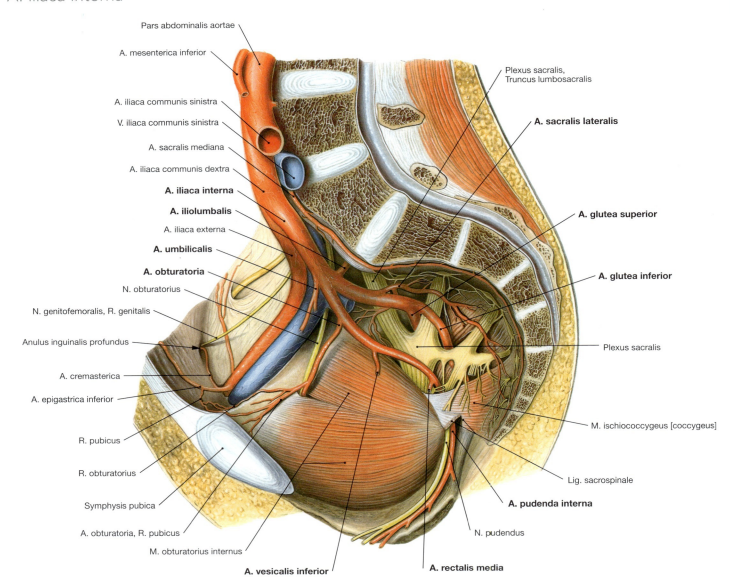

Fig. 7.110 A. iliaca interna; view from the left side.
In most cases (60%), the A. iliaca interna divides into an anterior and a posterior main branch. The sequence for the consecutive branching is highly variable. Thus, the arterial branches are categorised according to their perfusion area in **parietal branches** for the pelvic wall and the external genitalia and **visceral branches** for the pelvic viscera.

Fig. 7.111 Parietal branches of the A. iliaca interna.
- A. iliolumbalis: supplies the Fossa iliaca and the lumbar region
- Aa. sacrales laterales: to the sacral canal
- A. obturatoria: traverses the Canalis obturatorius
- A. glutea superior: exits through the Foramen suprapiriforme to the gluteal region
- A. glutea inferior: exits through the Foramen infrapiriforme to the gluteal region

For the visceral branches (different in men and women) → Figs. 7.112 and 7.113.

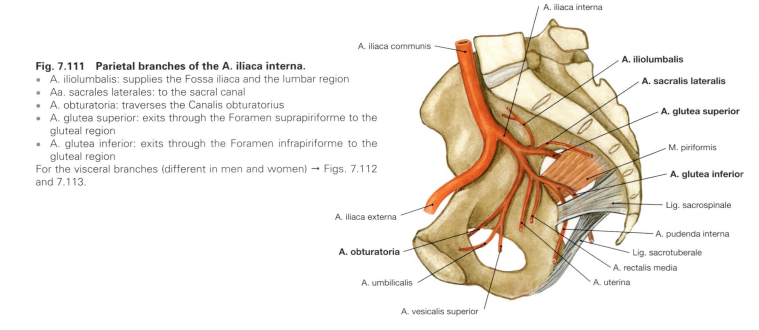

Efferent urinary system → Genitalia → Rectum and anal canal → **Topography** → Sections

Blood vessels of the male pelvis

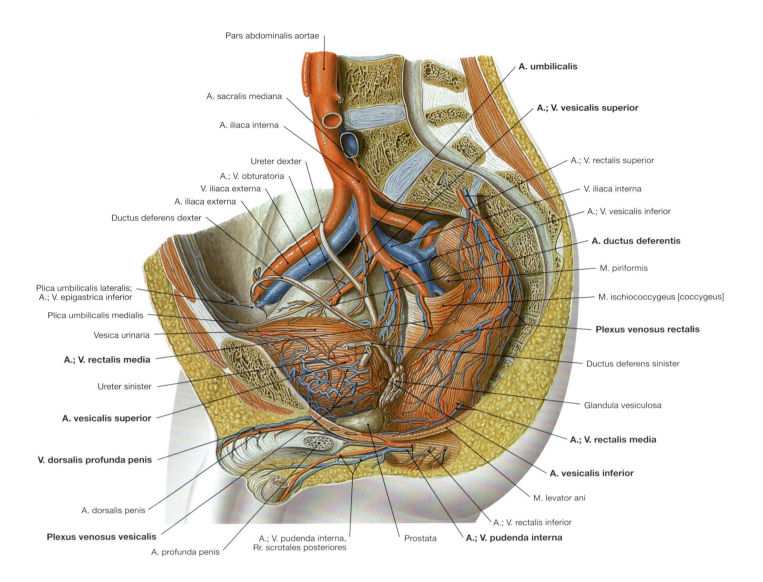

Fig. 7.112 Blood supply of the pelvic viscera in men; view from the left side.
The pelvic viscera are supplied by the **visceral branches** of the A. iliaca interna. The **parietal branches** for the pelvic wall are identical in men and women (→ Fig. 7.111).
Visceral branches of the A. iliaca interna in men:
- A. umbilicalis: gives rise to the A. vesicalis superior to the urinary bladder and often (here not shown) the A. ductus deferentis to the vas deferens before its obliterated part (Lig. umbilicale mediale) creates the Plica umbilicalis medialis.
- A. vesicalis inferior: to the urinary bladder, prostate gland, and seminal vesicle, occasionally (as shown here) gives rise to the A. ductus deferentis
- A. rectalis media: above the pelvic floor to the Rectum
- A. pudenda interna: passes through the Foramen infrapiriforme and successively the Foramen ischiadicum minus to the lateral wall of the Fossa ischioanalis (Canalis pudendalis, ALCOCK's canal). Here the A. rectalis inferior branches off to the inferior anal canal. The A. pudenda interna then divides into the superficial and deep terminal branches to supply the external genitalia. The superficial A. perinealis supplies the Perineum and provides Rr. scrotales posteriores to the Scrotum. The deep branches provide arterial blood to the cavernous bodies of the Penis (A. bulbi penis, A. dorsalis penis, A. profunda penis).

The venous blood drains into the **V. iliaca interna.** Its tributaries form communicating venous plexuses (Plexus venosi) around the pelvic viscera. These have to be removed during dissection to display the arteries and nerves of the pelvis:
- **Plexus venosus rectalis:** connected via the V. rectalis superior to the portal venous system and via the Vv. rectales media and inferior to the drainage system of the V. cava inferior (portocaval anastomosis)
- **Plexus venosus vesicalis:** at the base of the urinary bladder, also collects the venous blood from the accessory sex glands
- **Plexus venosus prostaticus:** drains not only the venous blood from the prostate gland, but also the blood from the Corpora cavernosa penis (V. dorsalis profunda penis). Connections to the venous plexuses around the vertebral column explain the frequently occurring vertebral metastases in patients with prostatic carcinoma.

→ *dissection link* 233

Pelvis and Retroperitoneal Space

Kidney and adrenal gland →

Blood vessels of the female pelvis

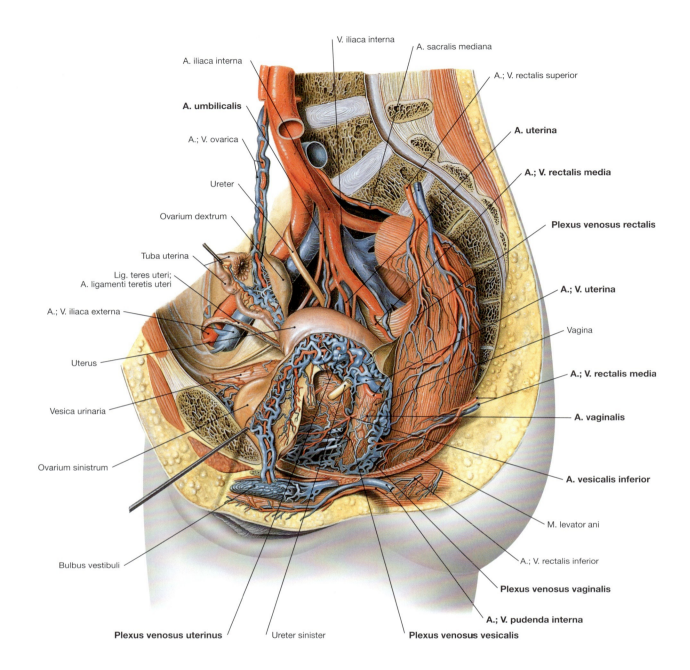

Fig. 7.113 Blood supply of the pelvic viscera in women; view from the left side.

The pelvic viscera are supplied by the **visceral branches** of the A. iliaca interna. The **parietal branches** for the pelvic wall are identical in men and women (→ Fig. 7.111).

Visceral branches of the A. iliaca interna in women:
- A. umbilicalis: gives rise to the A. vesicalis superior for the urinary bladder and the A. uterina before its obliterated part (Lig. umbilicale mediale) creates the Plica umbilicalis medialis.
- A. vesicalis inferior: to the urinary bladder and Vagina, may not be present and is then substituted by the A. vaginalis
- A. uterina: supplies the Uterus and has branches to the Tuba uterina, Ovarium, and Vagina
- A. vaginalis: occasionally substitutes the A. vesicalis inferior
- A. rectalis media: above the pelvic floor to the Rectum
- A. pudenda interna: passes through the Foramen infrapiriforme and successively the Foramen ischiadicum minus to the lateral wall of the Fossa ischioanalis (Canalis pudendalis, ALCOCK's canal). Here, the A. rectalis inferior branches off to the inferior anal canal. The A. pudenda interna then divides into the superficial and deep terminal branches to supply the external genitalia. The superficial A. perinealis supplies the perineum and provides Rr. labiales posteriores to the labia. The deep branches supply to the cavernous bodies of the Clitoris and vestibule (A. bulbi vestibuli, A. dorsalis clitoridis, A. profunda clitoridis).

The venous blood drains into the **V. iliaca interna.** Its tributaries form communicating venous plexuses (Plexus venosi) around the pelvic viscera. These have to be removed during dissection to display the arteries and nerves of the pelvis:
- **Plexus venosus rectalis:** connected via the V. rectalis superior to the portal venous system and via the Vv. rectales media and inferior to the drainage system of the V. cava inferior (portocaval anastomosis)
- **Plexus venosus vesicalis:** at the base of the urinary bladder, also collects the venous blood from the Corpora cavernosa clitoridis (V. dorsalis profunda clitoridis)
- **Plexus venosi uterinus and vaginalis:** drains the blood from Uterus and Vagina

→ dissection link

Efferent urinary system → Genitalia → Rectum and anal canal → **Topography** → Sections

Lymph vessels of the pelvis

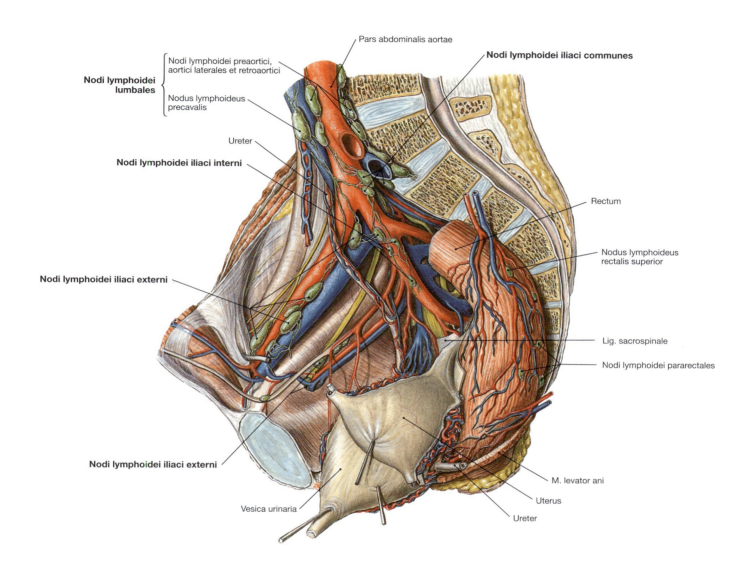

Fig. 7.114 Lymph nodes and lymph vessels of the pelvis (shown here in a woman); view from the left side.
The pelvis contains the Nodi lymphoidei iliaci interni and externi along the respective blood vessels and the Nodi lymphoidei sacrales at the ventral side of the sacrum. Due to their close proximity a strict separation between parietal lymph nodes at the pelvic wall and visceral lymph nodes around the pelvic viscera is not possible. Thus, the pelvic viscera (Rectum, urinary bladder, internal genitalia) drain into all groups of lymph nodes.
The lymph from the upper **Rectum** flows via the Nodi lymphoidei rectales superiores to the Nodi lymphoidei mesenterici inferiores in the retroperitoneal space and to the Nodi lymphoidei iliaci interni in the pelvis. However, the lymphatic drainage from the lower Rectum is directed into the Nodi lymphoidei inguinales superficiales. This explains why lymph node metastases from proximal rectal carcinomas are found in the retroperitoneal space and in the pelvis, but those from distal rectal carcinomas are found in the inguinal region.
The regional lymph nodes of the **urinary bladder** are predominantly the Nodi lymphoidei iliaci interni.
The lymphatic drainage pathways for the **female genitalia** (→ p. 213) and the **male genitalia** (→ p.195) are described in detail with the respective organs.
At last, the lymph passes through the Nodi lymphoidei iliaci communes and reaches the parietal lymph nodes of the retroperitoneal space which are collectively referred to as Nodi lymphoidei lumbales on both sides of the Aorta and the V. cava inferior.

→ dissection link

Pelvis and Retroperitoneal Space

Kidney and adrenal gland →

Male pelvis, median section

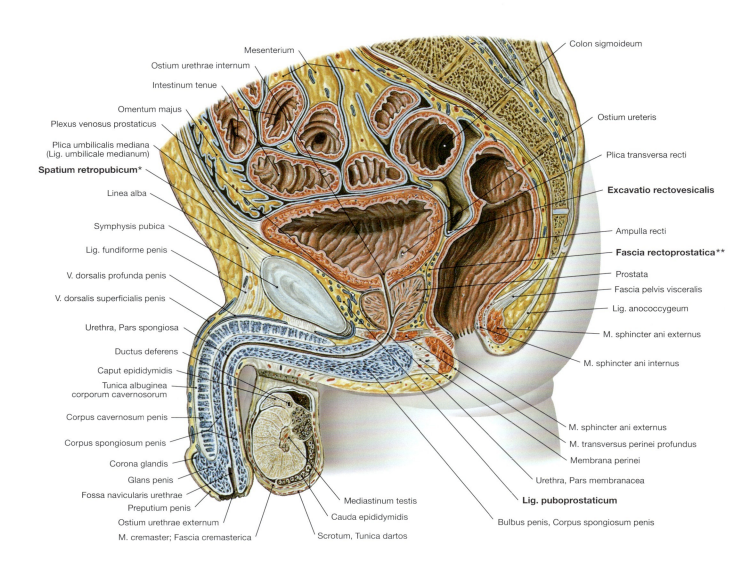

Fig. 7.115 Pelvis, Pelvis, of a man; median section; view from the left side.
The most inferior recess of the male peritoneal cavity is the **Excavatio rectovesicalis.** It is laterally confined by the **Plica rectovesicalis** containing the Plexus hypogastricus inferior. Caudal to this pouch, the **Fascia rectoprostatica** (*clinical term: DENONVILLIER's fascia) in the subperitoneal space separates the Rectum from the prostate gland.

The connective tissue space behind the pubic symphysis, the **Spatium retropubicum** (**clinical term: RETZIUS' space), contains the Lig. puboprostaticum which attaches the prostate gland and urinary bladder to the pelvic bone. In the inferior part of the Spatium retropubicum, the **V. dorsalis profunda** penis drains the blood from the Corpora cavernosa penis into the **Plexus venosus prostaticus** and further into the V. iliaca interna.

→ *dissection link*

Female pelvis, median section

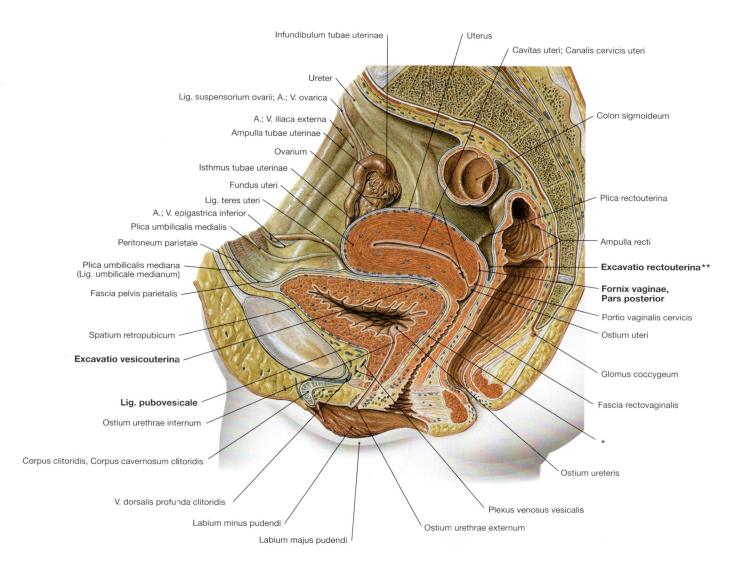

Fig. 7.116 Pelvis, Pelvis, of a woman; median section; view from the left side.

Because the Uterus is positioned between the Rectum and the urinary bladder the female peritoneal cavity has two caudal pouches. The most caudal pouch is the **Excavatio rectouterina** (** clinical term: pouch of DOUGLAS). This space is adjacent to the posterior Fornix vaginae and is confined laterally by the **Plica rectouterina** and the associated Plexus hypogastricus inferior. Caudally, the subperitoneal **Fascia rectovaginalis** separates the Rectum and the Vagina. The **Excavatio vesicouterina** between urinary bladder and Uterus is not as deep and covers the subperitoneal Septum vesicovaginale. The connective tissue space behind the pubic symphysis, the **Spatium retropubicum,** contains the thin Lig. pubovesicale which attaches the urinary bladder to the pelvic bone. In the inferior part of the Spatium retropubicum, the **V. dorsalis profunda clitoridis** drains the blood from the Corpora cavernosa clitoridis into the **Plexus venosus vesicalis** and further into the V. iliaca interna.

* clinical term: Septum vesicovaginale

Clinical Remarks

With **inflammations in the lower abdomen,** pus and fluids may accumulate in the pouch of **DOUGLAS**. The close vicinity to the posterior fornix of the Vagina enables the sampling of exudates through the Vagina.

7 Pelvis and Retroperitoneal Space

Male pelvis, transverse sections

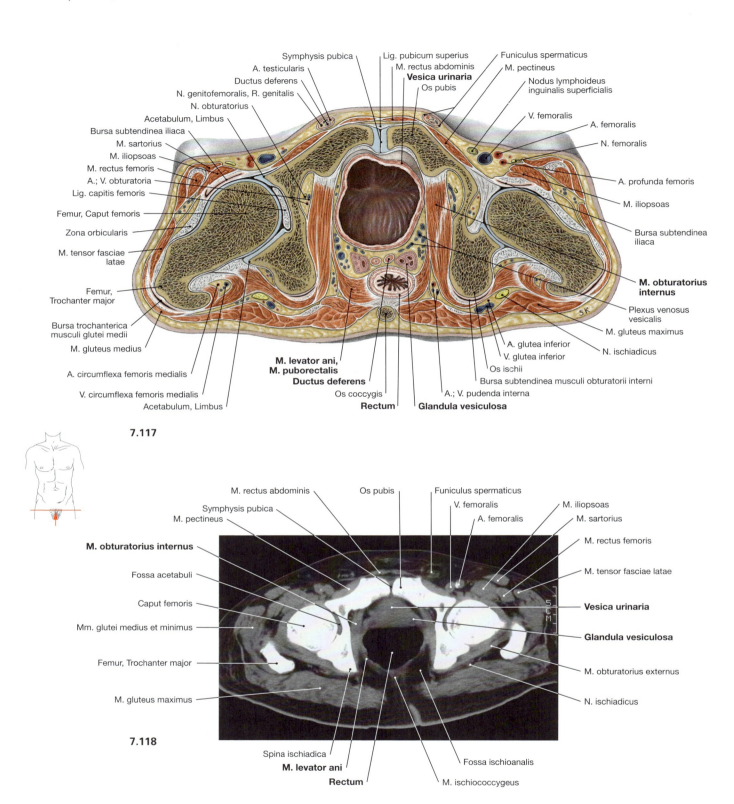

Fig. 7.117 and Fig. 7.118 Pelvis, Pelvis, of a man; transverse section at the level of the lesser pelvis (→ Fig. 7.117) and corresponding computed tomographic section (CT; → Fig. 7.118); caudal view. According to general convention, CT images are **always viewed from caudal.** The following pelvic viscera are recognizable: urinary bladder (Vesica urinaria), Rectum, and parts of the internal genitalia (vas deferens [Ductus deferens] and seminal vesicle [Glandula vesiculosa]). The transverse section is best suited to trace distinct muscles. Here, the M. puborectalis of the M. levator ani is shown, which forms a loop behind the Rectum and supports the perineal flexure. This mechanism contributes to the closure of the Rectum and is important for faecal continence. In addition, the complicated course of the M. obturatorius internus is visible: the muscle originates anteriorly from the inner aspect of the bony pelvis and courses dorsally until it bends around the ischium which serves as hypomochlion for the muscle. Finally the M. obturatorius internus inserts at the inner aspect of the Trochanter major.

Female pelvis, transverse sections

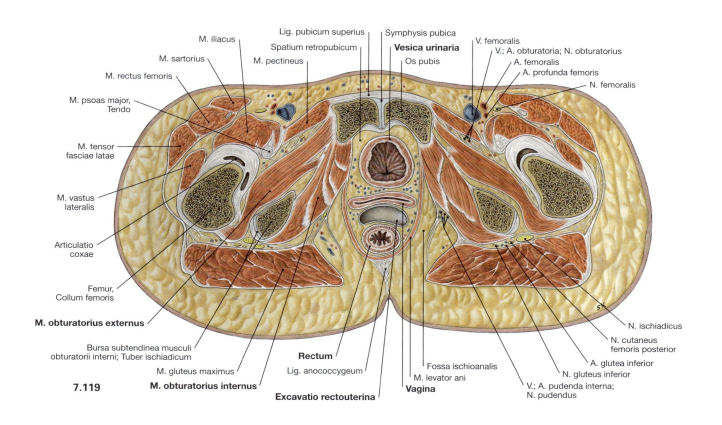

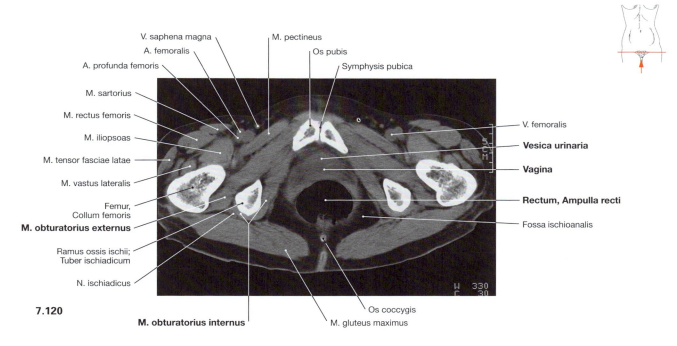

Fig. 7.119 and Fig. 7.120 Pelvis, Pelvis, of a woman; transverse section at the level of the lesser pelvis (→ Fig. 7.119) and corresponding computed tomographic section (CT; → Fig. 7.120); caudal view. The following pelvic viscera are visible: urinary bladder (Vesica urinaria), Rectum, and the Vagina in between the Rectum and bladder. The section also shows the Excavatio rectouterina (pouch of DOUGLAS) as the most caudal part of the peritoneal cavity. Compared to the section of the male pelvis (→ Fig. 7.117), the transverse section here is further caudal. Therefore, in addition to the M. obturatorius internus, the M. obturatorius externus at the opposite side of the pelvic bone is shown.

7 Pelvis and Retroperitoneal Space

Kidney → ... → Sections

Male pelvis, frontal section

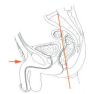

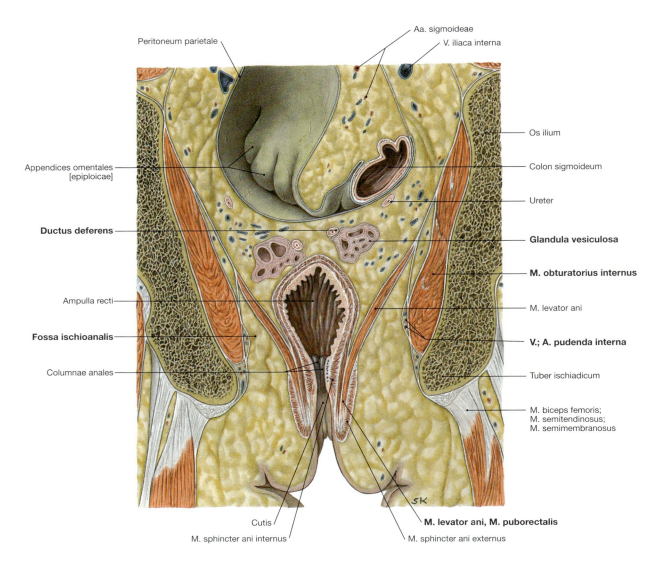

Fig. 7.121 Pelvis, Pelvis, of a man; oblique frontal section through the lesser pelvis.

The A. and V. pudenda interna course together with the N. pudendus within a duplicature of the M. obturatorius internus fascia (clinical term: ALCOCK's canal) to the Fossa ischioanalis.

240

Appendix

Picture Credits 243

Abbreviations, Terms, etc. 245

Index 247

Picture Credits

The editors sincerely thank all clinical colleagues that made ultrasound, computed tomographic and magnetic resonance images as well as endoscopic and intraoperative pictures available:

Prof. Altaras, Center for Radiology, University of Giessen (Figs. 2.18; 2.39; 2.40)
Prof. Brückmann and Dr. Linn, Neuroradiology, Institute for Diagnostic Radiology, University of Munich (Fig. 4.148)
Prof. Daniel, Department of Cardiology, University of Erlangen (Fig. 10.39)
Prof. Galanski and Dr. Schäfer, Department of Diagnostic Radiology, Hannover Medical School (Figs. 2.97; 5.3; 5.103; 6.31; 6.129)
Prof. Gebel, Department of Gastroenterology and Hepatology, Hannover Medical School (Figs. 6.73; 6.75; 6.76; 6.94; 6.95; 7.25)
Dr. Greeven, St. Elisabeth Hospital, Neuwied (Figs. 4.96; 8.96)
Prof. Hoffmann and Dr. Bektas, Clinic for Abdominal and Tranplantation Surgery, Hannover Medical School (Fig. 4.41)
Prof. Hohlfeld, Clinic for Pneumology, Hannover Medical School (Fig. 5.71)
Prof. Jonas, Urology, Hannover Medical School (Fig. 7.33)
Prof. Kampik and Prof. Müller, Ophthalmology, University of Munich (Fig. 9.66)
Dr. Kirchhoff and Dr. Weidemann, Department of Diagnostic Radiology, Hannover Medical School (Figs. 6.131; 6.133; 7.26)
Prof. Kleinsasser, Clinic and Polyclinic of Oto-Rhino-Laryngology, Plastic and Aesthetic Surgery, University Hospital Wuerzburg (Figs. 11.41; 11.42; 11.43)
PD Dr. Kutta, Clinic and Polyclinic for Oto-Rhino-Laryngology, University Hospital Hamburg-Eppendorf (Figs. 8.101; 10.16; 11.16)
Dr. Meyer, Department of Gastroenterology and Hepatology, Hannover Medical School (Figs. 6.22; 6.32; 7.104)
Prof. Pfeifer, Radiology Innenstadt, Institute for Diagnostic Radiology, University of Munich (Figs. 2.63–2.65; 2.67–2.70; 3.52; 3.54; 3.55; 4.97; 4.99; 4.100; 4.105; 4.106)
Prof. Possinger and Prof. Bick, Medical Clinic and Polyclinic II, Division of Hematology and Oncology, Charité Campus Mitte, Berlin (Fig. 2.141)
Prof. Ravelli †, formerly Institute of Anatomy, University of Innsbruck (Fig. 2.62)
Prof. Reich, Orofacial Surgery, University of Bonn (Figs. 8.60; 8.61)
Prof. Reiser and Dr. Wagner, Institute for Diagnostic Radiology, University of Munich (Figs. 2.71; 12.105; 12.106; 12.110; 12.111)
Dr. Scheibe, Department of Surgery, Rosman Hospital, Breisach (Fig. 4.79)
Prof. Scheumann, Clinic for Abdominal and Tranplantation Surgery, Hannover Medical School (Fig. 11.58)
Prof. Schillinger, Department of Gynaecology, University of Freiburg (Fig. 1.49)
Prof. Schliephake, Orofacial Surgery, University of Goettingen (Figs. 8.156; 8.157)
Prof. Schloesser, Center for Gynaecology, Hannover Medical School (Fig. 7.79)
cand. med. Carsten Schroeder, Kronshagen (Fig. 9.27)
Prof. Schumacher, Neuroradiology, Department of Radiology, University of Freiburg (Fig. 12.5)
Dr. Sel, University Hospital and Polyclinic for Ophthalmology, University Hospital Halle (Saale) (Fig. 9.64)
Dr. Sommer and PD Dr. Bauer, Radiologists, Munich (Figs. 4.101; 4.102)
PD Dr. Vogl, Radiology, University of Munich (Figs. 9.69; 9.70)
Prof. Witt, Department of Neurosurgery, University of Munich (Fig. 3.116)
Prof. Zierz and Dr. Jordan, University Hospital and Polyclinic for Neurology, University Hospital Halle (Saale) (Figs. 8.82; 12.151)

Additional illustrations were obtained from the following textbooks:
1 Benninghoff-Drenckhahn: Anatomie, Band 1 (Drenckhahn D., editor), 17. Aufl., Urban & Fischer 2008
2 Benninghoff-Drenckhahn: Anatomie, Band 2 (Drenckhahn D., editor), 16. Aufl., Urban & Fischer 2004
3 Benninghoff-Drenckhahn: Taschenbuch Anatomie (Drenckhahn D., Waschke, J., editors), Urban & Fischer 2007
4 Berchtold, R., Bruch, H.-P., Trentz, O. (editors): Chirurgie, 6. Aufl., Urban & Fischer 2008
5 Böcker, W., Denk, H., Heitz, P. U., Moch, H. (editors): Pathologie, 4. Aufl., Urban & Fischer 2008
6 Classen, M., Diehl, V., Kochsiek, K., Berdel, W. E., Böhm, M., Schmiegel, W. (editors): Innere Medizin, 5. Aufl., Urban & Fischer 2003
7 Classen, M., Diehl, V., Kochsiek, K., Hallek, M., Böhm, M. (editors): Innere Medizin, 6. Aufl., Urban & Fischer 2009
8 Drake, R. L., Vogl, A. W., Mitchell, A., Paulsen, F. (editors): Gray's Anatomie für Studenten, 1. Aufl., Urban & Fischer 2007
9 Drake, R. L., Vogl, A. W., Mitchell, A.: Gray's Anatomy for Students, 2nd ed., Churchill Livingstone 2010
10 Drake, R. L., Vogl, A. W., Mitchell, A.: Gray's Atlas der Anatomie, Urban & Fischer 2009
11 Fleckenstein, P., Tranum-Jensen, J.: Röntgenanatomie, Urban & Fischer 2004
12 Forbes, A., Misiewicz, J., Compton, C., Quraishy, M., Rubesin, S., Thuluvath, P.: Atlas of Clinical Gastroenterology, 3rd ed., Mosby 2004
13 Franzen, A.: Kurzlehrbuch Hals-Nasen-Ohren-Heilkunde, 3. Aufl., Urban & Fischer 2007
14 Garzorz, N.: BASICS Neuroanatomie, Urban & Fischer 2008
15 Kanski, J. J.: Klinische Ophthalmologie, 5. Aufl., Urban & Fischer 2003
16 Kanski, J. J.: Klinische Ophthalmologie, 6. Aufl., Urban & Fischer 2008
17 Kauffmann, G. W., Moser, E., Sauer, R. (editors): Radiologie, 3. Aufl., Urban & Fischer 2006
18 Lippert, H.: Lehrbuch Anatomie, 7. Aufl., Urban & Fischer 2006
19 Mettler, F. A. (editor): Klinische Radiologie, Urban & Fischer 2005
20 Moore, K., Persaud, T. V. N., Viebahn, C. (editors): Embryologie, 5. Aufl., Urban & Fischer 2007
21 Schulze, S.: Kurzlehrbuch Embryologie, Urban & Fischer 2006
22 Speckmann, E.-J., Hescheler, J., Köhling, R. (editors): Physiologie, 5. Aufl., Urban & Fischer 2008
23 Trepel, M.: Neuroanatomie, 4. Aufl., Urban & Fischer 2008
24 Welsch, U.: Sobotta Lehrbuch Histologie, 2. Aufl., Urban & Fischer 2005
25 Welsch, U., Deller, T.: Sobotta Lehrbuch Histologie, 3. Aufl., Urban & Fischer 2010
26 Welsch, U.: Atlas Histologie, 7. Aufl., Urban & Fischer 2005
27 Wicke, L.: Atlas der Röntgenanatomie, 7. Aufl., Urban & Fischer 2005
28 Rengier, F.: BASICS Leitungsbahnen, Urban & Fischer 2009

The following illustrators have developed the new illustrations:
Dr. Katja Dalkowski: Figs. 5.2, 5.5, 5.6, 5.7, 5.10, 5.20, 5.26, 5.28, 5.40, 5.41, 6.1, 6.2, 6.6, 6.64, 6.65, 6.66, 6.67, 6.92, 6.114, 7.6, 7.7, 7.8, 7.18, 7.19, 7.42, 7.43, 7.53, 7.72, 7.73

Sonja Klebe: Figs. 5.62, 5.64, 5.79, 5.95, 5.96, 5.97, 6.12, 6.13, 6.18, 6.19, 6.20, 6.28, 6.46, 6.47, 6.48, 6.50, 6.51, 6.71, 6.79, 6.80, 6.93, 6.115, 6.118, 7.61, 7.62, 7.85, 7.86, 7.90, 7.99

1. List of abbreviations

Singular:
A.   = Arteria
Lig. = Ligamentum
M.   = Musculus
N.   = Nervus
Proc. = Processus
R.   = Ramus
V.   = Vena
Var. = Variation

Plural:
Aa.   = Arteriae
Ligg. = Ligamenta
Mm.   = Musculi
Nn.   = Nervi
Procc. = Processus
Rr.   = Rami
Vv.   = Venae

♀ = female
♂ = male

Percentages:
In the light of the large variation in individual body measurements, the percentages indicating size should only be taken as approximate values.

2. General terms of direction and position

The following terms indicate the position of organs and parts of the body in relation to each other, irrespective of the position of the body (e.g. supine or upright) or direction and position of the limbs. These terms are relevant not only for human anatomy but also for clinical medicine and comparative anatomy.

General terms
anterior – posterior = in front – behind (e.g. Arteriae tibiales anterior et posterior)
ventralis – dorsalis = towards the belly – towards the back
superior – inferior = above – below (e.g. Conchae nasales superior et inferior)
cranialis – caudalis = towards the head – towards the tail
dexter – sinister = right – left (e.g. Arteriae iliacae communes dextra et sinistra)
internus – externus = internal – external
superficialis – profundus = superficial – deep (e.g. Musculi flexores digitorum superficialis et profundus)
medius, intermedius = located between two other structures (e.g. the Concha nasalis media is located between the Conchae nasales superior and inferior)
medianus = located in the midline (Fissura mediana anterior of the spinal cord). The median plane is a sagittal plane which divides the body into right and left halves.
medialis – lateralis = located near to the midline – located away from the midline of the body (e.g. Fossae inguinales medialis et lateralis)
frontalis = located in a frontal plane, but also towards the front (e.g. Processus frontalis of the maxilla)

longitudinalis = parallel to the longitudinal axis (e.g. Musculus longitudinalis superior of the tongue)
sagittalis = located in a sagittal plane
transversalis = located in a transverse plane
transversus = transverse direction (e.g. Processus transversus of a thoracic vertebra)

Terms of direction and position for the limbs
proximalis – distalis = located towards or away from the attached end of a limb or the origin of a structure (e.g. Articulationes radioulnares proximalis et distalis)

for the upper limb:
radialis – ulnaris = on the radial side – on the ulnar side (e.g. Arteriae radialis et ulnaris)

for the hand:
palmaris – dorsalis = towards the palm of the hand – towards the back of the hand (e.g. Aponeurosis palmaris, Musculus interosseus dorsalis)

for the lower limb:
tibialis – fibularis = on the tibial side – on the fibular side (e.g. Arteria tibialis anterior)

for the foot:
plantaris – dorsalis = towards the sole of the foot – towards the back of the foot (e.g. Arteriae plantares lateralis et medialis, Arteria dorsalis pedis)

3. Use of brackets

[ ]: Latin terms in square brackets refer to alternative terms as given in the Terminologia Anatomica (1998), e.g. Ren [Nephros]. To keep the legends short, only those alternative terms have been added that differ in the root of the word and are necessary to understand clinical terms, e.g. nephrology. They are primarily used in figures in which the particular organ or structure plays a central role.

( ): Round brackets are used in different ways:
- for terms also listed in round brackets in the Terminologia Anatomica, e.g. (M. psoas minor)
- for terms not included in the official nomenclature but which the editors consider important and clinically relevant, e.g. (Crista zygomaticoalveolaris)
- to indicate the origin of a given structure, e.g. R. spinalis (A. vertebralis).

Index

A

Abdomen 148–153
Abdominal cavity 70, 151
– transverse section 154–156
– – computed tomography 154–156
Abdominal viscera 69–156
– anastomoses of arteries 140
– arteries 140
– development 70
– projection onto the body surface 86
– topography 70
Abscess, Fossa ischioanalis 200
Absolute cardiac dullness 4
Accessory sex glands 183, 190
Acetabulum 238
Acinus(-i)
– pancreatici 123
– pulmonalis 38
– pulmonis 32
Acromion 68
ADDISON's disease 170
Adrenal gland 122, 166, 170
– in the retroperitoneal space 164
Adrenocortical insufficiency 170
– hypoglycaemic shock 170
Air conducting part, lower respiratory tract 32
ALCOCK's canal (Canalis pudendalis) 199–200, 217–218, 234, 240
Ampulla
– ductus deferentis 178, 186, 190, 201
– duodeni 77, 88–90
– hepatopancreatica 127
– recti 148, 180, 222, 225, 236–237, 239–240
– tubae uterinae 93, 206–208, 237
Anal canal 92, 222–223
– innervation 226
– projection onto the body surface 220
– rectoscopy 227
– sphincter muscles 223
– veins 225
Anal cancer 223
Anal fistula 223
Anal prolapse 223
Anastomoses, arteries of the abdominal viscera 47, 81, 106, 112, 140, 225
Anatomical dead-space, resuscitation 32
Androgens, adrenal glands 170
Angina pectoris 27
– coronary artery stenosis 23
Angle of HIS 75
Angustia (Oesophagus) 45
– aortica 45
– cricoidea 45
– diaphragmatica 45
Annular pancreas 121
Ansa subclavia 58, 61
Anteflexion, uterus 208
Anteversion, uterus 208
Anti-MÜLLERIAN hormone 163, 205
– differentiation of the MÜLLERIAN ducts 185
Antrum pyloricum 42, 75, 77, 85, 89, 153
Anulus
– fibrosus
– – dexter 16
– – sinister 16, 18
– inguinalis
– – profundus 232
– – superficialis 187, 191–192
– umbilicalis 93, 148
Anus 163, 199, 202, 217, 222, 224–226
– projection onto the body surface 86
Aorta 4, 15, 20, 24, 66, 68, 72, 103, 148, 155, 162
– abdominalis/thoracica See Pars abdominalis/thoracica aortae
– ascendens/descendens See Pars ascendens/descendens aortae
– branches 56
– overriding aorta 7
Aortic arch 6, 55
– branching variations of the great vessels 55
Aortic coarctation 7, 9
Aortic ring 16
Aortic valve 16, 19
– insufficiency 5
– projection onto the ventral thoracic wall 4
Aortic valve stenosis 5, 7, 9
– hypertrophy of the cardiac muscle 15
Apex
– cordis 4–5, 10, 12–13, 15, 17–18
– pulmonis 34–35, 40, 63
– vesicae 177–178
Appendicitis 73, 93, 95
– perforation, peritonitis 95
– pouch of DOUGLAS 237
Appendix(-ces)
– epididymidis 188, 191
– epiploicae [omentales] 94, 134, 240
– fibrosa hepatis 104–105
– projection
– – onto the body surface 86
– – onto the ventral thoracic wall 93
– testis 183, 188, 191
– vermiformis 74, 86, 92–93, 95–97, 101–102, 120, 128, 135–138, 143, 145–146, 161, 187, 208, 220
– vesiculosa 203
Arcus
– aortae 5–6, 8–9, 11–13, 24–25, 38, 41, 43–44, 48, 54–56, 62, 64, 68
– costalis 210
– tendineus musculi levatoris ani 196, 214–215
Area(-ae)
– cribrosa 167
– gastricae 77–78
– nuda 104–106, 148
Arrhythmia, ECG 22
Arteria(-ae)
– appendicularis 96–98, 140, 143, 146
– arcuata (Ren) 167, 169
– axillaris 60–61, 64, 68
– bulbi
– – penis 197, 200
– – vestibuli 216
– caecalis anterior 96–97, 146
– carotis
– – communis 6, 12–13, 38, 43–44, 46, 48, 51, 53–55, 58, 60–61, 63–64, 68
– – externa 55
– – interna 55
– caudae pancreatis 140
– cervicalis
– – ascendens 60–61
– – profunda 56
– circumflexa
– – femoris medialis 238
– – humeri posterior 68
– – scapulae 68
– colica
– – dextra 96–97, 140, 143, 145–146
– – media 96–97, 140, 143, 145–147
– – sinistra 97, 140, 145–147
– coronaria(-ae), 24
– – balanced or codominant perfusion type 26–27
– – dextra 12–13, 17, 19, 24–27, 62, 67
– – – branches 24
– – infarction pattern in the case of occlusion 27
– – left-dominant perfusion type 26–27
– – perfusion areas 27
– – right-dominant perfusion type 26–27
– – sinistra 13, 19, 24–27, 62, 67
– – – branches 24
– corticalis radiata 169
– cremasterica 191–193, 232
– cystica 80, 104, 110, 116, 118, 140, 142
– dorsalis
– – clitoridis 216, 218
– – penis 192, 197, 200, 233
– ductus deferentis 191, 193, 233
– epigastrica inferior 232–233, 237
– femoralis 238–239

Arteria(-ae)
– gastrica(-ae)
– – breves 80, 140, 142, 144
– – dextra 80, 83, 110, 140, 142
– – posterior 80, 142
– – sinistra 46, 80, 83, 96, 110, 125, 140, 142, 144, 150, 155
– – – branches 142
– gastroduodenalis 80, 83, 96, 110, 118, 122, 125, 140, 142, 144, 150
– gastroomentalis
– – dextra 80, 83, 110, 125, 140, 142, 144
– – sinistra 80, 83, 110, 140, 142, 144
– glutea
– – inferior 224, 232, 238–239
– – superior 224, 232
– helicinae 186
– hepatica
– – communis 80, 96, 110, 118, 122, 125, 140, 142, 144, 155
– – – branches 142
– – propria 80, 83, 96, 104, 108, 110, 118, 122, 125, 140, 142, 149–150, 155
– ileales 96, 140, 143, 145
– ileocolica 96–97, 140, 143, 145–146
– iliaca
– – communis 8, 148–149, 175, 215, 226, 228, 232
– – externa 8, 224, 232–234, 237
– – interna 8, 224, 232–234
– – – parietal branches 232
– – – visceral branches 232
– – – – in man 233
– – – – in woman 234
– iliolumbalis 232
– intercostalis 38, 67
– – posterior 52–53, 56–57
– – suprema 56, 60–61
– interlobaris (Ren) 167–169
– interlobularis 106
– jejunales 96, 140, 143, 145, 147, 150
– ligamenti teretis uteri 234
– lobaris superior 65
– lobi caudati 104
– lumbales 228
– mesenterica
– – inferior 97, 140, 146–147, 156, 162, 224, 226, 228, 232
– – – branches 146
– – – course 147
– – superior 80, 96–97, 110, 122–123, 125, 127, 140, 142–150, 156, 165, 228
– – – branches 98, 143
– – – course 145
– – – origin 144
– obturatoria 196, 215, 224, 232–233, 238–239
– ovarica 175, 206–208, 211–212, 228, 234, 237
– pancreatica
– – dorsalis 125, 140
– – inferior 125
– – magna 140
– pancreaticoduodenalis
– – inferior 96, 125, 140, 143–144, 147
– – superior 125
– – – anterior 96, 125, 144
– – – posterior 96, 125, 140
– pericardiacophrenica 11, 52–54
– perinealis 197, 200, 218
– phrenica inferior 171–172, 228
– profunda
– – cervicis 60–61
– – femoris 238–239
– – penis 186, 192, 198, 233
– pudenda
– – externa profunda 192
– – interna 197, 200–201, 218–219, 224–225, 232–234, 238–240
– pulmonalis(-es) 8–9, 38, 52
– – dextra 10–13, 15, 25, 35, 44, 62, 65
– – sinistra 6, 10–13, 25, 35, 44, 53

Index

Arteria(-ae)
- rectalis
  - – inferior 140, 200, 218, 224, 233–234
  - – media 193, 224, 232–234
  - – superior 97, 140, 146–147, 224–225, 234
- renalis 148–149, 156, 162, 164–167, 171–172, 175, 193, 228
  - – accessoria 164, 171
  - – course 171
  - – polaris
    - – – inferior 172
    - – – superior 172
  - – sinistra 165
- sacralis
  - – lateralis 232
  - – mediana 228, 232–234
- sigmoideae 97, 140, 146–147, 224, 240
- splenica [lienalis] 80, 83, 96, 110, 122, 125, 127, 129, 140, 142, 144, 150–151, 154–155
  - – branches 142
- subclavia 6, 12–13, 38, 43–44, 46, 48, 51, 54–56, 58, 60–61, 63–64
- subcostalis 57
- subscapularis 64
- supraduodenalis 140
- suprarenalis(-es) 172
  - – inferior 164, 166, 171–172, 228
  - – media 166, 171–172, 228
  - – superiores 166, 172
- suprascapularis 60–61
- testicularis 171, 187, 189, 191–194, 228, 238
  - – course 193
- thoracica interna 52, 54, 56, 60–61, 64, 66
- thoracodorsalis 64
- thyroidea
  - – ima 55
  - – inferior 46, 60–61
- transversa cervicis 60–61
- umbilicalis(-es) 8, 210, 232–234
- urethralis 192
- uterina 211, 232, 234
- vaginalis 211, 234
- vertebralis 46, 55, 60–61
- vesicalis
  - – inferior 193, 232–234
  - – superior 232–233

Articulatio(-nes)
- acromioclavicularis 68
- coxae 239
- humeri 68
- sacrococcygea 198

Ascending colon 101
ASCHOFF-TAWARA node (AV node, Nodus atrioventricularis) 20–21
Aspiration 28
- foreign bodies 28
Asthma bronchiale, left ventricular hypertrophy 15
Atrioventricular bundle (Fasciculus atrioventricularis, bundle of HIS) 16, 20–21, 24
Atrioventricular valves 16
- stenosis 16
Atrium cordis 6
- dextrum 4–10, 12–13, 15, 17, 21, 24–25, 41, 55, 62, 67, 149–150
- sinistrum 6–9, 13, 15, 18, 24–25, 55, 62, 66–67

Auricula
- dextra 12, 17, 19
- sinistra 5, 12–13, 15, 18, 24–25, 41, 55, 66

Auscultation, cardiac sounds 4
AV node (Nodus atrioventricularis, node of TAWARA) 20–21
Axilla 68
Axillary fossa 68
Azygos system, veins 57

B

BARTHOLIN's glands (Gll. vestibulares majores) 202, 204, 217, 219

Basis
- prostatae 190
- pulmonis 34–35
BAUHIN's valve (Valva ileocaecalis) 86, 95
Benign prostatic hypertrophy (BPH) 159, 190
- digital rectal examination (DRE) 221
Bifurcatio
- aortae 147
- tracheae 32–33, 41, 43–44, 62
- trunci pulmonalis 11
Bile concrement, pancreatitis 124
Bile ducts
- ERCP 127
- extrahepatic ducts 117
- – radiography 119
- intrahepatic ducts, radiography 119
- lymph vessels and lymph nodes 113
- malignant tumors 119
- variations 118
Biopsies, CT-controlled punctures 65
Borders of the right and left lungs
- midaxillary line 29
- midclavicular line 29
- paravertebral line 29
- projection
  - – onto the anterior thoracic wall 29
  - – onto the back 29
  - – onto the posterior thoracic wall 29
- scapular line 29
- sternal line 29
BPH (benign prostatic hypertrophy), digital rectal examination (DRE) 221
Bradycardia, ECG 22
Bronchial buds 31
Bronchial carcinoma 41
Bronchial trunk 31
Bronchioli 32
- respiratorii 38
- terminales 32, 38
Bronchopulmonary segments 36–37
Bronchoscopy 37
Bronchus(-i) 32–33, 41
- bronchoscopy 37
- lingularis
  - – inferior 32, 37
  - – superior 32, 37
- lobaris
  - – inferior 66
  - – – dexter 28, 32–33, 35
  - – – sinister 32–33
  - – medius 28, 32–33, 35, 66
  - – superior
  - – – dexter 28, 32–33, 35, 43, 65
  - – – sinister 28, 32–33, 37
- principalis
  - – dexter 28, 32–33, 35, 38, 41, 43–45, 52, 56, 58, 65
  - – sinister 28, 32–33, 35, 38, 41, 43–44, 53, 56, 58, 65
- segmentalis
  - – anterior 32, 37, 68
  - – apicalis 32
  - – apicoposterior 32, 37
  - – basalis
  - – – anterior 32, 37
  - – – lateralis 32, 37, 67
  - – – medialis 32
  - – – posterior 32, 37
  - – lateralis 32
  - – medialis 32
  - – posterior 32
  - – superior 32
BRUNNER's glands (Gll. duodenales) 89
Bulbus
- aortae 19
- penis 186, 201, 236
- vestibuli 202, 218–219, 234
Bundle of HIS (atrioventricular bundle, Fasciculus atrioventricularis) 16, 20–21, 24
Bursa
- omentalis 72, 132–133, 139, 148, 153–155
- – development 72

Bursa
- subtendinea iliaca 238
- – musculi obturatorii interni 238–239
- trochanterica musculi glutei medii 238

C

Caecum 92–93, 95–97, 101, 130, 134–138, 143, 145–146, 208
- projection onto the ventral abdominal wall 86
Calices renales 169
- majores 167, 174, 176
- minores 156, 167–168, 174, 176
CALOT's triangle (Trigonum cholecystohepaticum) 113
Canalis
- analis 92, 220, 222–223, 225–227
- – projection onto the body surface 86
- atrioventricularis 6
- cervicis uteri 207, 237
- inguinalis 187
- obturatorius 196, 214, 224–225
- pudendalis (ALCOCK's canal) 199–200, 217–218, 234, 240
- pyloricus 75, 77, 89, 124
Capsula
- adiposa (Ren) 151, 155, 164, 166, 171, 173
- fibrosa (Ren) 164, 166–168
Caput 187
- epididymidis 188–189, 191, 193, 236
- femoris 238
- humeri 63, 68
- longum (M. biceps brachii) 68
- medusae 112
- pancreatis 93, 120–124, 127, 144, 149–150
- – projection onto the ventral abdominal wall 86
Cardia (Pars cardiaca) 74–75, 77, 80, 131, 148, 153
Cardiac arrhythmias, ECG 22
Cardiac muscle 15
- dilation 13
- hypertrophy 5, 13, 15
Cardiac veins 25
Cardiac wall, structure 14
Carina tracheae 62
Cartilago(-ines)
- bronchiales 32
- costalis 65, 67
- cricoidea 32–33
- thyroidea 32–33
- tracheales 32–33, 62
Carunculae hymenales 202
Catecholamines, adrenal gland 170
Cauda
- epididymidis 183, 188–189, 193, 236
- equina 148, 156
- pancreatis 120–122, 124, 127, 138–139, 150, 155
- – projection onto the ventral abdominal wall 86
Cavernae corporum cavernosorum 186
Cavitas
- abdominalis 70, 151, 154–156
- extraperitonealis pelvis 201, 219
- glenoidalis 68
- nasi 28
- oris propria 42
- pericardiaca 62, 65
- peritonealis 70, 139, 148–150, 153–156
- – abdominis 158
- – pelvis 158, 201, 219
- pleuralis 40, 50, 52–53, 66, 154–155
- serosa scroti 189
- thoracis 62, 64–68, 151
- uteri 207–208, 219, 237
Central venous catheter (CVC) 35, 63
- pneumothorax 35
Centrum
- perinei 215
- tendineum (Diaphragma) 43, 52, 148, 152

Index

Cervical carcinoma 209
– lymph node metastases 213
Cervical constriction, oesophagus 45
Cervix uteri 206, 208–209, 211, 219
Cholecystitis 71
– referred pain in the right shoulder 54
Cholestasis 118–119
Chordae tendineae 17–19
Chronic obstructive pulmonary disease (COPD), hypertrophy of the right ventricle 15
Cisterna chyli 57, 99, 229
Clavicula 5, 54, 63, 68
Clitoris 202, 204, 212
Cloaca 162
Collecting duct 169
Colliculus seminalis 177–178
Collum
– femoris 239
– vesicae biliaris 88, 116–117, 119
Colon 74, 102, 120, 128, 161, 173, 220
– ascendens 81, 92–93, 95–98, 101, 111, 130, 134, 137–138, 146, 150, 176
– – projection onto the body surface 86
– descendens 81, 92–93, 97–98, 101, 111, 134, 137–138, 146–147, 150, 155–156, 176
– – projection onto the body surface 86
– sigmoideum 92–93, 97, 101, 130, 134, 136–139, 145–148, 150, 221, 224–225, 228, 236–237, 240
– – projection onto the body surface 86
– transversum 72, 92–93, 97, 101, 116, 130–131, 133–134, 136–138, 145–146, 148–150, 152–153, 155–156
– – positional variations 101
– – projection onto the body surface 86
Colonic carcinomas 101
– lymphatic drainage 99
Columnae
– anales 222–223, 225, 227, 240
– renales 167, 174
Commissura
– labiorum anterior 202
– – posterior 202
Complexus stimulans et conducente cordis 20–21
Computed tomography (CT) 65, 154
– abdominal cavity, transverse section 154–156
– kidney 173
– pelvis
– – of a man, transverse section 238
– – of a woman, transverse section 239
– thoracic cavity, transverse section 65
– thorax 3
Conducting system of the heart 20–21
Congenital cardial defects 7
Congenital inguinal hernia 185
Continence organ 223
Conus arteriosus 6, 12, 24
Cor 2, 12–13, 55, 66, 74, 102, 120, 128, 160–161
– bovinum 13
– position within the thorax 10
Corona glandis 186–187, 236
Coronary arteries 19
– See also Arteria coronaria dextra/sinistra
Coronary artery disease (CAD) 27
Coronary artery stenosis 23
Corpus(-ora)
– adiposum pararenale 173
– anococcygeum 198, 221
– cavernosum
– – clitoridis 202, 237
– – penis 178–179, 184, 186, 191–192, 194, 204, 236
– – recti 223–224
– clitoridis 237
– epididymidis 188–189
– gastricum 74–75, 77, 85, 130–132, 151
– luteum 207
– ossis pubis 149, 214
– pancreatis 120–124, 127, 133, 138, 144
– – projection onto the ventral abdominal wall 86

Corpus(-ora)
– penis 182
– pineale 160
– spongiosum penis 178–179, 184, 186, 191–192, 194, 199, 223, 236
– sterni 64–66
– uteri 206–208, 211, 219
– vertebrae 65, 155, 173
– vesicae 177–178
– – biliaris 88, 116–117, 119
Corpusculum renale 168
Cortex 170
– (Gl. suprarenalis) 170
– renalis 156, 167–168, 173–174
Costa 64–68
COWPER's glands (Gll. bulbourethrales) 160, 178, 183, 186, 190, 194, 197–199, 201, 221
Crista
– iliaca 29, 161, 231
– terminalis 17, 21
– urethralis 177–178
CROHN's disease 95
Crus
– clitoridis 202, 219
– dextrum
– – (Diaphragma) 155
– – (Fasciculus atrioventricularis) 20–21
– – (Pars lumbalis diaphragmatis) 57
– penis 186, 198, 201
– sinistrum
– – (Fasciculus atrioventricularis) 20–21
– – (Pars lumbalis diaphragmatis) 57, 154
Cryptorchidism 185
Cupula pleurae 29, 40–41, 63, 68
Curvatura
– major 75, 77, 130–132
– minor 75–77, 90, 131–132
Curvatures of the stomach, arteries 80
Cuspis
– anterior
– – (Valva atrioventricularis dextra) 16–17
– – (Valva atrioventricularis sinistra) 16, 19, 66
– commissuralis
– – dextra 16
– – sinistra 16
– posterior
– – (Valva atrioventricularis dextra) 16–17
– – (Valva atrioventricularis sinistra) 16, 18, 66
– septalis (Valva atrioventricularis dextra) 16–17
Cutis 187, 191
CVC (central venous catheter) 35, 63
– pneumothorax 35
Cystitis 180
Cystocele 214
Cystoscopy, ureteric orifice 177

D

DENONVILLIER's fascia (Fascia rectoprostatica) 190, 221, 236
Descensus
– testis 185
– Uterus/Vagina 214
Diabetes mellitus 123
– fatty liver 102
Diaphragma 5, 41, 43–46, 48, 52, 54, 58, 74, 79, 102, 104, 115–116, 120, 122, 128, 131, 148, 151, 155, 161, 173
– pelvis 158, 196, 198, 214–215
– urogenitale 158
Diaphragmatic constriction, oesophagus 45
Diastole 16
Digestive tract, overview 42
Digital rectal examination (DRE), prostata 221
Discus interpubicus 210
Diverticulum(-a)
– ampullae 178
– ilei 91
– of the oesophagus 45
Dorsal pancreatic bud 103, 121
Dorsum penis 182

DRUMMOND's anastomosis 97, 145–147
Ductuli
– efferentes testis 185, 189
– prostatici 177–178
Ductus
– arteriosus 6, 8
– – persisting 7, 9
– bilifer interlobularis 106
– choledochus (biliaris) 88, 103–104, 108, 110, 117–119, 121, 123–124, 127, 142, 149, 155
– – variation of the junction 124
– cysticus 88, 108, 110, 117–119, 122–123, 127, 155
– deferens 149, 160, 178, 183, 185, 187, 189–192, 194, 198, 233, 236, 238, 240
– ejaculatorius 177–178, 183
– excretorius (pancreas) 123
– glandulae bulbourethralis 178, 183, 197
– hepaticus
– – communis 88, 108, 110, 117–119, 122–123, 127
– – dexter 117, 119
– – sinister 117, 119
– lymphaticus 39, 60
– mesonephricus (WOLFFIAN duct) 162–163, 185, 205
– pancreaticus accessorius (SANTORINI's duct) 88, 117, 121, 124
– pancreaticus (duct of WIRSUNG) 88–89, 117, 121, 123–124, 127, 148–149
– – variations of the junction 124
– paramesonephricus (MÜLLERIAN duct) 163, 185
– thoracicus 2, 39, 53, 56–57, 59, 61, 64–67, 99, 151, 154–155, 229
– – junction 39
– venosus 8
– vitellinus 73
Duodenal ulcers 78
– duodenoscopy 90
Duodenoscopy 90
Duodenum 42, 58, 72, 74–77, 80–81, 85, 88–90, 93, 98, 102–103, 110–111, 116–124, 127–128, 135, 137–139, 142, 149–150, 161
– arteries 96
– divisions 88
– endoscopy 90
– inner relief 89
– projection onto the ventral abdominal wall 86, 120
– radiograph 90
– wall structure 89
Dysphagia lusoria 55

E

Echocardiography 3
– transoesophageal 62
Ejaculation, N. pudendus 194
Electrocardiogram (ECG) 3
– anatomical principles 22
– P wave 22
– Q wave 22
– R wave 22
– S wave 22
– T wave 22
Emission 194
– Sympathicus 194
Endocardium 14
Endocrine organs 160
Endometrial carcinoma 207
– lymph nodes metastasis 213
Endometrium 207
Endoscopy
– duodenum 90
– duodenal ulcers 78, 90
– gastric ulcers 78
Epicardium 11–12, 14, 17–18, 62
Epididymis 160, 183, 187–189, 191, 194
– blood vessels 189
Epigastrium
– abdominal surgery 133

Index

Epigastrium
- position of the viscera 130–132
- retroperitoneal organs 122

Epiorchium 187
Epiphrenic diverticula 45
Episiotomy 217
Epispadias 184
Epithelium
- (Gaster) 78
- (Intestinum tenue) 87, 94

ERCP (endoscopic retrograde Cholangiopancreaticography) 122
- bile ducts 127
- pancreas 127

Erection 194
- inhibitors of the enzyme phosphodiesterase 192
- parasympathetic system 194

Excavatio
- rectouterina (pouch of DOUGLAS) 138–139, 208–210, 237, 239
- – appendicitis 237
- – salpingitis 237
- rectovesicalis 138, 149, 181, 221–222, 236
- vesicouterina 139, 208–210, 219, 237

External female genitalia 202
- development 204
- lymph vessels and lymph nodes 213
- lymphatic drainage pathway 213

External male genitalia 182–183
- development 184
- lymph vessels and lymph nodes 195
- neurovascular structures 192

Extremitas
- acromialis (Clavicula) 68
- anterior
- – (Splen) 129
- inferior
- – (Ren) 173, 176
- – (Testis) 188
- posterior (Splen) 129
- superior
- – (Ren) 173
- – (Testis) 188
- tubaria (Ovarium) 206
- uterina 206

F

Facies
- anterior
- – (Gl. suprarenalis) 170
- – (Ren) 173
- colica (Splen) 129
- costalis
- – (Pulmo dexter) 34
- – (Pulmo sinister) 34–35
- diaphragmatica
- – (Cor) 10
- – (Hepar) 104–106, 131–132
- – (Pulmo) 35
- – (Splen) 129
- gastrica (Splen) 129
- medialis (Ovarium) 206, 208
- mediastinalis (Pulmo sinister) 35
- posterior
- – (Prostata) 178
- – (Ren) 173
- pulmonalis (Cor) 10
- renalis (Splen) 129
- sternocostalis (Cor) 10
- vesicalis 208
- visceralis
- – (Hepar) 105–106, 131
- – (Splen) 129

FALLOT's tetralogy 7
Fascia
- cremasterica 187–189, 191, 236
- obturatoria 199, 217
- pelvis
- – parietalis 237
- – visceralis 219, 236

Fascia
- penis 192
- – profunda 187, 191
- – superficialis 187, 192
- rectoprostatica (DENONVILLIER's fascia) 190, 221, 236
- rectovaginalis 237
- renalis (GEROTA's fascia) 152–153, 161, 164, 173
- spermatica
- – externa 187, 189, 191
- – interna 187–189, 191

Fasciculus
- atrioventricularis (atrioventricular bundle, bundle of HIS) 20–21, 24
- lateralis (Plexus brachialis) 68
- medialis (Plexus brachialis) 68
- posterior (Plexus brachialis) 68

Fatty liver
- alcohol abuse/diabetes mellitus 102

Fecal incontinence 214
Female genital system 203
Female genitalia, innervation 212
Female pelvis 180
Female urinary organs 203
Female urinary system 160
Femur 238–239
Fetal circulation 8
Fibrae obliquae (Tunica musularis, Gaster) 76
Fimbria(-ae)
- ovarica 206–207
- tubae uterinae 206–208

Fine needle aspiration biopsy (FNAB) 173
Fissura
- horizontalis (Pulmo dexter) 29, 34–35
- ligamenti teretis hepatis 104–105
- obliqua (Pulmo) 29, 34–35, 64–67
- umbilicalis 107

Flexura
- anorectalis 198
- coli
- – dextra 92, 101, 116, 134
- – sinistra 92, 101, 134
- duodenojejunalis 89–90, 120, 124, 136, 139, 150
- projection onto the ventral abdominal wall 86
- perinealis 220–222
- sacralis 220–222

Floating lung test 30
Folliculi ovarici 207
Foramen(-ina)
- infrapiriforme 196
- ischiadicum
- – majus 214
- – minus 196
- omentale 131–132
- ovale 6–9
- papillaria 167
- suprapiriforme 196
- venae cavae 43
- venarum minimarum 17
- vertebrale 65

Foregut 30
Foreign bodies in the oesophagus 45
Fornix
- gastricus 77, 148, 153
- vaginae 207, 209, 237

Fossa
- acetabuli 238
- ischioanalis 199–201, 217–219, 238–240
- – abscesses 200, 218
- – borders 199, 217
- – contents 200, 218
- jugularis 74
- navicularis urethrae 178–179, 236
- ovalis 17

Foveolae gastrica(-ae) 78
FRANKENHÄUSER's plexus (Plexus uterovaginalis) 212
Frenulum
- clitoridis 202

Frenulum
- labiorum pudendi 202
- ostii ilealis 95
- preputii 187

Fundus
- gastricus 75–77, 116, 131
- uteri 139, 206–208, 210–211, 237
- – position during pregnancy 210
- vesicae 139, 177
- – biliaris 88, 116–117, 130, 135, 138

Funiculus
- spermaticus 183, 188, 191–192, 198, 221, 238
- – coverings of the spermatic cord 187, 191

G

Gallbladder 117
- arteries 110
- developmental stages 103
- laparoscopic image 116
- projection onto the ventral abdominal wall 115
- radiograph 119
- – after intravenous application of contrast medium 119
- surgical removal, CALOT's triangle 118
- veins 111

Ganglion(-ia)
- aorticorenale 100
- cardiacum 23
- cervicale
- – medium 23, 58
- – superius 23
- cervicothoracicum (stellatum) 23, 58, 60–61
- coeliaca 84, 100, 155, 226, 231
- impar 231
- mesentericum
- – inferius 100, 226, 231
- – superius 100, 231
- pelvica 194, 212, 226
- stellatum See Ganglion cervicothoracicum
- thoracica 52–53, 58
- trunci sympathici 56–57, 194, 212, 226

Gaster 42–43, 46, 58, 72, 74–78, 80–85, 88, 90, 93, 98, 102–103, 110–111, 120, 128, 130–132, 138, 142, 148–150, 152–156, 160–161
- See also Stomach

Gastric canal 77
Gastric carcinomas 71
- lymph vessels and lymph nodes 82
- lymphatic drainage 48, 82
- perforation into adjacent organs 79

Gastric ulcer 78
- endoscopy 78
- perforation 79
- selective vagotomy 84
- total vagotomy 84

Gastritis 71
Gastro-(o)esophageal reflux disease (GERD) 42, 75
Gastroscopy 85
- biopsies 85

Genital tubercles 161, 163–164, 184, 204
- nephrectomy 164

GEROTA's fascia (Fascia renalis) 152–153, 161, 164, 173
- nephrectomy 164

Glandula(-ae)
- analis (proktodeal gland) 223
- bulbourethrales (COWPER's glands) 160, 178, 183, 186, 190, 194, 197–199, 201, 221
- duodenales (BRUNNER's glands) 89
- gastricae 78
- intestinales 87, 94
- mammaria 65–66
- oesophageae 44
- parathyroideae 160
- pinealis 160
- pituitaria 160

Index

Glandula(-ae)
- suprarenalis 79, 122, 139, 151, 155, 160–161, 164, 166, 170–171, 228
- – contact area on the posterior wall of the stomach 79
- thyroidea 48, 51, 54, 62, 160–161
- tracheales 33
- vesiculosa 148–149, 160, 178, 183, 185–186, 190, 194, 198, 201, 221, 233, 238, 240
- vestibulares
- – majores (BARTHOLIN's glands) 202, 204, 217, 219
- – minores 202

Glans
- clitoridis 202
- penis 178, 182, 184, 186–187, 194, 236

GLISSON's triad 106
Glomus coccygeum 237
Glucocorticoids, adrenal gland 170
Greater omentum 130
Gubernaculum testis 185

H

Haemorrhoidal knots 222, 227
Haemorrhoids 223, 227
Haustra coli 94–95, 101
HEAD's zones 42
Heart 2, 12–13, 55
- auscultation 4
- conducting system 20–21
- congenital cardial defects 7
- critical weight 13
- development stages 6
- fibrous skeleton 16
- innervation 23
- percussion 4
- position within the thorax 10
- projection onto the thorax 4
- radiograph of the right and left border 5
- stages of development 6
- ultrasound image 66

Heart contours
- postero-anterior radiograph 5
- projection onto the ventral thoracic wall 4

Heart murmurs 4, 16
Heart sounds 4, 16
- auscultation 4

Heart valves 16
- auscultation areas 4
- projection onto the ventral thoracic wall 4

Helicobacter pylori bacteria, production of gastric acid 84
Hepar 8–9, 42, 62, 72, 74, 81, 98, 102–107, 109–111, 114–116, 120–121, 127–128, 148–150, 152–156, 161, 173
- arteries 110
- contact areas 79
- development 72, 103
- laparoscopy 116
- lymph vessels and lymph nodes 82, 113
- of a fetus 8
- projection
- – onto the body surface 86
- – onto the ventral abdominal wall 86, 115
- sagittal section 106
- segments 107–109
- size, measurement 102
- sonography 114
- structure 106
- variations of the blood supply 110
- veins 111

Hepatic diverticulum 103
Hepatic lobules 106
Hepatitis 102
- sonography 114
- suspicious tumours 115

Hepatocytes 106
Hiatus
- analis 196, 214
- aorticus 43
- levatorius 214

Hiatus
- oesophageus 43–44, 48
- urogenitalis 196, 214

Hilar lymph nodes 39, 41
Hilum 166
- pulmonis 35
- renale 156, 166
- splenicum 129, 155

Hindgut 30
Hip, muscles 196
HIS, bundle of (atrioventricular bundle, Fasciculus atrioventricularis) 16, 20–21, 24
Horseshoe kidneys 162
Humerus 64
Hydrocele testis 185
Hymen 202
Hypertension
- increased sympathetic tonus 23
- insufficiency or stenosis of the mitral valve 5
- pulmonary hypertension 5, 15
- stenosis of the aortic valve 5

Hypogastrium
- inflammations 237
- positions of the viscera 134–136

Hypophysis 160
Hypospadias 184
Hypothalamus 160
Hysterectomies, ligation of the ureter during surgery 175

I

Ileocaecal valve (Valva ileocaecalis, BAUHIN's valve) 95
Ileum 74, 91–93, 95–96, 102, 120, 128, 130, 134–135, 138, 143, 145, 148–150, 161, 220
- arteries 96
- projection onto the body surface 86

Ileus, malrotation 73
Impotentia
- coeundi 194
- generandi 194

Impressio
- cardiaca
- – (Pulmo dexter) 35
- – (Pulmo sinister) 35
- colica (Hepar) 104
- duodenalis 104
- gastrica (Hepar) 104
- oesophagea 35, 104
- renalis 104
- suprarenalis 104

Incisura
- angularis 75, 77, 90
- cardiaca (Pulmo sinister) 29, 34–35, 40, 50
- cardialis 75, 77
- ligamenti teretis 104

Infundibulum tubae uterinae 203, 206–208, 237
Inguinal hernia 185
Inner female genitalia 203
- arterial supply 211
- development 205
- lymphatic drainage pathways 213
- lymph vessels and lymph nodes 213

Inner male genitalia 183
- blood vessels 193
- development 185
- lymph vessels and lymph nodes 195

Insulae pancreaticae 123, 160
Intermediate tubulus 169
Internal hernias 133
Internal organs, projection onto the body surface 74, 102, 120, 128, 161
Intestinal rotation 73
- malrotations 73

Intestinum 160
- crassum 42, 92, 94, 97–101, 137
- – *See also* Colon
- tenue 42, 72, 87, 98–100, 128, 136, 220, 236
- – *See also* Small intestine

Intracardiac injection 4
Intraperitoneal organs 70
Islets of LANGERHANS 123
Isthmus
- bursae omentalis 132
- tubae uterinae 206–208, 237
- uteri 206–207

J

Jejunum 74, 88–91, 96, 102, 120, 122, 127–128, 134–135, 137, 143, 145, 148, 150, 153, 155–156, 161
- arteries 96
- projection onto the body surface 86

Junctio (Linea) anorectalis 222

K

KEITH-FLACK, node of (sinu-atrial node, Nodus sinuatrialis) 20–21
KERCKRING's folds (Plicae circulares) 77, 89–91, 124
Kidney 122, 164, 166–167
- *See also* Ren
- arterial supply, variations 172
- ascensus 162
- computed tomography 173
- contact areas 165
- – on the posterior wall of the stomach 79
- course of renal arteries 169
- development 162
- physical examination, pain sensitivity 161
- position in the retroperitoneal space 164
- projection onto the dorsal body wall 161
- transverse section 168
- ultrasound image 173

Kidney lobes 167
KILLIAN's triangle 45
KOCH's triangle 17, 20
KRISTELLER's mucous plug 210

L

Labioscrotal folds 184, 202, 204
Labium
- anterius (Ostium uteri) 209
- majus pudendi 202, 204, 237
- minus pudendi 202, 204, 212, 217–219, 237
- posterius (Ostium uteri) 209

Lacunae urethrales 178
Lamina
- muscularis mucosae (Intestinum tenue) 78, 87, 94
- parietalis
- – (Pericardium serosum) 12–13, 62
- – (Tunica vaginalis testis) 187, 189, 191
- propria mucosae 78, 87, 94
- visceralis 18
- – (Pericardium serosum) 12–13, 17, 62
- – (Tunica vaginalis testis) 187, 189, 191

LANGERHANS, iselets of 123
LANZ's point 93
Laparoscopic image 116
- gallbladder 116
- liver 116

Large intestine 137
- *See also* Intestinum crassum
- arteries 97
- autonomic innervation 100
- conventional radiograph 101
- divisions 92
- lymph vessels and regional lymph nodes 99
- projection
- – onto the body surface 86
- – onto the ventral abdominal wall 86, 92
- regional lymph nodes and lymph vessels 99
- structure of the wall 94
- veins 98

Laryngotracheal primordium 31

Index

Larynx 28, 32–33, 45
Left ventricle 17–19
Left ventricular hypertrophy 15
Left-to-right shunt 7
Ligamentum(-a)
- anococcygeum 198–200, 217–218, 221, 236, 239
- anularia 32–33
- arteriosum 9–10, 12–13, 53, 55
- capitis femoris 238
- cardinale (Lig. transversum cervicis) 206
- coronarium 72, 104–106, 131, 139
- – development 72
- epididymidis
- – inferius 188
- – superius 188
- falciforme hepatis 103–105, 107–108, 118, 130–131, 138, 149, 154–155
- – development 72
- fundiforme penis 192, 236
- gastrocolicum 130–133, 144, 149, 153
- gastrophrenicum 139
- gastrosplenicum 72, 129, 131, 133, 139, 151, 153
- – development 72
- hepatoduodenale 108, 118, 131–132, 138–139, 155
- hepatogastricum 80, 131–132, 155
- inguinale 182
- latum uteri 206–208
- longitudinale anterius 57, 64
- ovarii proprium 203, 205–208, 211
- phrenicocolicum 131
- phrenicosplenicum 153
- pubicum
- – inferius 197, 216
- – superius 238–239
- puboprostaticum 177, 179, 198, 221, 236
- pubovesicale 237
- pulmonale 35
- rectouterinum (Lig. sacrouterinum) 206, 209
- sacrospinale 200, 232, 235
- sacrotuberale 199–200, 214, 217, 232
- splenorenale 72, 129, 151
- – development 72
- suspensorium
- – clitoridis 202
- – duodeni 89
- – ovarii (Lig. infundibulopelvicum) 205–206, 208, 211, 237
- – penis 187, 192
- teres
- – hepatis 9, 104, 107–108, 110, 115, 127, 130–132, 138, 142, 155–156
- – – development 72
- – uteri (Lig. rotundum) 203, 205–206, 208, 211, 234, 237
- transversum perinei 197, 216
- triangulare
- – dextrum 104
- – sinistrum 104, 139, 150–151
- umbilicale medianum 9, 177–178, 236–237
- venae cavae 104–105
- venosum 8–9, 104, 107
Limbus
- acetabuli 238
- fossae ovalis 17
Linea
- alba 154–155, 236
- anocutanea 222–223
- dentata (Linea pectinata, Canalis analis) 222–223
- terminalis 214
Lingula pulmonis (Pulmo sinister) 34–35, 40, 50
Liver See Hepar
Liver cirrhosis 102, 106, 112
- portal hypertension 98
- sonography 114
- suspicious tumours 115
Liver puncture
- position of the needle 115
- referred pain in the right shoulder 54

Lobuli testis 179, 188–189
Lobus
- anterior (Pulmo sinister) 64
- caudatus 104–105, 108–109, 132, 150, 155
- dexter
- – (Gl. thyroidea) 48
- – (Thymus) 51
- hepatis
- – dexter 82, 93, 104–105, 109, 115–116, 118, 130–132, 135, 138, 142, 150–152, 154–156, 173
- – sinister 80, 82, 104–105, 109–110, 115–116, 118, 127, 130–132, 138, 142, 148–149, 151, 153–156
- inferior
- – (Pulmo dexter) 28–29, 34–36, 40, 50, 54, 65–67, 149, 151–152
- – (Pulmo sinister) 28–29, 34–36, 40, 50, 67, 151, 153
- medius (Pulmo dexter) 28–29, 34–36, 40, 50, 66–67, 151
- prostatae
- – dexter 190
- – medius 190
- – sinister 190
- quadratus 104, 109, 155
- renalis 167
- sinister (Thymus) 51
- superior
- – (Pulmo dexter) 28–29, 34–36, 40, 50–51, 54, 64–65
- – (Pulmo sinister) 28–29, 34, 36, 40, 50, 54, 64, 66–67, 151
Lower intestinal tract
- haemorrhage 89
Lower respiratory tract
- air conducting part 32
Lung bud 30
Lung development
- alveolar period 31
- canalicular period 31
- pseudoglandular period 31
- stages 31
Lungs 2, 28, 40, 74, 102, 115, 120, 128, 161
- See also Pulmo
- acinus 38
- alveoles 38
- floating lung test 30
- lymph nodes 39
- lymph vessels 39
- mobility during respiration 29
- size 29
- Vasa
- – privata 38
- – publica 38
Lunula valvulae semilunaris 19
Lymph node metastasis
- cervical carcinoma 213
- endometrial carcinoma 213
- pancreatic carcinoma 126
- penile carcinoma 195, 213
- vulvar carcinoma 213
Lymph vessels
- bile system 113
- colon 99
- external and internal female genitalia 213
- external and internal male genitalia 195
- lungs 39
- peribronchial system 39
- rectum 235
- retroperitoneal space 229
- septal lymph system 39
- small intestine 99
- subpleural lymph system 39
Lymphatic drainage, carcinomas in the colon 99

M

Magnetic resonance imaging (MRI) 65
- thorax 3

Main bronchi, projection onto the anterior chest wall 28
Male genital system, innervation 194
Male pelvis 179
Male urinary organs 183
Male urinary system 160
Malrotation 73
- ileus 73
Mamma 67
Manubrium sterni 64
Margo
- anterior
- – (Pulmo dexter) 34–35, 40
- – (Pulmo sinister) 34–35, 40
- – (Testis) 188
- inferior
- – (Hepar) 104, 106
- – (Pulmo dexter) 34–35
- – (Pulmo sinister) 34–35, 40
- – (Splen) 129
- lateralis (Ren) 166
- liber 206
- medialis
- – (Gl. suprarenalis) 170
- – (Ren) 166
- mesovaricus 206, 208
- posterior
- – (Pulmo dexter) 34
- – (Pulmo sinister) 34
- – (Testis) 188
- superior
- – (Gl. suprarenalis) 170
- – (Ren) 166
- – (Splen) 129, 132–133
McBURNEY's point 93
MECKEL's diverticulum 73, 91
Mediastinum 2, 50, 52–53
- anterius 52–53
- inferius 52–53
- lymph nodes 59
- lymph vessels 59
- medium 52–54
- posterius 52–53
- – lymph nodes 48
- – nerves 58
- superius 52–53
- testis 188–189, 236
Medulla
- (Gl. suprarenalis) 170
- renalis 29, 152, 156, 167–168, 173–174
- spinalis 62–63, 154–155, 194, 212
Membrana perinei 197, 199, 202, 216–217, 236
Mesenteries 137
Mesenterium 70, 87, 91, 136–138, 236
- diverticuli 91
- dorsale 103, 121
- ventrale 103
Mesoappendix 135–139
Mesocolon
- sigmoideum 139
- transversum 94, 132–133, 135, 137, 139, 144–145, 147
- – contact areas on the posterior wall of the stomach 79
Mesogastrium dorsale 72, 103
Mesonephros 162–163
Mesosalpinx 206–208
Mesothelium epicardiale 14
Mesovarium 206, 208
Metanephros 162
MEYER-WEIGERT's rule, crossing of both ureters 176
Midaxillary line 29
- borders of the lungs 29
Midclavicular line 29
- borders of the lungs 29
Mineralocorticoids, adrenal gland 170
Mitral valve (Valva atrioventricularis sinistra) 4, 6, 16, 18–19, 66–67
- projection onto the ventral thoracic wall 4
- stenosis or insufficiency 5
Moderator band 17

Index

Mons pubis 202
MÜLLERIAN duct (Ductus paramesonephricus) 163, 185
– differentiation, anti-MÜLLERIAN hormone 185
Musculus(-i)
– biceps
– – brachii 68
– – femoris 240
– bulbospongiosus 198–202, 217–219, 223
– coracobrachialis 68
– corrugator ani 223
– cremaster 187–189, 191, 198, 236
– dartos 187, 191
– deltoideus 63, 68
– erector spinae 65, 68, 149, 152–156, 173
– gluteus
– – maximus 149, 196, 199–200, 217–218, 238–239
– – medius 238
– – minimus 238
– gracilis 199, 217
– iliacus 196, 231, 239
– iliococcygeus 149, 196, 214
– iliocostalis thoracis 155
– iliopsoas 238–239
– infraspinatus 63–65
– intercostales
– – externi 56, 64, 66–67, 115, 154–155
– – interni 56–57, 68, 115, 154–155
– ischiocavernosus 198–202, 217–219
– ischiococcygeus (coccygeus) 196, 214–215, 232–233, 238
– latissimus dorsi 66–67, 154–156
– levator ani 148–149, 196, 198–201, 214–215, 217–219, 221–226, 233–235, 238–240
– longissimus thoracis 155
– multifidi 155
– obliquus externus abdominis 154
– obturatorius
– – externus 238–239
– – internus 201, 214–215, 219, 224–225, 232, 238–240
– omohyoideus 63
– papillaris
– – anterior 17–19, 21
– – posterior 17–19
– – septalis 17
– pectinati 17
– pectineus 238–239
– pectoralis
– – major 63–67
– – minor 64
– pharyngis 45
– piriformis 149, 196, 215, 232–233
– psoas major 153, 164, 173, 176, 196, 230, 239
– pubococcygeus 148–149, 196, 214, 223
– puborectalis 223, 238, 240
– quadratus lumborum 152–153, 164, 230–231
– rectus
– – abdominis 130, 153–156, 238
– – femoris 238–239
– sartorius 238–239
– scalenus
– – anterior 54, 60–61, 63
– – medius 68
– semimembranosus 240
– semitendinosus 240
– serratus
– – anterior 63–68
– – posterior inferior 155
– sphincter
– – ampullae (ODDI) 117
– – ani
– – – externus 148, 198–200, 202, 217–218, 221–226, 236, 240
– – – internus 148, 222–223, 225, 236, 240
– – pyloricus 77, 89, 124
– – urethrae 221
– – – externus 181, 197–198, 216
– – urethrovaginalis 216

Musculus(-i)
– splenius capitis 68
– sternocleidomastoideus 63
– sternohyoideus 63
– sternothyroideus 64
– subclavius 63, 68
– subscapularis 64, 68
– supraspinatus 63, 68
– suspensorius duodeni (muscle of TREITZ) 89
– tensor fasciae latae 238–239
– teres major 64–65, 68
– trachealis 33
– transversus
– – abdominis 155, 230
– – perinei
– – – profundus 148, 181, 190, 197–199, 201, 216, 221, 223, 236
– – – superficialis 197, 199–200, 217–218
– – thoracis 67
– trapezius 63–66, 68
– vastus lateralis 239
Myocardial infarction 27
– coronary artery stenosis 23
Myocardium 14–15, 17–19
Myometrium 207

N

Nephrectomy, GEROTA's fascia 164
Nephrolithiasis, radiating pain 164
Nephron 169
Nervus(-i)
– anales 226
– anococcygei 200, 218
– axillaris 68
– cardiacus cervicalis
– – inferior 23, 60–61
– – medius 23
– – superior 23
– cavernosi 194
– clunium inferiores 200, 218
– cutaneus femoris
– – lateralis 230–231
– – posterior 200, 218, 239
– dorsalis
– – clitoridis 218
– – penis 192, 197, 200
– femoralis 230–231, 238–239
– genitofemoralis 164, 191–192, 230–232, 238
– gluteus inferior 239
– hypogastricus 100, 194, 212, 226
– iliohypogastricus 164, 230–231
– ilioinguinalis 164, 191–192, 230–231
– intercostalis 52–53, 56–58, 60–61, 64, 67, 154, 231
– ischiadicus 238–239
– labiales posteriores 212, 218
– laryngeus recurrens 10–11, 23, 51–54, 56, 58, 60–61
– obturatorius 196, 215, 230–232, 238–239
– pelvici 100
– perineales 200, 218
– phrenicus 2, 11, 51–54, 56, 60–61, 64–67
– – course 54
– pudendus 197, 200–201, 212, 218–219, 226, 232, 239
– – ejaculation 194
– rectales inferiores 200, 218
– sacralis 212
– scrotales posteriores 200
– splanchnicus(-i) 84, 239
– – lumbales 226
– – major 52–53, 56–58, 100, 151, 155, 230–231
– – minor 53, 56, 58, 100, 151, 155
– – pelvici 194, 212, 226
– subcostalis 164, 230–231
– suprascapularis 63
– thoracicus(-i) 52, 56–58, 155, 231
– – longus 64–66, 68

Nervus(-i)
– thoracodorsalis 68
– vaginalis 212
– vagus [X] 2, 10–11, 23, 51–54, 56, 58, 60–61, 63–67, 231
– – preganglionic parasympathetic neurons 100
NISSEN's fundoplication 75
Nodulus(-i)
– lymphoidei
– – aggregati (PEYER's plaques) 91, 95
– – solitarii 78, 87, 91, 94, 222
– valvulae semilunaris 19
Nodus(-i)
– atrioventricularis (AV node, node of TAWARA) 20–21
– lymphoideus(-i)
– – aortici 21
– – – laterales 235
– – axillaris, 64, 68
– – – apicalis 64
– – bronchopulmonales 39, 41, 65–67
– – cervicales profundi 48
– – coeliaci 83, 113, 126
– – colici
– – – dextri 99
– – – medii 99
– – – sinistri 99
– – cystici 113
– – gastrici 82–83
– – – dextri 82
– – – sinistri 82
– – gastroomentales 83, 155
– – – dextri 82
– – – sinistri 82
– – hepatici 82, 113, 126
– – ileocolici 99
– – iliaci
– – – communes 195, 213, 229, 235
– – – externi 195, 213, 229, 235
– – – interni 99, 195, 213, 235
– – – inguinales 99, 113, 213
– – – inferiores 229
– – – profundi 195, 213, 229
– – – superficiales 195, 213, 238
– – – – superomediales 229
– – intercostales 59
– – intrapulmonales 39
– – juxtaintestinales 99
– – juxtaoesophageales 48, 59, 67
– – lumbales 99, 195, 213, 235
– – – intermedii 229
– – mediastinales 67
– – – anteriores 10, 51, 59, 61
– – – posteriores 48, 151
– – mesenterici
– – – inferiores 99
– – – superiores 99, 126
– – mesocolici 99
– – pancreatici 156
– – – inferiores 126
– – – superiores 126
– – pancreaticoduodenales 126
– – paracolici 99
– – pararectales 235
– – parasternales 59
– – paratracheales 39, 59–60, 64, 68
– – pericardiaci 59
– – phrenici
– – – inferiores 59, 113, 229
– – – superiores 10, 59, 113
– – preaortici 235
– – precavalis 235
– – pylorici 82–83
– – rectalis 83
– – – superior 235
– – retroaortici 235
– – sacrales 195, 213
– – splenici 82–83, 126, 151, 155
– – supraclaviculares 59
– – tracheobronchiales 35, 53, 59, 68
– – – inferiores 35, 39, 48, 62, 67
– – – superiores 39, 48, 62

253

Index

Nodus(-i)
– sinuatrialis (sinu-atrial node, node of KEITH-FLACK) 20–21

O

Oesophageal atresia 30
Oesophageal carcinoma, lymph drainage 48
Oesophageal varices 47, 81, 112
– bleeding 49, 71
– – liver cirrhosis 112
– – portocaval anastomosis 112
– portal hypertension 49
Oesophagoscopy 49, 85
– oesophageal varices 49
Oesophagus 2, 30, 42–46, 48, 52–53, 56–58, 62–67, 74–77, 81, 85, 98, 111, 148, 151, 161, 231
– arteries 46
– cervical constriction 45
– diaphragmatic constriction 45
– diverticula 45
– foreign bodies 45
– lymph drainage 48
– oesophagoscopy 49
– projection
– – onto the body surface 86
– – onto the ventral thoracic wall 42
– structure of the wall 44
– thoracic constriction 45
– veins 46–47
Omentum
– majus 72, 80, 82, 93–94, 116, 130–138, 142, 148–149, 152–153, 155, 236
– – development 72
– – peritoneal duplicatures 130
– minus 72, 80, 103, 121, 131–132, 138, 155
Omphalocele 73
Orchis *See* Testis
Organa
– genitalia feminina
– – externa 202, 204
– – interna 160
– genitalia masculina
– – externa 182, 184, 192
– – interna 160, 183, 185
– urinaria 160
– urogenitalia
– – feminina 203
– – masculina 183
Oris 42
Os
– coccygis 148, 199, 217, 238–239
– ilium 150, 214, 240
– ischii 201, 238
– pubis 148, 150, 186, 198, 216, 221, 238–239
– sacrum 148–149, 214
Ostium
– abdominale tubae uterinae 206
– appendicis vermiformis 95
– atrioventriculare
– – dextrum 17
– – sinistrum 18–19, 66
– cardiacum 77, 138–139, 150–151, 153
– ileale 95
– primum 7
– pyloricum 89
– secundum 7
– sinus coronarii 17, 24
– ureteris 177, 179–180, 236–237
– urethrae 205
– – externum 178–180, 186–187, 202–203, 217–219, 236–237
– – internum 177–180, 186, 209, 236–237
– uteri 207, 209–210, 237
– uterinum tubae uterinae 207
– vaginae 202–203, 219
– venae cavae inferioris 21
Ovary (*Ovarium*) 93, 139, 160, 203, 205–208, 211–212, 234, 237

Ovary (*Ovarium*)
– inflammatory process 159
– peritoneal duplicatures 206, 208

P

Pancreas 42, 72, 74, 82, 102, 120–124, 126–128, 132, 135–136, 142, 147–148, 151, 155–156, 161
– anulare 121
– arteries 125
– contact area onto the posterior wall of stomach 79
– development 121
– divisum 121
– ERCP 127
– excretory duct system 124
– histology 123
– inflammation 120
– lymphatic drainage 126
– projection
– – onto the surface of the body 86
– – onto the ventral abdominal wall 86, 120
– ultrasound image 127, 155
Pancreatic buds 103, 121
– fusion 121
Pancreatic carcinoma 119
– lymph node metastases 126
Pancreatic diseases 124
Pancreatitis 71, 120, 123
– bile concrements 124
– ultrasound image 155
Papilla
– duodeni
– – major (ampulla of VATER) 88–89, 117–118, 124
– – – endoscopy 122
– – minor 88, 117, 124
– mammaria 67
– renalis 167–168, 174, 176
Papillary muscles 17, 19
Paracystium 209
Paradidymis 183
Parametrium 209
Paraproctium 209
Parasympathetic nervous system
– effect on the heart 23
– erection 194
– perfusion of the intestines 100
– sacral division 100, 231
Paravertebral line 29
– borders of the lungs 29
Paries
– anterior (Gaster) 85, 131–132
– membranaceus (Trachea) 33, 62
– posterior (Gaster) 85
Pars
– abdominalis
– – aortae (Aorta abdominalis) 9, 43, 56, 58, 114, 127, 140, 147–148, 151, 156, 165, 172–173, 193, 226, 228, 230, 232–233, 235
– – – branches 228
– – oesophageae 45–46, 58, 75, 77
– – – arteries 46
– – (Oesophagus) 43
– anterior
– – (Facies diaphragmatica, Hepar) 106
– – (Fornix vaginae) 209
– ascendens
– – aortae (Aorta ascendens) 10, 13, 17, 21, 24–25, 55–56, 58, 62, 65–66
– – duodeni 88–90, 93, 117, 120, 124, 137
– – – projection 86
– – – – onto the body surface 86
– – – – onto the ventral abdominal wall 86
– cardiaca 43, 75
– cervicalis (Oesophagus) 43–44, 46, 48, 62
– – arteries 46
– – veins 46

Pars
– convoluta
– – (Tubulus distalis) 169
– – (Tubulus proximalis) 169
– costalis
– – diaphragmatis 114, 152–156
– – (Pleura parietalis) 40, 52–53, 64, 152–156
– descendens
– – aortae (Aorta descendens) 13, 45, 48, 55, 65–67
– – duodeni 75, 77, 88–90, 93, 117, 120, 122–124, 127
– – – projection
– – – – onto the body surface 86
– – – – onto the ventral abdominal wall 86
– diaphragmatica (Pleura parietalis) 11, 40, 54, 151, 154–156
– horizontalis (Duodenum) 88–90, 117, 120, 122–124, 135, 137, 139
– – projection
– – – onto the body surface 86
– – – onto the ventral abdominal wall 86
– intramuralis (Urethra masculina) 178–179
– intrasegmentalis 68
– laryngea pharyngis 28, 42
– lumbalis diaphragmatis 43, 56–57, 62, 114, 142, 148–149, 151, 154–156
– mediastinalis (Pleura parietalis) 11, 35, 51–52, 65
– membranacea
– – (Septum interventriculare) 6–7, 19
– – (Urethra) 178–179, 186, 236
– muscularis (Septum interventriculare) 6–7, 17–18
– nasalis pharyngis 28
– oralis pharyngis 28, 42
– posterior (Fornix vaginae) 209, 237
– profunda (M. sphincter ani externus) 223
– prostatica (Urethra) 177–179, 190
– pylorica (Pylorus) 58, 74–77, 80, 85, 88–90, 130, 133, 138, 153
– recta
– – (Tubulus distalis) 169
– – (Tubulus proximalis) 169
– spongiosa (Urethra) 178–179, 192, 236
– sternalis diaphragmatis 62
– subcutanea (M. sphincter ani externus) 202, 223
– superficialis (M. sphincter ani externus) 223
– superior (Duodenum) 75, 77, 88–90, 116–117, 120, 123, 138–139, 150
– – projection
– – – onto the body surface 86
– – – onto the ventral abdominal wall 86
– terminalis ilei 95, 135
– thoracica
– – aortae (Aorta thoracica) 7, 38, 43–46, 53, 55–56, 58, 64, 122, 154
– – – branches 56
– – (Ductus thoracicus) 53, 56–57
– – (Oesophagus) 43–46, 48, 53, 56–58, 62, 151
– uterina 207
Pecten analis (Canalis analis) 222–223
Pelvic floor
– function 196
– in man 198
– muscles 196
– in woman 214–215
Pelvic floor insufficiency 214
Pelvic kidneys 162
Pelvic viscera
– in man, blood supply 233
– in woman, blood supply 234
Pelvis 148–150, 179–180, 235–239
– female 180, 237
– – lymph nodes and lymph vessels 235
– – transverse section 239
– – – computed tomography 239
– male 148–150, 179, 236
– – oblique frontal section 240
– – transverse section 238

Index

Pelvis male
– – computed tomography 238
– renalis 160, 166–168, 173–174, 176, 183, 203
Penis 182–183, 185–187, 192
– cavernous bodies 186
Perfusion of the intestines
– parasympathetic influence 100
– sympathetic influence 100
Pericardial cavity 30, 72
Pericardial effusion 11
Pericardial tamponade 11
Pericarditis 11
Pericardium 2, 11, 13, 40, 44, 50, 54, 153
– fibrosum 11, 48, 51–53
– serosum 2, 11–13, 17–18, 62
Perimetrium 207
Perineal muscles
– in man 197–198
– in woman 216
Perineal region
– in man 199
– – vessels and nerves 200
– in woman 217
– – vessels and nerves 218
Perineal space
– deep 197, 199, 201, 217, 219
– in man 201
– superficial 197, 199, 217, 219
– in woman 219
Perineal tears 217
Perineum 199, 202, 217
Periorchium 187
Peritoneal carcinosis 133
Peritoneal cavity 70, 72, 148, 158
– dorsal wall 139
– recesses 139
Peritoneum 105
– parietale 70, 116, 130, 148, 154–156, 181, 201, 219, 221–222, 237, 240
– viscerale 70, 87, 148, 152, 154–155
Peritonitis 133
– appendicitis, perforation 95
PEYER's plaques (Noduli lymphoidei aggregati) 91, 95
Pharynx 28, 42, 85
Phimosis 186
– circumcision 186
Phosphodiesterase, enzyme inhibitors, erection 192
Physiological umbilical hernia 73
Placenta 8, 210
Pleura
– parietalis 11, 35, 40, 51–54, 63–65, 151–156
– visceralis (pulmonalis) 40, 63–64, 68, 152–153
Pleura borders, projection
– onto the anterior thoracic wall 29
– onto the posterior thoracic wall 29
Pleural cavitaty 2, 40, 50, 52–53
Pleural cupula, transverse sections at the level of the shoulder joint 63
Pleural effusions 29, 40
Plexus
– aorticus
– – abdominalis 226, 231
– – thoracicus 11, 53, 58
– brachialis 51, 60–61, 63–64, 68
– cardiacus 23, 53–54, 58
– coeliacus 100, 226, 231
– deferentialis 191, 194
– hepaticus 100
– hypogastricus
– – inferior 100, 194, 212, 226
– – superior 100, 194, 212, 226, 231
– intermesentericus 100, 231
– lumbalis 164, 230
– – branches 230
– mesentericus
– – inferior 100, 231
– – superior 100, 231

Plexus
– oesophageus 52, 58, 231
– ovaricus 212
– pampiniformis 187, 189, 191–193
– prostaticus 194
– pulmonalis 52–53
– rectalis 226
– renalis 100
– sacralis 212, 226, 231–232
– splenicus 100
– testicularis 191, 194
– uretericus 100
– uterovaginalis (FRANKENHÄUSER's plexus) 212
– venosus
– – prostaticus 193, 201, 233, 236
– – rectalis 225, 233–234
– – submucosus 47, 112
– – uterinus 234
– – vaginalis 234
– – vertebralis internus (posterior) 62–63
– – vesicalis 201, 219, 233–234, 237–238
Plica(-ae)
– caecalis vascularis 135
– circulares (KERCKRING's folds) 77, 89–91, 124
– duodenalis inferior 137, 139
– gastricae 77, 85
– gastropancreatica 132–133, 139
– hepatopancreatica 132–133, 139
– ileocaecalis 135, 139
– interureterica 177
– longitudinalis duodeni 124
– mucosae (Vesica biliaris) 117
– rectouterina 206, 237
– rectovesicalis 236
– semilunares coli 94–95, 101
– spiralis (HEISTER) 88, 117, 119
– transversa recti 148, 180, 222–223, 236
– umbilicalis
– – lateralis 233
– – medialis 208, 233, 237
– – mediana 236–237
Pneumothorax 29
– central venous catheter (CVC) 35, 63
Porta hepatis 104
Portal hypertension 47, 81, 106, 225
– liver cirrhosis 98
– oesophageal varices 49
– portocavale anastomoses 49
Portal system, hypertension 98
Portal tracts 106
Portal vein 81, 141
– increased blood pressure 81
– tributaries 141
– ultrasound image 114
Portio
– supravaginalis cervicis 207
– vaginalis cervicis 207, 209–210, 237
Portocaval anastomoses 46–47, 81, 98, 106, 112, 225
– bleedings of esophageal varices 112
– portal hypertension 49
Posterior myocardial infarction (PMI) 10, 27
Postnatal circulation 9
Pouch of DOUGLAS (Excavatio rectouterina) 138–139, 208–210, 237, 239
– appendicitis 237
– salpingitis 237
Preganglionic parasympathetic neurons 100
Preganglionic sympathetic neurons 100
Prenatal circulation 8
Preputium
– clitoridis 202
– penis 182, 186–187, 236
Primary intestinal loop 73
Primitive laryngeal inlet 31
Primordial gut, development 72
Primordial ovary 163
Primordial testis 163
Processus
– articularis superior 154
– coracoideus 68

Processus
– papillaris 155
– spinosus 63–64, 67, 173
– transversus 65
– uncinatus 123–124, 144, 149
– xiphoideus 62, 67, 74, 154, 210
Proctodeal glands (Gll. anales) 223
Promontorium 148
Pronephros 162
Prostate (Prostata) 148–149, 160, 177–178, 181, 183, 185–186, 190, 194, 198, 201, 221, 223, 233, 236
– digital rectal examination (DRE) 221
– zones 190
Prostatic carcinoma 159, 190
– digital rectal examination (DRE) 221
Pubes 182
Pulmo 2, 40, 74, 102, 115, 120, 128, 161
– dexter 11, 28, 34–36, 40, 50–51, 54, 63–67, 149, 151–152
– sinister 11, 28, 34–36, 40, 51, 54, 63–64, 66–68, 151, 153
Pulmonary circulation 2
Pulmonary emboli, right ventricular hypertrophy 15
Pulmonary hypertension 5
– right ventricular hypertrophy 15
Pulmonary ring 16
Pulmonary valve 16
– projection onto the ventral thoracic wall 4
Pulmonary valve stenosis 7
– right ventricular hypertrophy 15
Pulmonary veins 18
Pulpa splenica 129
Pyelonephritis, referred pain 164
Pylorus (Pars pylorica) 58, 74–77, 80, 85, 88–90, 130, 133, 138, 153
Pyramides renales 167–168, 173–174

R

Radiograph(s)
– after intravenous application of contrast medium 119
– colon 101
– duodenal ulcers 90
– duodenum 90
– extrahepatic bile ducts 119
– gallbladder 119
– heart contours 5
– intrahepatic bile ducts 119
– left border of the heart 5
– renal pelvis 176
– right border of the heart 5
– thoracic cage 5, 41
– thoracic viscera 5, 41
– thorax 3, 5
– ureter 176
– – variations 176
Radix
– mesenterii 139
– parasympathica 194, 212, 226
Ramus(-i)
– anterior
– – (A. pancreaticoduodenalis inferior) 96, 125
– – (A. renalis) 166
– – (V. portae hepatis) 114
– atriales
– – (A. coronaria dextra) 26
– – (A. coronaria sinistra) 26
– atrioventriculares
– – (A. coronaria dextra) 26
– – (A. coronaria sinistra) 26
– bronchiales
– – (Aorta) 38, 52, 56
– – (N. vagus) 56, 58
– cardiacus(-i)
– – cervicalis inferior (N. vagus) 23
– – thoracici
– – – (N. vagus) 23, 52–54
– – – (Truncus sympathicus) 53

Index

Ramus(-i)
- circumflexus (A. coronaria sinistra) 13, 24–26
- coeliacus (Truncus vagalis) 84
- colicus (A. ileocolica) 96–97, 143, 146
- communicantes (Truncus sympathicus) 52, 58, 194, 212
- coni arteriosi
- – – (A. coronaria dextra) 24, 26
- – – (A. coronaria sinistra) 24
- dexter
- – – (A. hepatica propria) 155
- – – (V. portae hepatis) 114, 141, 150, 154–155
- femoralis (N. genitofemoralis) 230
- gastrici anteriores (Truncus vagalis anterior) 58, 84
- genitalis (N. genitofemoralis) 191–192, 230, 232, 238
- helicini (A. uterina) 211
- hepatici (Truncus vagalis) 84
- ilealis (A. ileocolica) 96, 143
- inferior ossis pubis 186, 216
- interganglionaris (Truncus sympathicus) 212
- interventricularis(-es)
- – – anterior (A. coronaria sinistra) 12, 19, 24–27, 67
- – – posterior (A. coronaria dextra) 13, 24, 26–27
- – – septales
- – – – (A. coronaria dextra) 26
- – – – (A. coronaria sinistra) 24, 26
- labiales posteriores (A. pudenda interna) 218
- lateralis (R. diagonalis, A. coronaria sinistra) 24, 26–27
- marginalis
- – – dexter (A. coronaria dextra) 24, 26
- – – sinister (A. coronaria sinistra) 24, 26
- nodi
- – – atrioventricularis (A. coronaria dextra) 20, 24, 26
- – – sinuatrialis
- – – – (A. coronaria dextra) 20, 24, 26
- – – – (A. coronaria sinistra) 24
- obturatorius (A. epigastrica inferior) 232
- oesophageales
- – – (A. gastrica sinistra) 46, 140
- – – (A. thyroidea inferior) 46
- – – (N. laryngeus recurrens) 56, 80
- – – (Pars thoracica aortae) 46, 56
- – – (V. cava inferior) 47
- – – (V. portae hepatis) 47
- omentales
- – – (A. gastroomentalis dextra) 80
- – – (A. gastroomentalis sinistra) 80, 142
- ossis ischii 197, 216, 239
- ovaricus (A. uterina) 211
- pancreatici (A. splenica) 125
- pericardiacus (N. phrenicus) 54
- perineales (N. cutaneus femoris posterior) 200, 218
- phrenicoabdominales (N. phrenicus) 54
- posterior
- – – (A. pancreaticoduodenalis inferior) 96, 125
- – – (A. renalis) 166
- – – (V. portae hepatis) 114, 154
- – – ventriculi sinistri (A. coronaria sinistra) 24, 26
- posterolateralis dexter (A. coronaria dextra) 24, 26
- pubicus
- – – (A. epigastrica inferior) 232
- – – (A. obturatoria) 232
- scrotales
- – – anteriores (V. dorsalis profunda penis) 192
- – – posteriores
- – – – (A. perinealis) 200
- – – – (A. pudenda interna) 233
- – – – (V. pudenda interna) 233
- sinister (V. portae hepatis) 114, 127
- splenici (A. splenica) 144
- subendocardiales 20
- superior ossis pubis 196, 216

Ramus(-i)
- tubarius (A. uterina) 211
- vaginales (A. uterina) 211

Raphe
- perinei 199, 202, 217
- scroti 187, 189, 191

Recessus
- axillaris 68
- costodiaphragmaticus 5, 29, 40–41, 50, 54, 152–154, 156
- costomediastinalis 4, 40, 50, 64, 67
- duodenalis
- – inferior 136, 139
- – superior 136, 139
- ileocaecalis
- – inferior 135–137, 139
- – superior 135, 137, 139
- inferior (Bursa omentalis) 132–133
- intersigmoideus 136, 139
- phrenicomediastinalis 40
- pneumatoentericus 72
- sigmoideus 139
- splenicus (Bursa omentalis) 132–133, 139, 155
- superior (Bursa omentalis) 132, 139, 155
- vertebromediastinalis 40, 64, 66

Rectal prolapse 223
Rectocele 214
Rectoscopy, anal canal 227
Rectum 74, 81, 92, 97–98, 101, 111, 120, 137–138, 146–147, 149, 161, 181, 196, 198, 208–209, 215, 219–226, 230, 235, 238–239
- arteries 224
- innervation 226
- lymph nodes and lymph vessels in a woman 235
- in the male pelvis 221
- projection onto the body surface 86, 220
- veins 225

Red pulp, spleen 129
Referred pain 115
- in the right shoulder
- – – cholecystitis 54
- – – liver biopsies 54

Regio
- analis 158, 199, 217
- perinealis 158, 199, 201, 217–219
- – – in man 199–200
- urogenitalis 158, 199, 217

Relative cardiac dullness 4
Ren (Nephros) 74, 102–103, 120, 122, 127–128, 131, 136, 138–139, 147, 151–153, 155–156, 160–168, 171, 173, 175–176, 183, 185, 193, 203, 205, 228
- See also Kidney

Renal biopsy 173
Renal calices 167
Renal cell carcinoma 171
Renal concrements 175
Renal corpuscle 169
Renal cortex 167
- microscopy 168
Renal infarction 165
Renal medulla 167
Renal pelvis 167, 174
- radiograph 176
Renal pyramids 167
Renal segments 165
Renal tumours, obstruction of the venous drainage 193
Renal veins 169
Respiratory distress syndrome (RDS) 30
Resuscitation, anatomical dead-space 32
Rete testis 163
Retroflexion of the uterus 208
Retroperitoneal organs 70, 138
Retroperitoneal space 70, 158, 228
- autonomic nervous system 231
- lymph nodes 229
- lymph vessels 229
- somatic nerves 230
Retroversion of the uterus 208
RETZIUS' space (Spatium retropubicum) 209–210, 236–237, 239

Right and left branches of the artioventricular bundle (Crus dextrum and sinistrum, bundle of TAWARA) 17, 20
Right ventricle 17
Right ventricular hypertrophy 7, 15
Right-to-left shunt 7
Rima oris 42
RIOLAN's anastomosis 97, 140, 143, 145–147
Rugae vaginales 207, 209

S

Saccus aorticus 6
Salpingitis, pouch of DOUGLAS 237
Salpinx (Tuba uterina) 139, 160, 203, 205–208, 211–212, 234
SANTORINI's duct (Ductus pancreaticus accessorius) 88, 117, 121, 124
Scalene gap 60
Scapula 5, 63–65, 68
Scapular 29
- borders of the lungs 29
Scrotum 182, 184, 187, 236
Segmental bronchi 36
- bronchoscopy 37
Segmentum(-a)
- anterius
- – (Hepar) 107
- – inferius
- – – (Hepar) 108
- – – (Ren) 165
- – (Pulmo dexter) 36
- – (Pulmo sinister) 36
- – superius
- – – (Hepar) 108
- – – (Ren) 165
- apicale (Pulmo dexter) 36
- apicoposterius (Pulmo sinister) 36
- basale
- – anterius
- – – (Pulmo dexter) 36
- – – (Pulmo sinister) 36
- – laterale
- – – (Pulmo dexter) 36
- – – (Pulmo sinister) 36
- – mediale (cardiacum) (Pulmo dexter) 36
- – posterius
- – – (Pulmo dexter) 36
- – – (Pulmo sinister) 36
- bronchopulmonalia 36–37
- inferius (Ren) 165
- laterale
- – inferius (Hepar) 107–108
- – (Pulmo dexter) 36
- – superius (Hepar) 107–108
- lingulare
- – inferius (Pulmo sinister) 36
- – superius (Pulmo sinister) 36
- mediale
- – inferius (Hepar) 107–108
- – (Pulmo dexter) 36
- – superius (Hepar) 107–108
- posterius
- – inferius (Hepar) 107–108
- – (Pulmo dexter) 36
- – (Ren) 165
- – superius (Hepar) 107–108
- renalia 165
- superius
- – (Pulmo dexter) 36
- – (Pulmo sinister) 36
- – (Ren) 165
Seminal vesicle (Gl. vesiculosa) 178, 183, 190
Seminiferous tubules 188
Septula testis 188–189
Septum
- atrioventriculare (Pars membranacea) 7
- interatriale 17–18
- interventriculare 6–8, 17–20, 66
- – (Pars membranacea) 7
- – (Pars muscularis) 7

Index

Septum
- oesophagotracheale 31
- – development 31
- penis 192
- primum 7
- scroti 187, 189, 191
- secundum 7
- spurium 7
- transversum 72
- vesicovaginale 237

Septum formation, developmental steps 7
Shoulder joint 68
Sinu-atrial node (Nodus sinuatrialis, node of KEITH-FLACK) 20–21

Sinus
- anales (anal crypts) 222–223, 227
- aortae 19, 67
- coronarius 13, 15, 25
- epididymidis 188
- obliquus pericardii 11, 13
- paranasales 28
- prostaticus 177
- renalis(-es) 156, 167–168, 173–174
- transversus pericardii 11, 13, 62, 66
- trunci pulmonalis 15
- urogenitalis 163
- venarum cavarum 25

Sinus septum 7
Sinus valves 7

Situs
- cordis 10
- inversus 73
- viscerum 130–136

Small intestine
- *See also* Intestinum tenue
- autonomic innervation 100
- cross-section 87
- mesenteries 137
- projection onto the ventral abdominal wall 86
- regional lymph nodes and lymph vessels 99
- tumors 71
- veins 98
- wall structure 87

Sonography *See* ultrasound image(s)

Spatium
- epidurale 154
- extraperitoneale 70, 158
- – pelvis 70, 158
- profundum perinei 197, 199, 201, 217, 219
- retroperitoneale 70, 158
- retropubicum (space of RETZIUS) 209–210, 236–237, 239
- retrorectale 209
- subarachnoideum 63
- superficiale perinei 197, 199, 201, 217, 219

Spermatic cord *See* Funiculus spermaticus

Spina
- iliaca
- – anterior superior 74, 93, 182, 210
- – posterior superior 161
- ischiadica 238
- scapulae 29, 63

Spinal cord injuries 54
Spleen (Splen, Lien) 72, 74, 80–81, 93, 98, 102–103, 110–111, 120–121, 128–129, 131–133, 139, 142, 151, 153–155, 161
- contact area on the posterior wall of the stomach 79
- infarction 129
- peritoneal duplicatures 129
- rupture 71, 129

Spontaneous breathing 30
Sternal line, borders of the lungs 29
Sternum 51, 62, 65, 67, 74, 210
Steroid hormones, adrenal gland 170
Stomach 30, 75, 77, 85
- *See also* Gaster
- arteries 80
- autonomic innervation 84
- contact areas 79
- – of the anterior wall 79
- – of the posterior wall 79

Stomach
- development 72
- exit 77
- inner muscle layers 76
- lymph nodes and lymph vessels 82
- lymphatic drainage stations 83
- parasympathetic fibres 84
- projection
- – onto the body surface 86
- – onto the ventral abdominal wall 74
- regional lymph nodes 83
- sympathetic fibres 84
- veins 81
- wall 78

Stratum
- circulare
- – recti 223
- – (Tunica muscularis, Duodenum) 89
- – (Tunica muscularis, Gaster) 76, 78
- – (Tunica muscularis, Intestinum crassum) 87, 94
- – (Tunica muscularis, Intestinum tenue) 87
- – (Tunica muscularis, Oesophagus) 44
- longitudinale
- – recti 222–223
- – (Tunica muscularis, Duodenum) 89
- – (Tunica muscularis, Gaster) 78
- – (Tunica muscularis, Intestinum crassum) 87, 94
- – (Tunica muscularis, Intestinum tenue) 87
- – (Tunica muscularis, Oesophagus) 44

SUDECK's point 224

Sulcus
- aorticus 35
- arteriae subclaviae 35
- coronarius 12–13, 15, 25
- interventricularis
- – anterior 12, 15
- – posterior 12–13, 15, 25
- terminalis 13
- venae brachiocephalicae 35

Superior thoracic aperture, neurovascular structures 60–61
Suprarenal arteries 172
- variations 172
Suprarenal glands 122, 166, 170
- in the retroperitoneal space 164
Suprarenal veins 172
- variations 172
Surfactant 30
Sympathetic innervation
- emission 194
- perfusions of the intestines 100
Sympathetic tonus, increased
- heart rate 23
- hypertension 23
- tachycardia 23
Sympathetic trunk 2, 58
Symphysis pubica 74, 150, 181, 196–197, 202, 209–210, 214, 216, 232, 236, 238–239
Systemic circulation 2
Systole 16

T

Tachycardia
- ECG 22
- increased sympathetic tonus 23

Taenia
- libera 94–95, 130, 134
- mesocolica 94–95
- omentalis 94–95, 130

TAWARA, node of (Nodus atrioventricularis) 20–21

Tela
- submucosa
- – (Duodenum) 89
- – (Gaster) 78
- – (Intestinum crassum) 94
- – (Intestinum tenue) 87
- – (Oesophagus) 44
- – (Peritoneum viscerale) 87

Tela
- subserosa
- – (Gaster) 78
- – (Ileum) 91
- – (Intestinum crassum) 94
- – (Intestinum tenue) 87
- – (Jejunum) 91
- – (Peritoneum viscerale) 87

Terminal ileum 95
Testicular cancer 185, 194
- lymph node metastases 195
- transscrotal testicular biopsy 195
Testis (Orchis) 160, 183, 185, 188–189, 191, 194
- coverings 187, 191
- lobules (Lobuli testis) 188
- primordial 163
Testosteron 183
- WOLFFIAN ducts, differentiation 185
Thigh, muscles 196
Thoracic aorta 43–44
Thoracic cage
- inferior 151
- postero-anterior radiograph 5
- radiograph 41
Thoracic cavity 62, 68
- radiograph 5, 41
- transverse section 64–67
- – computed tomography 65
Thoracic constriction, oesophagus 45
Thoracic viscera 1–68
- radiograph 5, 41
Thoracic wall, layers 115
Thorax
- computed tomography 3
- conventional radiograph 5
- MRI 3
Thymus 40, 50–53, 160
- of an adolescent 51
- in a newborn 51
TODARO's tendon 16–17, 20
Trabecula(-ae)
- carneae 18
- septomarginalis 17, 21
- splenicae 129
Trachea 2, 5, 28, 30–33, 38, 43, 45–46, 48, 51, 54, 56–58, 60, 62–64, 161
- projection onto the ventral thoracic wall 28
Tracheo-oesophageal fistula 30
Traction diverticula 45
Transoesophageal echocardiography 66
Transposition of the great vessels 7
Transscrotal testicular biopsy 195
Transurethral catheter, positioning 180
Transverse colon *See* Colon transversum
TREITZ hernias 136
TREITZ, muscle of (M. suspensorius) 89
Tricuspid valve (Valva atrioventricularis dextra) 4, 6, 16–17, 62, 67
- projection onto the ventral thoracic wall 4
Trigone of the bladder (Trigonum vesicae) 177
Trigonum
- cholecystohepaticum (CALOT's triangle) 118
- fibrosum
- – dextrum 16
- – sinistrum 16
- pericardiacum 4, 40
- thymicum 40, 50
- vesicae 177
Truncus(-i)
- arteriosus 6
- brachiocephalicus 12–13, 43–45, 48, 51, 54–56, 62, 64
- bronchomediastinalis 39, 48, 60–61
- coeliacus 46, 80, 96, 103, 110, 122, 125, 140, 142, 144, 165, 226, 228, 231
- – branches 142
- – origins 144
- costocervicalis 56, 60–61
- inferior 60–61
- intestinalis 48, 99, 229
- jugularis 48, 60

257

Index

Truncus(-i)
- lumbalis(-es) 99, 229
- – dexter 229
- lumbosacralis 230–232
- pulmonalis 5–6, 8–10, 12–13, 15, 19, 24–25, 41, 55, 65–66
- subclavius sinister 61
- sympathicus 2, 52–53, 56–58, 60–61, 64–65, 67, 100, 151, 154, 156, 194, 230–231
- thyrocervicalis 60–61
- vagalis
- – anterior 58, 84, 100, 231
- – posterior 84, 100, 231

Tuba uterina (Salpinx) 139, 160, 203, 205–208, 211–212, 234
- peritoneal duplicatures 206, 208

Tuber ischiadicum 199, 202, 217, 239–240
Tuberculum pubicum 202
Tubulus
- distalis 168–169
- proximalis 168–169

Tunica
- adventitia
- – (Intestinum crassum) 94
- – (Oesophagus) 44
- – (Trachea) 33
- albuginea
- – corporum cavernosorum 186, 191–192, 236
- – (Testis) 188–189
- dartos 187, 189, 191, 236
- fibrosa (Splen) 129
- mucosa
- – (Gaster) 78
- – (Intestinum crassum) 94
- – (Intestinum tenue) 87
- – (Oesophagus) 44
- – (Trachea) 33
- – (Uterus) 207
- – (Vesica biliaris) 117
- – (Vesica urinaria) 177
- muscularis
- – (Duodenum) 89
- – (Gaster) 76, 78
- – (Intestinum crassum) 94
- – (Intestinum tenue) 87
- – (Jejunum) 91
- – (Oesophagus) 44, 76
- – (Rectum) 222
- – (Uterus) 207
- – (Vesica urinaria) 177–178
- serosa
- – (Gaster) 78
- – (Ileum) 91
- – (Intestinum crassum) 94
- – (Intestinum tenue) 87
- – (Jejunum) 91
- – (Lobus hepatis dexter) 105
- – (Lobus hepatis sinister) 105
- – (Oesophagus) 44
- – (Perimetrium) 206
- – (Splen) 129
- – (Uterus) 207
- – (Vesica biliaris) 117
- vaginalis testis 187–189, 191

U

Ulcus
- duodeni 90
- – endoscopy (duodenoscopy) 90
- – radiograph with contrast imaging 90
- ventriculi 71, 78

Ultrasound image(s)
- kidney 173
- liver 114
- liver veins 114
- pancreas 127
- pancreatitis 155
- portal vein 114
- Vv. hepaticae 114

Umbilical cord 9

Umbilical hernia 73
Umbilicus 182
Upper abdominal situs
- abdominal surgery 133
- development 72
- position of the viscera 130–132
- retroperitoneal organs 122

Upper intestinal tract, haemorrhage 89
Upper respiratory tract 28, 32–33
- development 30

Ureter 139, 160, 162–167, 171, 174–176, 178, 180, 183, 185, 194, 198, 203, 205–206, 208–209, 221, 228, 233–235, 237, 240
- common variations, radiographs 176
- constrictions 175
- course 175
- crossing, MEYER-WEIGERT's rule 176
- duplex 176
- fissus 176
- irreversible damage, hysterectomy 175
- parts 175
- radiograph 176

Ureteric bud 162
Ureteric colic, renal concrements 175
Ureteric orifice 163
- cystoscopy 177

Urethra 179, 186, 190, 204, 216, 236
- bends 179
- feminina 160, 180–181, 203, 210, 216, 219
- masculina 160, 177–178, 181, 190, 192, 194, 197

Urethral folds 184, 204
- incomplete fusion 184

Urethral groove 184
Urinary bladder See Vesica urinaria
Urinary incontinence 214
Urinary organs
- development 163
- in man 183
- in woman 183

Urinary pole 168
Urinary system 160
Urogenital folds 184
Uterine neck 209
Uterus 93, 160, 203, 205–210, 216, 234–235, 237
- anteflexion 208
- anteversion 208
- connective tissue spaces 209
- descensus 214
- duplex 205
- with foetus 210
- ligaments 209
- peritoneal duplicatures 206, 208
- position 208
- prolapse 214
- retroflexion 208
- retroversion 208
- septus 205
- subseptus 205

Utriculus prostaticus 177
Uvula vesicae 177

V

Vagina 160, 180, 203–205, 207–208, 210–211, 215–216, 219, 234, 239
- descensus 214
- musculi recti abdominis 155
- position 208
- prolapse 214

Vagotomy, selective proximal or total, gastric ulcer 84

Valva(-ae)
- aortae 4, 6, 16, 19, 62, 66–67
- atrioventricularis
- – dextra (Valva tricuspidalis) 4, 6, 16–17, 62, 67
- – sinistra (Valva mitralis) 4, 6, 16, 18–19, 66–67
- cordis 16

Valva(-ae)
- ileocaecalis (ileocaecal valve, BAUHIN's valve) 86, 95
- trunci pulmonalis 4, 6, 16

Valvula(-ae)
- anales 222–223
- foraminis ovalis 7, 18
- semilunaris
- – anterior 16
- – dextra
- – – (Valva aortae) 16, 66
- – – (Valva trunci pulmonalis) 16, 19
- – posterior (Valva aortae) 16, 19, 62, 66
- – sinistra
- – – (Valva aortae) 16, 19, 66
- – – (Valva trunci pulmonalis) 16
- sinus coronarii 7, 17, 21
- venae cavae inferioris 7, 17, 21

Varicocele 171, 193
Vas(-sa)
- lymphatica 87, 191
- privata (Pulmo) 38
- publica (Pulmo) 38
- recta 169

Vena(-ae)
- appendicularis 111, 141
- arcuata (Ren) 169
- atriales 25
- axillaris 60–61, 64, 68
- azygos 46–48, 52, 56–57, 64–67, 112, 155
- brachiocephalica 40, 50, 52–53, 60
- – dextra 13, 51, 54, 57
- – sinistra 13, 46, 51, 54, 57, 61–62
- bronchiales 52, 57
- bulbi
- – penis 197
- – vestibuli 218
- cardiaca(-ae) (cordis)
- – magna 12–13, 18, 25, 67
- – media (V. interventricularis posterior) 13, 25, 62
- – minimae (Vasa THEBESII) 25
- – parva 12, 25
- cava
- – inferior 5–6, 8–9, 11, 13, 15, 17, 20, 25, 46–47, 55, 57, 72, 81, 98, 104–105, 107–108, 111–112, 114, 122, 127, 141, 144, 149–150, 154–156, 164–165, 171–173, 193, 225, 228–230
- – – tributaries 228
- – superior 4–6, 8–13, 15, 17, 21, 25, 44, 46, 48, 51–52, 54–55, 57, 64–66
- centralis
- – (Gl. suprarenalis) 170
- – (Hepar) 106
- cephalica 68
- circumflexa femoris medialis 238
- colica
- – dextra 98, 111, 141, 145
- – media 98, 111, 141, 145, 147
- – sinistra 98, 111–112, 141, 145, 147
- cordis 25
- corticales radiatae 169
- cremasterica 191–192
- cystica 98, 111, 116, 141–142
- dorsalis
- – profunda
- – – clitoridis 216, 237
- – – penis 192, 197, 233, 236
- – superficialis penis 192, 236
- epigastrica
- – inferior 112, 233, 237
- – superficialis 112
- femoralis 238–239
- gastrica(-ae)
- – breves 80–81, 98, 111, 141
- – dextra 80–81, 98, 111, 141
- – sinistra 46–47, 80–81, 98, 111–112, 141–142, 150, 155
- gastroomentalis 80
- – dextra 80–81, 98, 111, 141–142, 144
- – sinistra 46, 80–81, 98, 111, 141–142, 144

Index

Vena(-ae)
- glutea
  - – inferior 225, 238
  - – superior 225
- hemiazygos 46–47, 53, 57, 62, 112, 155
  - – accessoria 46, 53, 57
- hepatica(-ae) 8–9, 98, 105–106, 111–112, 141, 228
  - – dextra 108, 149, 154
  - – intermedia 108
  - – sinistra 108, 149–150
  - – ultrasound image 114
- ileales 98, 111, 141, 145
- ileocolica 98, 111, 141
- iliaca
  - – communis 112, 148–149, 175, 215, 225, 228, 232
  - – externa 225, 233–234, 237
  - – interna 112, 225, 234, 240
- intercostales posteriores 46, 52–53, 56–57, 66–67
- interlobaris (Ren) 169
- interlobularis 106
- interventricularis
  - – anterior 12, 25
  - – posterior (V. cardiaca [cordis] media) 13, 25
- jejunales 98, 111, 141, 145, 147
- jugularis interna 39, 44, 46, 54, 60–61, 68
- lumbalis(-es) 228
  - – ascendens 57
- marginalis
  - – dextra 25
  - – sinistra 25
- mediastinales 57
- mesenterica
  - – inferior 81, 98, 111–112, 141, 147, 225
    - – branches 98, 111
    - – course in the retroperitoneal space 147
  - – superior 81, 96, 98, 111–112, 122–123, 141, 144–145, 147–150
    - – branches 111
    - – course 145
- obliqua atrii sinistri 25
- obturatoria 196, 215, 225, 233, 238–239
- oesophageae/oesophageales 46–47, 57, 81, 98, 111–112, 141
- ovarica(-ae) 112, 175, 206–208, 228, 234, 237
  - – dextra 165
  - – sinistra 165–166, 171
- pancreaticae 98, 111, 141
- pancreaticoduodenalis(-es) 98, 111
  - – superior posterior 141
- paraumbilicales 111–112
- pericardiacae 57

Vena(-ae)
- pericardiacophrenica 11, 51–54
- perinealis 197
- phrenica inferior 46–47, 112, 171, 228
- portae hepatis 8–9, 47, 80–81, 98, 104, 108, 110–112, 114, 118, 122–123, 127, 141–142, 144, 149–150, 154–156
- pudenda(-ae)
  - – externa 191
  - – – profunda 192
  - – interna 197, 200–201, 218, 225, 233–234, 238–240
- pulmonalis(-es) 38, 41, 52
  - – dextra(-ae) 10, 13, 15, 18, 25, 35, 44
  - – – inferior 11, 66
  - – – superior 11, 66
  - – sinistra(-ae) 9, 13, 15, 25, 44, 53, 62
  - – – inferior 10–11, 18, 35, 62, 66–67
  - – – superior 10–11, 18, 35, 62, 65
- rectalis(-es)
  - – inferiores 112, 141, 225, 233–234
  - – mediae 141, 225, 233–234
  - – superior 98, 111–112, 141, 147, 225, 234
- renalis(-es) 156, 164–168, 171, 175, 193, 228
  - – course 171
  - – dextra 148–149, 165, 172–173
  - – sinistra 112, 127, 165, 172
- sacralis mediana 225, 228
- saphena magna 239
- sigmoideae 98, 111–112, 141, 147, 225
- splenica (lienalis) 81, 98, 111–112, 122–123, 127, 129, 141, 144, 147, 151, 154–156
  - – branches 111
- stellata (Ren) 169
- subclavia 44, 51, 54, 57, 63
  - – dextra 39, 46, 54, 60
  - – sinistra 39, 61
- subcostalis 57
- suprarenalis(-es) 166, 172
  - – dextra 164, 171–172, 228
  - – media 164
  - – sinistra 164–165, 171–172, 228
- testicularis 112, 165–166, 171, 192–193, 228
  - – course 193
- thoracica interna 40, 50–51, 64
- thyroidea inferior 46, 51
- umbilicalis 8, 103, 210
- uterina 234
- ventriculi
  - – dextri anteriores 25
  - – sinistri posteriores 25
- vertebralis 46
- vesicalis inferior 233
Ventral pancreatic bud 103, 121
Ventricular septal defect 7

Ventriculus
- dexter 4, 6, 8–10, 12–13, 15, 17, 25, 55, 66–67, 150
- sinister 4–10, 12–13, 15, 17–19, 25, 41, 44, 55, 66–67
Vertebra
- lumbalis 155–156
- thoracica 63–68, 154
Vesica
- biliaris (fellea) 8, 42, 80–81, 93, 98, 102–104, 107–108, 110–111, 115–119, 121, 127, 131–132, 142, 156
  - – projection onto the body surface 86
- urinaria 8, 93, 137–139, 148–149, 160, 162, 177–178, 181, 183, 185–186, 190, 194, 203, 205, 208–210, 216, 219, 221, 223, 233–235, 238–239
  - – lymph nodes 235
  - – in man 181
  - – in woman 181
Vestibule (Vestibulum vaginae) 202
Vestibulum
- bursae omentalis 132–133
- nasi 28
- oris 42
- vaginae 180, 202
Villi intestinales 87
Visceral surgery, liver segments 108
Vortex cordis 15
Vulvar carcinoma, lymph node metastases 213

W

White pulp, spleen 129
WIRSUNG's duct (Ductus pancreaticus) 88–89, 117, 121, 123–124, 127, 148–149
- variations of the junction 124
WOLFFIAN duct (Ductus mesonephricus) 162–163, 205
- differentiation, testosteron 185
WOLFF-PARKINSON-WHITE syndrome, ECG 22

Z

ZENKER's diverticula 45
Zona
- alba (Canalis analis) 222
- columnaris (Canalis analis) 222–223
- cutanea (Canalis analis) 222–223
- orbicularis 238